CHILDREN'S LANGUAGE DISORDERS

AN INTEGRATED APPROACH

Robert D. Hubbell

California State University, Sacramento

PRENTICE-HALL, INC., ENGLEWOOD CLIFFS, NEW JERSEY 07632

Library of Congress Cataloging in Publication Data

HUBBELL, ROBERT D   (date)
    Children's language disorders.

    Bibliography: p.
    Includes index.
    1. Language disorders in children.   2. Children—
Language.   I. Title.   [DNLM: 1. Language disorders—
In infancy and childhood.   WM 475 N876c]
RJ496.L35H8   618.92′855   80-39591
ISBN   0-13-132001-7

Editorial production/supervision
and interior design by *Edith Riker*
Cover design by *Wanda Lubelska*
Manufacturing buyer *Edmund W. Leone*

Ask not what you can do for language;
ask what language can do for you.

10   9   8   7   6   5   4   3   2   1

Prentice-Hall International, Inc., *London*
Prentice-Hall of Australia Pty. Limited, *Sydney*
Prentice-Hall of Canada, Ltd., *Toronto*
Prentice-Hall of India Private Limited, *New Delhi*
Prentice-Hall of Japan, Inc., *Tokyo*
Prentice-Hall of Southeast Asia Pte. Ltd., *Singapore*
Whitehall Books Limited, *Wellington, New Zealand*

CONTENTS

7049714

TO

Bobby, Mike, Brian, Danny, Lyle, Tracy, Jean, Chris, Chad,

Matt, Trina, Jonathan, Jared,

Karla, Margaret, Charlie, Eric, Marie, Eddie, . . .

ACKNOWLEDGMENTS

For several years I taught courses in linguistics, children's language acquisition, and children's language disorders. At the same time I supervised a clinical program for language impaired youngsters. In the process of doing all these activities concurrently, I had a beautiful opportunity to study how these various areas relate in children's language disorders. It was from those experiences that this book was born.

In writing these acknowledgments, I am reminded of a history teacher I once knew who emphasized how each figure in history stood on the shoulders of those who had gone before. My writing is in the same mold, because I have taken ideas from practically everyone. To use a different metaphor, creativity is sometimes defined as seeing old things in new relationships. This book fits at least the first half of that definition, because indeed most of the ideas are not new with me.

There are some people that I must recognize individually, because of their contributions to my growth, and to my understanding of children. They are: Ida MacDonald, Harvey Reddick, Maryjane Rees, Oliver Skalbeck, Peg Byrne, Jim Stachowiak, Bob Douglass, Ralph Shelton, Georgia Foster, and Jim Chalfant; also, a special thanks to Sue Seitz. There are other individuals who have taught me much, although I have never met them. You will see their names cited over and over in the pages of this book. Finally, I thank the students that I've known for their enthusiasm, ideas, and penetrating questions, as well as their patience with my abstractions and word games.

I have learned the most from the children that I have had the opportunity to work with. While I changed their names as I wrote about them, their presence in the book is very real to me. I take this opportunity to express my deep gratitude and affection to each of them.

The editors at Prentice-Hall provided a superior combination of guidance and support: Brian Walker with the early development of the manuscript and John Busch who worked with me through the last two-thirds of the book. I also owe a large debt to Prentice-Hall's editoral consultants. These anonymous reviewers contributed more to the book than they realize in awakening me to my blind spots, providing new directions, and forcing me to confront my own muddy thinking. I hope I meet these reviewers sometime . . . perhaps I already have. Additionally, I would like to thank Vicki Bellino, who should enter the typewriter olympics. She produced draft after draft with her own charming blend of patience, efficiency, and hard work. To all of these people, I give my thanks for support unfailing and criticism unflailing.

Finally, I thank my beloved wife and children, Nancy, Ann, and Greg, who sacrificed three summer vacations and many weekends so that Pa could write his book.

R.D.H.

INTRODUCTION

Language is at the heart of human experience. It involves all three of the great spheres through which we interact with the world: the sensate, the rational, and the emotional. It is sensate because it depends on and guides perception, the receiving and recognizing of information through the senses. It is rational both because it is a coherent linguistic system and because logic and reason depend on language. Finally, it is emotional, not only because we use language to express emotions, but because language use both forms human relationships and derives from human relationships. Childhood is the crucible in which these three ways to know the world develop in each individual. The study of children's language disorders is thus of value at two levels. First, we can explore the question of how best to serve language-impaired children and their families. Second, because disorders of language highlight the human processes in which they occur, we can learn a little more about ourselves. Let us begin.

I see four factors that are of special importance in children's language development and language disorders. The first is conceptual development. The child's conceptual repertoire forms the pool of knowledge and meaning that underlies language. If language could not represent knowledge, there would be little to talk about. At the same time, language contributes to the development of concepts and knowledge in general.

A second factor is the child's information-processing skills. Included here are sensory systems, attention, intermodal connections, memory, and cognitive strategies. It is through these functions that we take in information, both linguistic and nonverbal, and that we express ourselves. Also, these processes are the bases for specific skills, such as auditory memory span, that are of concern to professionals working with language-disordered children. It is clear that conceptual development depends on the child's information-processing capacities. As we will see, information-processing skills are themselves influenced by conceptual development. The two come together in the area of problem solving.

The third factor in language development and disorders is the nature of language itself. We will take a brief look at linguistic theory, both structural and transformational. Particular emphasis will be given to the relationship between language structure and how language conveys meaning. We will focus on the development of language as a means to communicate, rather than the development of linguistic structure *per se*.

Communication does not occur in a vacuum, however. The fourth factor is human relationships. One cannot communicate without entering into a human relationship to some extent. Thus, the use of language is inseparable from participation in such relationships. This observation is of obvious importance because clinical work and teaching are human relationships. In addition, study of this fourth factor leads directly to the study of the family system and working with parents.

Language learning, then, is based on all four of these factors, each influencing all the others. Language intervention schemes need to recognize this complexity. Fortunately, there are some general principles that can be derived from this intersection of disciplines. The development of these principles will be one of several themes running through this book.

Another theme is individual differences.

If each child is a product of the interaction of many factors, no two cases of language impairment are going to be quite the same. It follows that the mode of treatment will vary with the child's situation. With some children the most efficient strategy might be to work almost entirely with the parents. Other children need highly structured training. Still others may need a more flexible regimen, perhaps with the focus more on relationship contexts than on structural elements of language. In many cases the clinician or teacher may wish to implement more than one treatment strategy with the same child.

A third theme is that language learning should involve the active participation of the child. Children think while they learn, and we should take advantage of that fact. Thus, we will focus on cognitive strategies, problem solving, and decision making by the child as related to language use. Both comprehension and expression will be viewed as problem-solving tasks.

Finally, I will approach parent involvement from a family theory perspective. There is a great deal of evidence that the family functions as a system. Change in one family member, either in a child or in a parent attempting to help that child, is best viewed in terms of the family system. If we understand something of how a child functions in a family, we are better able to help both the child and the family.

In this book, then, I will be concerned with the integration of these many factors. No such integration can be complete or entirely satisfactory, but we can only learn from the attempt. As a subscriber to general systems theory, I believe that no one of the factors in language development is independent of the others and that change in one

area leads to change in others. Before embarking on this tour, let me discuss the nature of language and children's language disorders a little more specifically.

LANGUAGE

Language has both cognitive and social aspects. It may be seen as having two major functions. First, language is representational. We use language to represent our knowledge of reality, both concrete things and events and abstract thoughts and theories. Second, language is a communicative medium. We use language to exchange information with other human beings. Language is often viewed from one or the other of these perspectives, for instance, in studies of the relation between language and perception or in studies of language and social behavior. An appreciation of the dual nature of language, however, is essential to approaching children's language disorders. The representational function is related to perception, the development of concepts, logical thinking, and other areas of cognition, and is the avenue of most school learning. The communicative function is also involved in learning but is in addition a major mechanism in the conduct of our daily lives and ultimately a fundamental means of participating in human relationships.

This duality of language, however, has a circular quality to it which, at a deeper level, unites these two functions. We represent what we know with language. When we communicate, we communicate this representation, rather than any "pure" knowledge or facts (Bandler and Grinder 1975). At the same time, much of what we know is acquired through communication, and much of that through language (Watzlawick 1976). Thus, the two functions are inseparable in language. We develop our representation of the world largely through language and other communication, but we communicate through language only that which we represent with language.

Let us look at how language accomplishes this dual function. It is a code in which information such as perceptions, ideas, and feelings are represented by linguistic elements, such as words and grammatical features. This representational process may be called symbolization (Chafe 1970). The elements of language are combined in various ways to create different messages, but there is a consistency in how they are combined. In other words, language is a system. The combinations that occur are predictable. In fact, languages are often described with sets of rules that specify just which combinations can occur. Linguists use the term "lexicon" to refer to the collection of symbols or the vocabulary pool and the term "grammar" to refer to the rules for the construction of utterances.

If language is to succeed as a code, various users of any particular language will have to apply the items in the lexicon and grammar in very similar ways. We all agree to some extent on what different words mean, and we use approximately the same set of rules for constructing utterances. At a higher level, though, language is arbitrary. There is no inherent relation between a word and what it symbolizes. Any combination of sounds can represent any idea, as long as the speakers of a language associate the same combination with the same idea. This arbitrariness of language seems so apparent as to be trivial in our culture with its many communication technologies, but it may not be at all apparent or trivial in cultures where words have magical power or, perhaps, for young children, who appear to treat a word as somehow the same as, or as having control over, what it represents.

Language is structured in a way that contributes to its efficiency as a code. There is a finite number of speech sounds in each language. In English there are about forty-six, depending on how many dialectical variants you count. These sounds are combined into an enormous number of words, around half a million. Hockett (1960) has used the term "duality of patterning" to refer to this process of combining and recombining a certain number of elements into many different items. Thus, we form the many words of English by different patterns of the same sounds, and similarly we can produce literally an infinite number of sentences through different patterns of words. This tremendous variety underscores again the importance of the regularity of the language code. It is hard to imagine anyone being able to learn a code that did not exhibit such regularity. It is this regularity of expression, the grammar of the language, that the child must learn, as well as the lexical items and their associated meanings.

CHILDREN'S LANGUAGE DISORDERS

A language disorder may be thought of as a significant impairment in the use of language, whether in its representational-cognitive function, its communicative-relationship function, or both. Clearly this statement is too broad to function as a definition. Virtually everyone, at one time or another, has difficulty that could be called significant in using language. You may freeze up while asking for a raise; a child may not comprehend a remark from an adult; a student may not remember names or dates on a test or fail a test because of misinterpreting some of the questions. A language disorder must be more serious than these occasional difficulties that we all encounter.

Consider adult aphasia, the impairment of language function caused by brain damage. Aphasics may report that they know what they want to say but cannot get the words out. Some aphasics retain reading or writing skills better than auditory or vocal skills; some show other patterns. The overall picture is of impairment of language function *per se*.

Using the model of adult aphasia is not entirely satisfactory when viewing children's language disorders, although, of course, there are children with true aphasia. In aphasia there is a specific etiology, or cause, whereas in children's language disorders there may, in many cases, be no identifiable etiology. The individual with adult aphasia had already learned language before the impairment occurred, whereas in a child impairment occurs concomitant with the development of language. This factor makes it difficult to sort out language impairment from learning or cognitive impairment.

Language disorders in children encompass all areas of language, including vocabulary, meaning, sentence structure, details of grammar such as plurals and tenses, and the ability to use language in learning and in other forms of communication. Both receptive and expressive skills may be involved. Disorders range from language delay, in which the child is significantly behind chronological age norms in language development, to impairments in the use of grammatical structures in older children. In language delay both the representational and communicative functions are affected. The older child may have a more subtle disability that permits successful functioning in

everyday communicative situations but becomes a major obstacle in classroom learning.

Children's language disorders may occur in association with a number of other aspects of developmental impairment, or they may be present in children who seem otherwise relatively intact. Hearing loss obviously has a powerful effect on language development, although hearing-impaired children are not usually considered as having a language disorder *per se*. Children may present symptoms of retardation, emotional disturbance, or learning disabilities as well as impairments in the use of language. It is often difficult to sort out these various problem areas. In fact, the relations between language disorders and retardation, emotional disturbance, and learning disabilities are perhaps more important than the differences between them. Each disorder area is not necessarily a clear-cut entity, separate and distinct from other areas of developmental impairment.

Finally, children's language disorders are specific to each impaired child. Cultural groups that demonstrate difficulty with language in the classroom should not be thought of as demonstrating language disorders. For example, in certain Amerind groups, children do not answer immediately after they are spoken to by adults. Such an answer would be impulsive and would not reflect respect and careful thought. Similarly, large numbers of children do not speak the same dialect or even the same language as that used in the classroom. These groups of children do not manifest any pathology in using language. I do not mean to imply that the difficulties these children may encounter are not real or important, only that they should not be regarded as pathological or disordered.

In summary, a language disorder is a

disability in the use of language specific to a particular child. This disability is severe enough to cause significant impairment in the child's language functioning in the representational domain, the communicative domain, or both. Because of the central importance of language in cognitive activity, learning, socialization, and the human experience in general, a language impairment can have profound effects on the course of a child's life.

Working with language-disordered children is a problem-solving process. We try to figure out how best to enhance the language skills of each different child. This book is an attempt to provide a framework for making those decisions. The first five chapters concentrate on areas that are fundamental for language learning and use. We will begin with concepts and rules. These ideas will then be placed in the context of information processing and perception. With that background we can look more directly at language itself. Finally, in Chapter 5, language will be considered from the perspective of human relationships and communication. The next three chapters will continue to integrate this information but will stress the more specific clinical concerns of causation, assessment, and language sampling. The remaining chapters are devoted to intervention. After presenting a general perspective in Chapter 9, the succeeding chapters will focus on different aspects of intervention. The representational and communicative functions of language will be brought together in developing ways to help children learn to use specific aspects of language, such as vocabulary items and grammatical structures. Next we will consider human relationship contexts in which that learning is enhanced. Chapter 12 will expand this theme by approaching human relationships in the larger perspective of family processes. Finally, the last chapter will focus on clinicians and trainers themselves and the problem-solving strategies they engage in.

1

CONCEPTS, RULES, AND METARULES

One way we can think of language is as a way to represent reality. Both speakers and listeners interpret language as referring to various aspects of reality. If I say to a child, "Put your bubble gum in the garbage can," and the child does so, then my words represent aspects of reality, such as *bubble gum* and *garbage can,* to both me and that child. Language is the system that links the sounds I uttered to those items of reality. But reality isn't limited to the physical world. I can also use language to talk about past events, dreams of the future, and many other phenomena whose existence is entirely mental. Reality is truly infinite.

If language is going to represent specific aspects of this infinite range of possibilities, then reality must be constituted in such a way that this type of representation is possible. Bolinger (1975) has described some aspects of reality that are necessary for language to function in this way. First, reality must be segmentable. We have to be able to identify various components of reality and to separate them from other aspects of reality. Thus, the word *dog* has no meaning unless we are able to differentiate dogs from cats and other furry critters. If we cannot separate a particular segment of reality from other aspects of reality, we cannot identify or recognize that segment. In addition, these segments of reality are generally repeatable. We recognize many furry animals as dogs, and we recognize the same dog in different instances. Our knowledge of reality is based partially on the consistency of that reality. Finally, these segments of reality must have some element of ambiguity built into them. We have to be able to recognize tall dogs and short dogs, furry dogs and hairless dogs, brown dogs and white dogs, shaggy dogs and manicured dogs with ribbons and rhinestones, all as

belonging to the category *dog*. Our segments cannot be so specific that they do not allow any variation within a segment.

These segments of reality are perhaps best viewed as concepts. Definitions of the term "concept" vary, but in general concepts involve categorization (That is a dog, not a cat) and generalization (That, too, is a dog). Moreover, as Bruner, Goodnow, and Austin (1956) point out, concepts go beyond generalization and categorization. A concept is a network of inferences by which one goes beyond the properties used to identify and classify an object or event to inferences about unobserved properties and functions of that object or event. Thus, if we see a furry animal with the appropriate configuration of body, head, and other features, we classify that animal as a dog, but in addition we know that that animal can bark, bite, learn tricks, carry objects in its teeth, jump, run, perhaps carry a flask around its neck, and do many other things.

Concepts, then, represent our knowledge about reality. In turn, they are the subject matter about which we talk. When we say that language represents reality, we really mean that language represents our conceptions of reality. In fact, language, communication, and reality interact in fascinating ways. In the preceding paragraphs reality was discussed as if it were absolute and independent of our knowledge of it. In truth, however, it appears that we construct our knowledge of reality (Ornstein 1972), that is, each person develops an individual representation of reality. This personal construction of reality is heavily influenced by the culture of which we are a part, and culture in turn is based on communication. As Olson (1970a) put it, we learn to interpret reality—to perceive selectively—and language plays an important role in directing our perceptions. Expanding that focus, Watzlawick (1976) has argued convincingly that what we know as reality is dependent upon communication rather than upon transcendent truths of some sort. Thus, reality, concepts, communication, and language are all overlapping and mutually interdependent. Language does not develop in a vacuum, nor does it develop to fit reality. Rather, children's language and their construction of reality develop together in the context of communication and culture.

We will explore aspects of this phenomenon as we proceed through this book. Our focus now is on concepts, rules, and metarules. What follows is not at all intended as a description of a developmental progression of various stages in conceptual development. Rather, it is an attempt to describe various types of concepts and rules in ways that I hope will be useful in understanding their relations to language and language training.

CORE CONCEPTS

A concept may be defined according to its functions or according to its perceptual attributes. That is, one may define a ball according to what it is used for or according to what it looks like. Nelson (1973) proposed that many early concepts develop first in terms of function. For example, a child first learns about cups by using them. Nelson calls these concepts "core concepts." There are several components to the development of a core concept. First, the child must identify a cup as an individual whole. It must be separated from other things in the environment. At this stage, however, it is not

necessary for the child to analyze the cup into its component attributes, such as round, open on the top but closed on the bottom, and having a handle.

Functional Relations

Now that the child is aware of a cup as an entity, awareness of the functional relations of that cup develops. The child learns that the cup holds liquids, is used for drinking, that its contents can spill out, and so forth. These things are learned through actual experience with the cup. Nelson states that these functions are learned in the defining context for cup. That is, one learns about the functions of cup by experiencing cups in the context in which they are used. It is much more difficult to learn the functions of cup by looking at cups on a shelf or using a cup as a building block. Thus, the term "functional relation" represents the idea that the child learns how the cup functions in relation to its defining context, which would include such things as people, food and liquids, and other eating implements. The core concept as described so far could become established with only one exemplar of cup. This concept broadens as the child begins to experience other cups in similar defining contexts and a more generalized core concept develops.

The development of a core concept is based on knowledge of one's acts on an object or class of objects. For this reason core concepts are more likely to develop for objects that the child can grasp or manipulate, such as cup, ball, or toy car, than for objects that cannot be manipulated, such as tree, sofa, or floor. The young child's life contains many recurring experiences that would lend themselves to the development of core concepts, such as opening doors, eating with a spoon, putting on clothes, and playing with blocks.

Language and Core Concepts

Nelson believes that language is not necessary for the development of core concepts. They depend on the discovery of functional relations through motor activity and therefore would be classified as sensory-motor in Piaget's formulation. It should be added, though, that motor behavior can be learned through imitating a model (Bandura 1969). That is, a child may begin to eat with a spoon after seeing a sister use one. In addition, language may play a role in calling attention to the object or to the model.

The importance of core concepts for the language clinician is twofold. First, many children will demonstrate knowledge of core concepts for which they do not know the appropriate words. This observation may be particularly important in working with severely impaired children who appear to know few words, if any at all. These children may demonstrate knowledge of core concepts such as sock, shoe, shirt, wash, eat, cup. This information is very useful in deciding where vocabulary training should begin. The process involved in the acquisition of core concepts is important in a second way: the clinician can use functional relations presented in appropriate defining contexts to teach a child certain types of concepts where verbal explanations might be beyond the child's comprehension.

CONCRETE CONCEPTS

Obviously, objects do not occur only in their defining contexts. Cups appear, not only when there is something to drink, but also on store shelves, in boxes of junk, on automobile dashboards, and many other places. In these cases one cannot recognize a cup by its functional relationships, because they are not apparent outside the defining context. Rather, one recognizes a cup by its perceptual attributes, such as its shape, hollow configuration, and handle. Nelson emphasizes that it is not appropriate to think of this as a second "stage" in the development of a concept. For most concepts, a child is becoming aware of perceptual attributes concurrently with the development of functional relations.

Criterial Attributes

For much of the remainder of our discussion of concepts and rules, we will use the terminology proposed by Gagné (1970). He refers to concepts based on perceptual attributes as concrete concepts. "Concrete" refers to the fact that they are ultimately verifiable through the senses. In other words, if an object has the perceptual attributes associated with a particular concept, then it is an exemplar of that concept. If one doesn't have an exemplar of a particular concrete concept available, in principle at least, one can go and find such an exemplar. Because an object is categorized as belonging to a particular concrete concept if it has a specific configuration of attributes, these characteristics are sometimes called "criterial attributes." A criterial attribute is some characteristic that an item must have if it is to be a member of a particular concept. For example, a triangle must have three straight sides, all joined together at the ends. If one side is not straight, it isn't a triangle; if it has four sides, it isn't a triangle.

The learning of concrete concepts, then, depends primarily on perception rather than motor activity. In this perceptual activity the child learns to recognize various configurations of criterial attributes as being associated with various concrete concepts. Frequently such concepts develop and become refined over time. A young child may develop concrete concepts that contain some, but not all, of the criterial attributes, for example, a child who refers to all large domesticated mammals as *cow* or who calls all men *daddy*. It is again impossible accurately to partial out the influence of language in these situations. Does a child "see" cows, horses, donkeys, and sheep as being the same or merely use the same word for them? Similarly, might that child be aware of attributes that differentiate among those animals but at the same time not consider them criterial?

Core Concepts and Concrete Concepts

It can be seen that typically neither core concepts nor concrete concepts are complete in themselves. Consider a concept like *ball*. We identify objects as belonging to this category both on the basis of criterial attributes, such as "round," and in terms of function, such as "rolls" and "is used for play." Different objects may be classified for different reasons. A piece of paper that has been crunched up may be classified as a ball because of its roundish appearance and because it's being thrown around the classroom. A ball bearing may be classified as a ball because it is nearly perfectly round, but a round lamp globe would not be considered a ball. If we could not classify objects on both perceptual and functional bases, our concepts would not be nearly as finely differentiated or as rich as they are.

Gagné argues that the acquisition of concrete concepts cannot be explained on the basis of simple stimulus-response learning. In his view the effect of acquiring a concrete

concept is to free the individual from control by specific stimuli with regard to that particular concept. This type of generalization is what gives concrete concepts their tremendous power. As mentioned at the beginning of this chapter, knowing a concept entails a whole set of inferences that may go far beyond the physically present stimuli (Bruner, Goodnow, and Austin 1956). In like fashion, this versatility adds to the power and flexibility of language because one function of language is to represent such concepts.

Target Areas

Not all scholars view perceptually based concepts in terms of criterial attributes. Chafe (1970) suggests that concepts function as "target areas." That is, each concept is manifested in a central focus and then a gradual fading away from that focus. The color spectrum presents a good example of this idea. There are some colors that are very definitely blue and would be recognized as blue by anyone in our culture. These blues are in the central focus of the concept *blue*. There are other blues that one would classify as being bluish but not right on target. Fading further away, there are some colors that may be categorized as either blue or green by different individuals. They are on the very periphery of the concept. Finally, there are many colors that virtually no one would identify as blue. Rosch (1973) has made a proposal that is similar in many ways. A perceptual category is organized around the "best examples" of that category, which she calls "focal examples." Other exemplars of the category approximate the focal examples to greater or lesser degrees. Thus, in either Chafe's or Rosch's view, a child would identify the central focus of a concept after some experience with that concept, the amount of experience varying with the concept and the child. The child would then categorize other objects in terms of how "close" they are to the focal examples.

Concepts and Language

There has been a great deal of study concerning the relationship between conceptual development and language development with regard to the types of concepts discussed so far. Must a concept be present before its corresponding word can be acquired, or does a word provide a focus around which a concept can develop? Gagné notes that concrete concepts, by definition, can be acquired without language; they are based on perception. Language, he feels, makes the acquisition of these concepts much easier, but not through any explanation or definition of a particular concept. Rather, language directs perception and provides a vehicle for making associations. Suppose, for example, you want to teach a young child what *hollow* means. You can show a child things that vary greatly in appearance, such as a piece of pipe, a balloon, and an empty jar, but by indicating that each is hollow you direct the child to the feature that is the same about each object. At the same time, you provide a symbol to associate with that feature.

Other scholars have explored the relation between concepts and language in broader perspectives. Piaget and Inhelder (1969) argued that conceptual development is primary. Language represents concepts, but it is not a major influence in their development. Bruner (1966), on the other hand, argues that with increasing maturity the child's conceptual system conforms more and more to the structure represented by the language of the culture. Beilin (1976) proposed that both the language and the con-ceptual systems are derived from a more general and abstract set of structures.

It may be that the ultimate truth in this matter will never be uncovered or perhaps doesn't even exist in the terms that have been used to explore the question. It makes sense to me that concepts, language, and the social milieu interact and are mutually influential in complex ways. Further, there is no reason to assume that all concepts are dealt with in the same way by all children. It may be that some children have a tendency to develop central focus concepts while others attend more to specific perceptual attributes. Further, different concepts may lend themselves to different types of formulation. Concepts in a continuously varying medium, such as color or smell, may encourage the development of central focus concepts, while others may not. Certainly it would be easier to develop a core concept for *book* than for *ceiling*. Similarly, children may vary in the degree to which their perceptions are directly influenced by the language they hear. The degree of individual differences in the development of concepts by children has not been explored systematically. Wherever individual differences in cognitive processing have been the focus of study, however, they have indeed been found. We will return to this matter in the next chapter.

It is noteworthy that in the vast majority of vocabulary work with language-disordered children, the focus is on concrete concepts. We test children and train children primarily through the use of picture stimuli. For the most part these stimuli allow the child access to the concept only through perceptual attributes—and at one level of abstraction away from the real objects at that. Pictures have two advantages. They are compact and easy to handle, and with them clinicians can depict a greater range of concepts than can be done with genuine exemplars of those objects. It is difficult, to say the least, to bring a house or a car into a clinic room. On the other hand, I have worked with children who did not respond appropriately when I asked them to point to a picture of a ball or a toy car but demonstrated very clearly that they possessed the appropriate core concepts when I offered them a car or ball to play with. We should not be seduced by the convenience of picture stimuli to use such stimuli without first attempting to determine what type of stimuli will be most effective with a particular child.

RELATIONAL OR ABSTRACT CONCEPTS

There are many concepts that cannot be identified through perceptual attributes. They can be identified only in terms of relationships with other concepts. Gagné calls such concepts abstract concepts, in contrast to concrete concepts. He suggests, however, that they might better be termed relational concepts because they always contain a relation. Consider the following line:

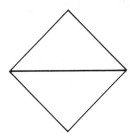

You would not be inclined to call this line a diagonal, but if I put it in the appropriate context, it would then be a diagonal:

Diagonal, then, is a relational concept. You cannot identify this relational concept in the same way you identify a concrete concept. A relational concept has no perceptual attributes embodied in it. It is identifiable only in terms of its relationships with other concepts. In this case those concepts are *straight line, rectangle,* and *opposite corner.* It is the relationship between the straight line and the opposite corners of the rectangle that defines the straight line as a diagonal. There is nothing inherent in the line itself that indicates that it is a diagonal.

Varieties of Relational Concepts

There appear to be several varieties of relational concepts. These varieties may be aligned on a continuum according to how they are apprehended. Some may be observed directly. For example, relational concepts like *in, on, third,* and *diagonal* can be identified in any one instance. Note again the character of these concepts. *On* indicates a position in space some object may have relative to something else. *Third* only has meaning relative to other ordinal positions. Obviously, while these concepts can be identified in one instance, it may have taken many instances for them to have been learned in the first place.

Other relational concepts may be observed but not on the basis of one instance. *Miles per gallon* would be an example. One cannot determine miles per gallon by observing how much gas is in the tank and what the mileage of the car is. Rather, one must keep a record over time of both gasoline consumption and miles traveled. *Reinforcement* would be another example. Giving candy to a child cannot be defined as reinforcement *a priori.* Rather, one must keep a record over time to see if the repeated presentation of candy systematically influences the way the child behaves.

Finally, there are relational concepts that apparently can never be identified through observation. *Democracy* would be an example. Gagné calls such relational concepts "defined concepts" because they must be learned by definition. Other examples of defined concepts would be *uncle* and *president*. It can be seen, then, that relational concepts vary greatly in degree of abstraction. In addition, the component concepts in a relational concept may be concrete, as in the case of *lid*, or they may themselves be relational, as in the case of *family*.

Relational Concepts and Language

With some exceptions, such as those related to physical position in space, relational concepts are intimately bound to language. Typically they are learned with the aid of language. Many, particularly defined concepts, literally cannot be learned without language. Could one learn the concept of *formula* without language? *Sociology? Pun? Abstraction? Perception?*

At the same time, grammatical categories are themselves relational concepts. Subject, verb, and object are described by linguists as basic grammatical relations. Verb tenses similarly are relational in nature. *The* doesn't mean anything except in relation to other words. The use of pronouns and the whole area of what linguists call "deixis"— the orienting features of language relative to place and time and shifts in speaker-listener roles (Lyons 1968)—are all based on relational concepts. Training children to use grammatical categories, then, presents an ironic challenge. According to Gagné, the best way to teach relational concepts is through language. But attempts to explain to a young child when to use *I* and when to use *me* are notoriously unsuccessful. Such grammatical categories must be presented to children in ways that highlight their relational qualities.

RULES

Relational concepts turn out to be a special case of a more general phenomenon, which Gagné calls "rules." A rule is a combination of concepts. Rules show relationships between concepts. This definition of rule is broader than the conventional idea of a rule as a prescription for behavior, as in "Keep to the right," "Right turn permitted after stop," or "No smoking." A rule merely specifies a relationship between certain concepts.

Consider a simple rule: *Ice cream melts.* Any young child who leaves an ice-cream parlor with a nice new strawberry cone and arrives home with red nose, red chin, and a drippy red hand and elbow is coming to know this rule. What makes this statement a rule is that it specifies a relationship between two concepts, *ice cream* and *melt*. Before truly possessing this rule the child will know these two concepts and the relationship between them. Here is another rule: *Blocks can be stacked.* To understand this rule the child must first know *blocks* and *stack*. The *can* suggests that other things as well may be done with blocks and is at least partly an artifact of English usage. It's a little awkward to say simply, *Blocks stack.* One more: *Turning the doorknob opens the door.* Note again that in order to function with this rule, the child must know *turn, doorknob, open,* and *door*.

Characteristics of Rules

There are several characteristics that these rules share. First, as has been mentioned, an individual needs to know the component concepts in order to know the rule. Second, rules generally contain at least one relational concept. Recall that a rule is a relation between concepts. That relation is often embodied in a relational concept. *Melt, stack, turn,* and *open* are all such concepts. The rules we have used have all contained concrete concepts as well, but that doesn't have to be the case, as in *Melting can be stopped.* Third, rules vary greatly in their complexity. While the rules in the preceding examples have been very simple, any one could be expanded to a more complex rule: *Ice cream melts quickly on a hot day if you don't lick it up speedily.* We now have a richer and more complicated set of relations between concepts. Rules can get inordinately complex, as in many statements in textbooks (surely not this one!) and the classic example, published governmental regulations.

Some clarification may be needed concerning the difference between a relational concept and a rule. They are formally the same: relationships between concepts. The difference is in their applications. As Gagné puts it, in a relational concept one is defining the relation involved; in a rule one is applying the relation. Thus, in defining the relational concept of *diagonal* what is important is that we note the relation between the line and its surrounding rectangle. In applying the rule *The thermostat controls the room temperature,* what is important is that we apply the relation between the thermostat and the temperature.

Rules and Language

Two other aspects of rules need more extensive discussion. The first is the interplay between language and rules. Each of the preceding rules was presented as a grammatical statement. Language, however, is not necessary for the acquisition of all rules. Any young child who looks up at a light fixture while flicking a light switch is evidencing knowledge of a rule concerning the relation between lights and light switches, with

or without the words for it. Stated more forcefully, knowing a verbal statement of a rule is not always the same as knowing the rule itself. The rule statement may be memorized as a verbal chain without the accompanying knowledge of the rule. Being able to recite a particular formula in math or statistics, for example, is not the same as being able to solve problems related to that formula. Similarly, "simple, clear" directions for assembling a kit may prove frustratingly difficult when one is actually trying to put the thing together. Gagné also cites evidence showing that while the verbal statement of a rule may be forgotten rather quickly, "rule-governed behavior" is often retained at a high level.

This phenomenon is apparent in language learning and language use. Almost no one but a linguist can tell you the order in which different types of adjectives appear before a noun in English, but we all conform to that order in talking. Many speakers of English cannot state the rule *Use the subjunctive in cases contrary to fact,* but they use that construction appropriately. On the other hand, many students are taught that rule and can recite it but do not demonstrate it in their use of English.

Summarizing, we must be careful to separate the statement of a rule from the knowledge of that rule. Gagné argues, however, that language is often very important in the learning of rules. Verbal statements may function as cues to aid rule learning. As with relational concepts, language may direct perception and provide key associations. In some cases a verbal statement may be enough to teach a rule. (If this were not the case, the entire higher education enterprise might be out of business.) Obviously the effectiveness of teaching rules through verbal statements depends on both the nature of the rule and the sophistication of the listener. In language training we are faced with the fascinating complication of using language to teach language.

The Reality of Rules

A final consideration in our discussion deals with the nature of rules themselves. Gagné states that a rule is an inferred capability. When we say that children's behavior is rule governed, we mean that they act as if they know the rules relevant to the situation. To say, then, that a child in clinic "has the rule for plurals" or "knows the rule for past tense" is reification. To reify is to treat an abstraction as if it were a thing. Thus, to say that a child knows certain linguistic rules because that child's verbal behavior can be described with those rules is to reify or impute a reality to those rules in the child's head. But linguistic rules are developed by linguists, not by children. We simply do not know how information about language structure is coded in the minds of language users. The term "linguistic rule," then, when used to refer to aspects of a speaker's knowledge of language, is a metaphor. It is a convenient fiction used to represent the void in our knowledge about how people actually store and process language. This metaphor is convincing because the scientific community of Western culture has been describing many phenomena with rules for a long time and linguists have been describing languages with rules for a long time. However, returning to Gagné's formulation, a rule is an inferred capacity. Although a child behaves in a way that can be described with a rule, we do not know that the child organized that behavior with a rule. Most important, as suggested by Miller (1964), we do not know that the child organized that behavior with the same rule that we used to

describe it. I am not arguing against the psychological reality of rules. In fact, I will use the concept of rules frequently myself. I am simply saying that we should be cautious in imputing to children the knowledge of specific linguistic rules, such as "the passive transformation rule" or the "subject-verb agreement rule."

In spite of their somewhat nebulous character, rules are extremely important. They represent the relations between concepts that are expressed in the relations between words and sentences. Whatever the ultimate psychological reality of linguistic rules, they are a major means for analyzing and describing the structure of language. At the same time they are very abstract. Grammatical rules describe relations between other grammatical rules and the relational concepts embodied in grammatical classes. Bruner (1966) has commented on the remarkable fact that young children demonstrate fairly competent knowledge of the abstract rules and categories of language but do not demonstrate a comparable level of dealing with abstraction in other areas of intellectual development. As children mature and enter school, rule learning becomes a major component, if not the dominant aspect, of classroom learning.

Rules and Behavior

I have emphasized an interpretation of rules as specifying relations between concepts. Linguistic rules were seen as a special case of this phenomenon. It should be emphasized that, in addition, rules do indeed govern and organize behavior. In fact, the function of social groups, from individual families to entire cultural groups, may be described with sets of rules. Rules of this type still specify relations between concepts, but the concepts involved relate more directly to behavior as well as the conceptual categories that represent that behavior. Thus, rules may have a conceptual or intellectual manifestation and, in addition, a behavioral or social manifestation.

RULE HIERARCHIES AND METARULES

In many cases a great many different rules can be used to describe the same phenomenon. Consider, for example, a situation in which a clinician is using contingency management techniques in training a child to produce certain types of grammatical structures. At the very least there are rules involved in the contingency management procedure, there are rules involved in other aspects of the interpersonal relationship, and there are rules involved in the grammatical structures themselves. Or consider the rules involved in solving a complicated multiplication problem. There are rules representing the individual arithmetic facts, such as $9 \times 4 = 36$ and $6 + 3 = 9$, and there are rules about what to multiply by what, where to add, and so forth. In either of these examples there are lower-level rules associated with relatively small aspects of the whole situation and there are higher-level rules associated with more global aspects of the situation. Two terms are important in this connection. The first is "rule hierarchy." A rule hierarchy is a system of rules on a continuum between lower-level rules and higher-level rules. The second term is "metarule." A metarule is a higher-level rule, or a rule about rules.

Rule Hierarchies

Let us explore these two terms more fully. Any complex behavior can be described with a rule hierarchy. Take a card game, for example. There is a set of relational concepts that identify the individual cards. Then there are rules specifying the relationships among the cards. There are rules indicating how many people may play and in what orders they may participate. Then there are rules governing the behavior of individual players, such as the moves a player can make. The rule hierarchy as described so far is similar to what one might find in a printed set of rules for that particular card game. But there are additional levels of rules, sometimes written and sometimes not, related to strategies for winning and for playing the game with appropriate etiquette. These rules may vary, depending on whether one is playing with friends or strangers and on whether the game is being played for fun or for money. Finally, there may be rules regulating when and where the game can be played at all. For example, card playing or gambling may not be permitted in certain locales. All of these rules together, and doubtless other sets of rules, comprise the rule hierarchy associated with that particular game. The same principle would apply to chess, bowling, or ticktacktoe. Some of these rules clearly exist in explicit form, such as the rules that regulate the moves a player can make. Others are of a more tenuous nature, such as those regulating the human relationships involved.

Language is very definitely organized in a fashion that suggests a rule hierarchy. Bruner (1966) commented on this phenomenon from a psychological viewpoint. Bolinger (1975) made similar observations from a linguistic perspective. From either viewpoint there are rules governing the formation and combination of elements at each level of language and rules relating the various levels. Language consists of sets of categories (relational concepts) and sets of rules (rule hierarchies) for nesting or organizing those categories.

Metarules

The second term to be discussed is "metarule." Some of the rules in the preceding examples occur at higher levels than others. For example, if card playing is not permitted in some situation, all the other rules about card playing become irrelevant in that situation. Or, if you choose a particular strategy of play in a card game, this choice will organize many of the lower-level rules concerning the types of moves you can make. These higher-level rules, or metarules, govern the use of lower-level rules. They specify which lower-level rules may apply, and they specify the relationships between lower-level rules.

Suppose you are multiplying fractions. The metarule is that you multiply the numerators together, then you multiply the denominators together, and then you divide the numerator by the denominator, if possible. That metarule governs your use of the individual multiplication rules (multiplication facts) and the relational concepts of numerator and denominator. You need all these levels of knowledge before you can multiply fractions. Or, imagine a situation in which a young child says loudly, "I gotta go!" during a church service and the mother responds with a "Shush." That child's utterance may be described with linguistic rules, and the production of that utterance results from the application of a metarule, "Tell your mother when you have to go"; but the mother is applying a higher-level metarule, "We don't holler things like that out loud in polite society."

This last example illustrates another point. A rule can be identified as being a metarule only in relation to some other rule

or rules. That is, "metarule" is itself a relational concept. Thus, rules within a rule hierarchy will be "meta" to lower-level rules but will in turn be lower-level rules to other metarules at still higher levels. Further, it can be seen that the ideas of rule hierarchy and metarule are interlocking and interdependent. The existence of a rule hierarchy always implies the presence of metarules; but the existence of metarules is only possible in the context of a rule hierarchy.

It may not always be important to determine whether a particular rule is or is not "meta" to some other rule. What is important is that regular predictable behavior, such as talking, may be described with rules, and the use or application of these rules may in turn be regulated or governed through metarules. In general, social interaction involves at least two major rule hierarchies: one governing the structure of language and the other governing the use of language in communication. This statement has profound implications for the understanding and treatment of children's language disorders. I will develop this topic more fully in Chapter 9.

PROBLEM SOLVING

We face many situations in which we have to make decisions or choices. In many of these situations we do not have all the information necessary to be entirely confident of what choice to make. Working through such situations may be viewed as a problem-solving process. The essence of a problem is that we have some information, perhaps quite a bit of information, but we aren't sure how to put it together. There is a gap in our knowledge. Stated in the terms that have been developed in this chapter, we lack one or more of the necessary relations or metarules.

Acquiring New Metarules

One may acquire new metarules in two ways. First, one may be taught a rule. This process is a basic component of instruction and a very common occurrence in most classrooms. In learning to work with algebraic equations, for example, a student may be taught that the two sides of the equation have to balance. Lower-level rules for determining and maintaining this balance may also be taught. As another example, a child may be told that mixing blue and yellow paints will produce green and then be given paints to try out this relation. The other way in which new metarules may be acquired is by discovery. Through trial and error, intuition, or whatever, one discovers independently the metarule specifying a particular relation. By mixing different paints the child may find without instruction that blue and yellow make green. Following Gagné, this discovery process will be called problem solving. In the abstract, then, problem solving involves developing new rules, usually new metarules.

Let us consider some examples. The fundamental principle in working a jigsaw puzzle is that all the pieces must interdigitate with each other to form a coherent whole. One may proceed by simply attempting to fit various pieces together. Such a procedure represents a fairly low-level rule. One may notice that a number of the pieces are roughly the same shade of blue and hypothesize that the picture contains some sky or a body of water. One might then sort out all the blue pieces and work with them separately. This process would illustrate problem solving and the concomitant development of a metarule. Assuming that no

one had told the person working on the puzzle to sort the pieces by color, that person discovered or worked out that procedure independently. The result of this "solution" is a metarule that organizes or governs the application of the lower-level rule, namely, trying to fit various pieces together. Obviously there are other metarules that could be invoked in working jigsaw puzzles, such as "Complete the entire border first." Again, the effect would be to organize how the individual works with the pieces of the puzzle. Choosing among these metarules would be another instance of problem solving.

For a more complicated example, imagine a child's first day at school. The child has many different behaviors that could apply but is lacking at least some of the metarules. That is, the child doesn't know specifically which behaviors are appropriate in the classroom. Some of these metarules will be provided through instruction by the teacher, such as those governing general behavior. Others the child will discover independently, dealing with such things as how best to approach the teacher, how to participate in free play activities, and how to make friends. The child could use various means to develop these metarules, such as imitation of other children or trial and error. The point is that the child will develop consistent ways to organize and regulate ongoing activity, that is, a set of metarules. It may be added that there is no choice in the matter. Physical presence in the situation means that the child is behaving in some fashion or other. Thus, the problem solving involves choices in the child's behavior relative to the interests and contingencies in the situation.

Once one has learned a metarule, one may merely apply that rule in similar conditions in the future. Stated less abstractly, once one develops a technique or set of behaviors for functioning in a particular type of situation, one uses those behaviors when that situation recurs. One does not need to solve the same problem over and over, although, of course, one may develop better solutions or adapt with changing circumstances. At the same time, the metarules that an individual develops for a particular circumstance may not be optimal for that situation, as with a child who hits to express needs or a child who elects not to talk in situations where talking would be appropriate and effective.

Variation in Problem Solving

It should be obvious by now that my conception of "problem" is very broad. A problem is involved in any situation in which an individual has to make a decision. The degree of problem solving involved depends on the novelty of the decision to be made. Thus, in very routine decisions, ones with very well-established metarules, one chooses an option with little thought. I do not debate about how to spell my name when I sign a letter (although I do have to decide whether to use my whole name or just my first name). I do not have to do a lot of problem solving to know that the ice is in the freezer (although once in a while it is not). Similarly, competent speakers construct most of their sentences without difficulty. If, on the other hand, one is making a decision in a novel or difficult situation, one engages in more vigorous problem solving. Examples would include deciding how to talk to a friend about a delicate personal matter or first learning how to drive a car. Similarly, a child learning to use a particular grammatical structure is engaged in active problem solving.

It should also be noted that the way a problem is solved varies with the individual and with the type of problem. The individual's style of problem solving interacts with the type of problem in determining how the problem will ultimately be solved. The solution of a problem may come quickly or it may involve many trials. When the solution does arrive, it may appear suddenly (what Gestalt psychologists call an "aha experience"), or it may evolve bit by bit. In addition, some problems will be solved very well and others with varying degrees of success.

Problem solving in purest form, then, means developing or discovering new rules and metarules. In concert with Winitz and Reeds (1975), it is my contention that problem solving is a fundamental component of the child's language learning. The child employs problem solving both in learning rules of language structure, as in choosing appropriate forms of utterance, and in learning the metarules of language use, as in learning how to deal with other people through language.

CONCLUSIONS

The purpose of this chapter has been to develop a perspective on different kinds of concepts and rules and how they relate to each other. The order in which they have been presented is not meant to represent a developmental sequence. Rather, the progression has been from more concrete and specific to more abstract and general. This framework is not perfect; the categories overlap and doubtless there are inconsistencies. What I am striving for is a working model from which we can view the relations among concepts, rules, and language.

It seems to me there are at least four kinds of relations in this regard. First, language symbolizes concepts. Concepts are a result of our attempts to understand reality. We use language to refer to these concepts and thus to communicate about reality. Similarly, language symbolizes rules by specifying the relations among various concepts. Language development, then, cannot be separated from conceptual development. Second, language functions in the formation and processing of concepts and rules. Relatively concrete concepts and rules can develop without language but, typically, language contributes to their development by directing perceptions, providing associations, and expanding their use. More abstract concepts and rules are heavily dependent on language, and some have no existence at all outside of language. Third, language is itself a particular set of concepts and rules. An understanding of the nature of concepts and rules, therefore, helps in understanding the nature of language. At the same time, there is a paradoxical flavor to our understanding of language. We cannot step outside language to view language; ultimately our only tool in the study of language is language itself. Fourth, the use of language is governed by higher-level rules. Thus, the selection of particular utterances is always influenced by metarules concerning how one should talk in any particular instance. This focus on the selection of utterances leads directly to viewing the use of language as a series of problem-solving tasks. It is in this light that we will approach clinical intervention.

Finally, it was seen that the interdependent ideas of rule hierarchy, metarule, and problem solving are very general. We will use these ideas to help organize our understanding of cognitive processing, interpersonal communication, the family system, and the clinical process itself.

2

HUMAN INFORMATION PROCESSING

In the previous chapter we considered language as a representation of reality. The focus was on the relations among concepts, rule hierarchies, and language. With this perspective as background let us now look at how the human organism might process complex information such as that embodied in language.

THE HUMAN INFORMATION-PROCESSING SYSTEM

It might be helpful to begin by imagining that we wanted to build a device that could function as a language user. What would have to be included in such a device? My approach to this question owes much to the overview of the human information-processing system provided by Simon (1972). First, it will have to have mechanisms to receive input, that is, sensory systems. These systems will have to be able to handle information in all sensory modalities. Second, it will have to have mechanisms for attention. Typically there are many stimuli available to the organism at any one time. We will need a means of directing attention selectively to only certain of these stimuli. Third, we will need a means of relating information in one modality to that in others, so that we can relate what is seen with what is heard and touched, and so forth. That is, we need a system of intermodal connections. Fourth, we will need systems of memory, so that information can be retained over time. Some material will need to be retained permanently, but other information needs retention for only limited periods of time. Finally, we need a means of organizing and controlling our information-processing activities. We may consider this aspect of the system as a hierarchy of cognitive strategies,

of routines and programs for handling information.

These five functions form the basis of the human information-processing system. The description so far might suggest four components or "structures" that information may pass through and a fifth that organizes the other four. It should be emphasized, however, that all are active, interrelated functions that operate together in the processing of information. None should be viewed as a static structure or "box" that merely registers the presence of information as it passes through.

It can be seen that we are back in the land of metaphor. This description of human information processing does not stem directly from neuroanatomy. Rather, this view was developed primarily by analogy from computer simulations of cognitive processes (Apter 1970; Newell and Simon 1971) and other theoretical work in information processing. The logic is simply that we have to carry out the functions in this model somehow, or we couldn't use language and perform other intelligent behavior as we do. To describe these functions is not to state precisely how they are carried out in the nervous system.

Let us consider each aspect of the human information-processing system separately. My purpose will not be to plumb each function of the system in great depth, but to present an overall perspective on how we process language.

SENSORY SYSTEMS

A fundamental requirement of any complex information-processing system is the capacity to receive input. In humans the input functions are accomplished by the sensory systems. This input information is our contact with the environment. As Simon (1969) puts it, the sensory systems are an interface between the individual and the environment. This contact provides the stimuli upon which we act and the data from which concepts are formed and language develops.

There are several sensory systems in the human organism, often listed as auditory, visual, haptic, olfactory, and gustatory. Hearing and vision have been studied most extensively, perhaps partly because their respective stimuli are more easily controlled for scientific study, and partly because of their high cultural relevance. That is, they often appear to be our dominant senses because they are capable of processing such a variety and such fine gradations of stimuli, but our culture emphasizes just such detailed analysis. A good introduction to audition and vision is included in Lindsay and Norman (1972).

"Haptic" refers to sensations of touch and body movement (Chalfant and Scheffelin 1969) and includes a number of subcategories such as temperature, pain, kinesthesis, and balance. In addition to receiving stimuli from the environment, the haptic system receives a great deal of information from the body itself, which is used in monitoring continuing bodily activity such as movement, position in space, and balance. Obviously, it should be added, all sensory modes contribute to this monitoring. The channels of smell and taste have not been studied thoroughly. Along with parts of the haptic system, they do not appear to lend themselves to precise differentiation of very large numbers of stimuli, as hearing and vision do. At first glance they may not seem as culturally relevant either, until you think of the numbers of deodorant and junk-food ads we are exposed to each week.

Sensory Systems and Language

We may ask how the sensory systems relate to language. In an obvious way hearing is the dominant channel for language. The basic medium for language is sound. In our technological and literate culture it is sometimes hard to realize that the majority of the languages in the world do not have any written form at all. It is also true, however, that the majority of the people in the world speak a language that does have a written form, emphasizing the importance of vision as well as audition. At the same time, children normally learn language through the auditory medium before they begin any real contact with reading and writing. In another way, though, language depends on other sensory modalities as well as hearing, because the other modalities provide much of the input that is the basis for the role of language as a representation of reality. That is, core and concrete concepts, which are represented by words, are formed by interpreting input from various sensory channels. In addition, the referent(s) for any particular utterance may be apprehended by different channels, as in, "That cake smells luscious." There would be nothing for language to represent if input from the several sensory channels were not available. Finally, face-to-face communication involves input through various senses. The words we hear spoken are accompanied by visual stimuli and sometimes other sensory stimulation as well. As will be discussed in Chapter 5, these nonlinguistic stimuli complement and enhance the verbal message.

The neurological mechanisms underlying the sensory systems are complex. In general they involve sensing stimuli from the environment, recoding those stimuli as nerve impulses, and transmitting them to the higher centers of the nervous system. The process involves transforming the information somewhat at each relay station and progressively reducing the amount of information (number of neurons firing) as the information travels increasingly higher in the system. Ultimately the nature of the medium in which the stimuli are received and the structure of the sensory receptors determine how the information will be coded in the nervous system. For example, auditory stimuli are linear to a much greater degree than visual stimuli are. The sensory systems seem to be particularly attuned to detecting changes in whatever stimuli are present.

Summary

My purpose in this section has been simply to point out that human information processing is dependent on the sensory systems for the reception of information. I will defer discussion of perception and specific sensory-related language functions such as auditory discrimination until after the other aspects of human information processing have been presented. It is worth stressing that impairment in sensory function affects proficiency in information processing and that certain types of sensory impairment have profound effects on language skill. Hearing is the most apparent example, but the language of children with other sensory impairments may also suffer. A child with a visual impairment, for example, may not get the nonverbal cues that accompany talking. In addition, that child's conceptual development may not be as rich as that of a child with all sensory systems functioning normally.

ATTENTION

In most situations there is an incredible array of stimuli available to us through the various sensory channels. Typically we focus on only a few of these stimuli, those we are interested in at the moment. It is through the mechanisms of attention that we accomplish this focus. Attention implies selection. We actively select certain information to process at any one time, allowing other stimuli to remain on the periphery or perhaps to be out of conscious awareness completely. As will be discussed in the section on memory, we seem capable of processing only limited amounts of information at any one time. The mechanism of attention selects that information and thus enables it to enter our information-processing system.

Levels of Attention

Attention may be viewed as occurring on a continuum. At one end there is a general level of attention that involves focusing on a particular task. This mechanism is sometimes referred to as a set to attend, or an orienting response. The idea is that the child is ready to take in information emanating from a particular source. A child who is described as having a poor attention span normally is having difficulty with this kind of attention. Thus, a child in school may not be able to stay at any one task for more than a minute or two, or a child in clinic may not be able to finish even a brief test in one sitting.

At the other end of the continuum, attention involves selecting specific stimuli within a task. For example, in viewing geometrical forms of various colors, three-year-olds are more likely to attend to the color, whereas children around six years of age often show a preference for the form of these stimuli (Gotts 1973). Similarly, some elementary-school–aged children are described as attending primarily to the global outlines of objects while others may attend to feature details within objects (Messer 1976). In clinic this level of attention is illustrated by the child who sits cooperatively and attends to the clinician but who does not attend to the particular aspects of the situation which are the clinical focus. A child may repeat sentences, for example, without apparent awareness of grammatical structures they contain. Similarly, a child may respond to an auditory discrimination test without attending specifically to the same-different distinctions contained in the test.

Determinants of Attention

A key concept in the phenomenon of attention is what is referred to as "saliency." A salient stimulus is noticeable; it is "attention grabbing." Obviously, then, the more salient an activity or a particular stimulus is to an individual child, the more it is likely to attract the child's attention. In the same manner, salient items are likely to hold a child's attention for greater periods than are stimuli of less salience.

Considerable research has been done on the determinants of attention. At a general level two attributes of a stimulus contribute to its saliency: energy and change (Anderson 1975). We are attracted to stimuli with high levels of energy, such as loud noises, bright lights, and powerful odors. In the same vein, we attend to stimuli that are large, close, or present in large numbers. We also attend to stimuli that change in some way—an object that moves or a fluctuating light. Research such as that reviewed in

Pick, Frankel, and Hess (1975) has identified a variety of things that influence the saliency of various stimuli to children, such as pointing to the item, naming or discussing it, or minimizing other stimuli, as well as characteristics such as shape and color mentioned earlier.

One can argue, however, that ultimately the determinants of attention are within each person. Salient means attention-grabbing for the individual and is related to characteristics such as survival value and meaningfulness, which are really in the child's head, as well as physical characteristics. Thus, in clinical work one has to determine just what types of stimuli are salient for each individual child. Research findings and clinical experience provide guidelines but not every child responds in the same ways.

Exploration and Search

As the child develops, there is a trend toward increased specificity in attention and in other aspects of information processing as well. Wright and Vlietstra (1975) have described this process as a progression from exploration to search. In exploration the young child is heavily influenced by the perceptual salience of external stimuli. In a toy store the child darts from one thing to the next with little organization. In search the child's attention is more influenced by internal cognitive processes; it is task oriented. Salience is redefined as relevance to the task at hand. In Wright and Vlietstra's (1975) formulation, search develops out of exploration. The relevance of language and cognitive strategies is apparent in the task-oriented nature of search activity. While attention in mature individuals is frequently related to search, we employ exploration when appropriate, such as in "people watching" at a beach or cocktail party.

Summary

Attention, in summary, is a complex phenomenon. It is difficult to study because it cannot occur by itself. It always involves sensory systems, memory, and cognitive strategies; it involves perception, which is in turn related to conceptual development; it can be influenced by verbal directions and by reinforcement contingencies. In addition, attention varies within the same individual. Children who are generally fleeting in attention may attend for long periods to stimuli that they find particularly salient, such as a schoolchild who cannot stay with math problems for more than thirty seconds but who will watch television for an hour or more. As a practical matter, the sources of attention should be sought in the environment rather than in the child. That is, one can manipulate the stimuli in the environment but one cannot manipulate the child's head. The challenge to the clinician is to present stimuli to children in ways that those children will find salient.

INTERMODAL CONNECTIONS

In spite of the process of attention, we do not receive information from only one sensory channel at a time, and in fact we often focus attention on input from multiple modalities simultaneously. Thus, a function of human information processing is to integrate information from this variegated input. Integration is a form of synthesis. It is a process in which the individual organizes and relates information of different types and from different sources.

This integrative process is extremely common in human experience. We are almost constantly relating different kinds of input. We hear a sound and we look at the source of that sound. We see something soft and we reach out to touch it. In exploring a new substance a small child may touch it, smell it, see it, and taste it all at once. In addition, the parent may name it. The same happens with adults: Consider the sensory information you integrated the last time you ate a piece of celery. In all of these situations, a principal activity of human information processing is to integrate the information received from the various sensory modalities.

A great deal is still unknown about the specifics of intermodal connections, both as psychological and as neurological phenomena. Babies demonstrate evidence of such connections in that they look toward the source of a sound and reach for objects they can see. At the same time, kindergartners show difficulty with laboratory tasks requiring intermodal integration. In general there seems to be considerable development of integration among the visual, haptic, and auditory modalities between the ages of five and seven (Birch and Lefford 1963; Birch and Belmont 1965). However, research in this area is open to many interpretations.

As Torgeson (1975) points out, changes in intermodal integration may be due to a number of factors. They may be due to complex maturational changes in the nervous system. Involved here are aspects such as hemispheric specialization and the differences between processing linear information, such as that in the auditory channel, and primarily gestalt information, such as that in the visual mode. Memory constraints may also be involved, because the information that is to be integrated must be held in memory long enough for that integration to occur. Changes in intermodal integration may also be due to the development of abstract cognitive skills independent of particular sensory systems. It may well be that all of these factors are involved in the development of intermodal connections.

In any case, intermodal connections are of fundamental importance in language learning. We constantly relate words to input from any of the senses. More generally, our knowledge of reality is based on syntheses of information from all sensory modalities. It can be seen that intermodal connections add greatly to the richness of concept formation. *Fudge,* besides its general property of being a candy, has a texture, a look, a smell, and a taste. Similarly, most language training is integrative. We show children pictures and ask them to name them. We say words for children and ask them to point to appropriate pictures. We may ask children to act out what we're saying. Some children respond better to multisensory input in training, whereas others appear to function more efficiently when the variety of stimuli is limited.

MEMORY

Memory is the cornerstone of our information-processing capacities. Memory is at the very heart of language learning and use. Most accounts of the psychological processes in language assume the presence of a set of rules, stored in memory, and a lexicon or vocabulary, also stored in memory. Similarly, memory is paramount in learning. In fact, one way to look at learning is in terms of getting information into permanent memory—and out again at appropriate

times. The child's memorial processes, then, are a key factor in language learning and remediation. In this section we will consider three different distinctions that have been prominent in memory research.

Types of Information in Memory

The first aspect relates to the nature or quality of the information being stored. The distinction here is between "episodic memory" and "semantic memory" as described by Brown (1975). My discussion follows her presentation closely.

Episodic Memory

In episodic memory an item is remembered as a whole, with little analysis of its component parts or structure. Specific events are retained whether or not they are meaningful. Because the material is not analyzed, this type of memory does not include inference or generalization, but is rather a copy of the event involved. Many of the tasks used in memory research are episodic, such as remembering lists of unrelated words. If, in clinic, children are asked to repeat sentences that they don't comprehend (perhaps unbeknownst to the clinician), the task is primarily episodic. Similarly, auditory discrimination and auditory memory span tests typically focus on episodic memory.

Semantic Memory

Semantic memory, on the other hand, is independent of any specific event. It is stored knowledge about the concepts and rules discussed in the previous chapter and the words and meanings that relate to them. Brown uses the terms "reconstructive" and "imaginative reproduction" in characterizing semantic memory. A reproduction from semantic memory is a reconstruction of the event, focusing on the gist of that event, rather than a holistic copy, as in episodic memory. Semantic memory ". . . consists of our comprehension of rules and relationships involved in events, a comprehension which permits us to regenerate past experience in a suitable form for the needs of the moment" (Brown 1975, p. 113). There is an irresistible parallel between this statement and many views of language. Surely our knowledge of the lexicon and rule hierarchies of language must be stored in this form.

The distinction between episodic memory and semantic memory is not a dichotomy. It should be viewed as a continuum. Further, I do not mean to imply that there are two memory systems in the head. I simply mean to say that we retain some information in specific form (episodic) and some in generalized form (semantic), and that these two types of remembering overlap. The important conclusion I would draw so far is that language use and language learning are not based on episodic memory, the retention of specific utterances, but on semantic memory. Similarly, a child cannot truly learn language by being taught to produce certain utterances in episodic fashion. Parrots do that. To learn language a child must be able to reconstruct sentences, not merely recite them.

Attitude of the Individual Toward Remembering

A second dimension is concerned with the attitude of the individual who is doing the remembering. I continue to draw from Brown (1975) in this discussion. The distinction now is between "deliberate" or "in-tentional" memory and "involuntary" or "automatic" memory.

Intentional Memory

Intentional memory is often episodic in nature, as in committing to memory your social security number, the words to a song, or material that you will have to recite on a test. Intentional memory typically involves the use of mnemonic devices or memory aids. Rehearsal is an example of such a device—one repeats the information to be remembered over and over again. Other mnemonic devices include organizing the material, relating it to something else, self-testing, and disattending unimportant aspects of the material. There are also retrieval strategies for helping recall the material after it's been committed to memory, such as visualizing an outline and recalling related items together. Brown (1975) suggests that the intent to remember has no effect on the actual ability to remember in either children or adults. The activity of the individual does make a difference, however, and in adults the intent to remember produces appropriate activity, such as the mnemonic devices just mentioned.

Involuntary Memory

Involuntary memory, in contrast, is the retention of information without specific intent to do so. It is ". . . the involuntary product of our continuous interactions with a relatively meaningful environment" (Brown 1975, p. 113). Involuntary memory is primarily semantic rather than episodic in character. If an experience is meaningful to an individual, it is likely to be retained, but typically in generalized rather than mirror-image form. That person can reconstruct the gist of that event. This phenomenon has received considerable attention as it applies to memory for sentences, where it is referred to as "semantic integration." Brown (1975) and also Hagen, Jongeward, and Kail (1975) have reviewed studies in this area. Children and adults retain sentences as holistic semantic relations rather than as strings of words and particular grammatical structures.

Young children rarely seem to show intent to remember. It seems probable that intentional memory has little ecological validity for a young child. That is, there are relatively few occurrences where a child has to remember something that is inherently nonmeaningful or that requires episodic reproduction. On the other hand, children can remember specific information when it is important to a meaningful activity, as demonstrated by Yendovitskaya (1971). Jenkins (1971), in discussing memory research with adults, made a related point. Adults function much more efficiently in meaningful memory tasks than in meaningless ones. As Brown (1975) points out, if Jenkins's statement is true of adults, who have the abstract attitude necessary to participate in a meaningless task when asked to do so, then it must apply even more profoundly to children, who do not have any such abstract perspective.

Again it should be pointed out that intentional memory and involuntary memory are best seen on a continuum rather than as two distinct categories. The importance of this dimension of memory to language learning is that children do not learn language because they want to; they do not manifest an intention to remember language. Rather, they learn language because they experience it in contexts that are meaningful to them. Language enters semantic memory because it has ecological validity in the child's in-

teractions with the world. The child's attitude toward language learning seems to be summed up by Roger Brown's (1973) observation that children who are learning language talk as if they assume they will be understood: They don't learn language in an active, purposeful sense; they use it.

Duration of Retention

The third dimension of memory relates to time. It is concerned with the duration for which information is retained. Various types of memory have been posited in this regard. The briefest may be called the sensory store. This is the literal retention of sensory input momentarily. For a second or two we can "hear" an auditory stimulus or "see" a visual stimulus after that stimulus has been removed. Next is short-term memory (STM), in which information is retained for a relatively short period, several seconds or longer, but has been transformed to symbolic form from the literal sensory images of the sensory store. Finally, there is long-term memory (LTM), in which information is retained permanently. The kinds of information that I have described as semantic memory would be stored in LTM. They are permanent knowledge. Many of the items relating to episodic memory do not get to LTM. They are used and forgotten. Some, of course, do remain in LTM. I still remember my Army serial number, although I haven't had any need for it in twenty years. There is an obvious question in comparing STM and LTM: How long is short? Most estimates of STM run in seconds, rather than hours or days, but the estimates vary widely, and some authors have even suggested a middle-term memory. In the following discussion I will concentrate on STM and the retention of information.

Short-Term Memory

The idea of STM is intuitively appealing because indeed there are many things that we retain for only brief periods of time. You look up a number in the phone book and retain it only long enough to get it dialed. If the call doesn't go through, you'll probably have to look the number up again. There are many other examples of this type of phenomena, such as addresses and ZIP codes, ordering for several people at a fast food emporium (three double burgers with everything, one with no onions, one regular burger plain, two milks, a strawberry shake, and two coffees, one with cream). We retain this information long enough to use it and then dismiss it. Some aspects of STM are not quite so obvious. It seems that in comprehending a spoken sentence, you have to retain that sentence long enough to identify its structure before you can interpret it. Similarly, in producing a sentence you have to retain the beginning of that sentence as the end comes by if you want to make sense. Obviously, though, this detailed knowledge does not end up in LTM for the vast majority of the sentences we process.

Limits on Short-Term Memory

Much of my discussion of STM will be based on Simon (1969). From an information-processing view, the basic problem is to get information into permanent store (LTM). STM is a bottleneck in this process because there are limits on its capacity. Simon describes two such limits. The identification of these phenomena comes from research on episodic, intentional memory and from computer simulations. The first limit is that it takes time to transfer something from STM to LTM. If you have

ever had to study vocabulary in a foreign language or memorize the names of the cranial nerves, you know this is true. Based on his knowledge of the literature, Simon (1974) estimates that the time involved may be around five to ten seconds per item for adults. As you know from the memorizing you have done, this time is not spent idly but is used to employ cognitive strategies such as the mnemonic devices mentioned earlier. Transferring information from STM to LTM in this fashion is work, in terms of both time and effort.

The second limit Simon describes is on the number of items that can be held in STM at one time. This topic has received a great deal of study. Miller (1956) summarized this research and concluded that, for adults, the number of items that can be retained in STM was approximately seven, give or take two. More recently, Simon (1974) argued that the number is between five and seven, and Anderson (1975) put it at five. This range of figures is probably a good estimate for adults. The corresponding parameters have not been conclusively established for children.

The major point from this theoretical view, however, is that such limits on information processing do exist and that no one can escape them. We all process language and other information within these limits. I must emphasize again that the primary data on these limits come from the study of intentional, episodic memory in psychological experiments in which subjects typically memorize lists of words or the like and then recall them. The memory span is the number recalled, not the number taken in. Obviously there is no precise way to measure the amount of information taken in except through some sort of recall test. Clearly, however, this type of memory task is different from the STM functions in comprehending a sentence. For one thing, what one remembers from comprehending a sentence is semantically coded rather than episodically coded. In addition, the items in sentences are related to each other in systematic ways, as will be discussed in the next two paragraphs.

Chunking

So far I have used the term "item" in referring to what is retained in STM. Suppose that I ask you to remember a sequence of six words. Is each word an item, or is each sound in each word an item? Miller (1956) observed that we group information into familiar units, which he termed "chunks." Thus, each word in the sequence would be a grouping of sounds into a chunk. Simon defines a chunk as a ". . . maximal familiar substructure of the stimulus" (1969, p. 38). Paralleling his example, *KOH* must be retained as three separate letters, because they are the maximal familiar substructures available in that stimulus. Thus *KOH* contains three chunks in this context. *DOG,* on the other hand, can be retained as one chunk because the letters do form a familiar grouping. It can immediately be seen that chunking is a great boon to retention in STM. By chunking items together into groups we can greatly expand the amount of information that can be retained within the limited span of STM, because we retain chunks, not individual items.

There is an interesting interplay between chunking and language. Chunking is typically done on the basis of relationships between items; related items are grouped together.[1] At the same time, the fundamental function of grammar is to show the relationships between items in the sentence (Bolinger 1975). Thus, language is a "natural chunker." It chunks sounds together into words, as in the example above, and it chunks words together into longer structures, such as *the quick brown fox* in "Watch out for the quick brown fox," and *after I've finished my lunch* in "After I've finished my lunch we'll go to the park." Thus, chunking and language are mutually supportive and interrelated. Language provides a framework for chunking through its structure and through rhythm and intonation patterns, and chunking provides a means for processing language efficiently.

Menyuk (1969) presented data that support this view. She studied preschoolers' and kindergartners' abilities to repeat sentences ranging from two to nine words in length and varying in grammatical complexity. She found that the ability to repeat sentences in correct order depended on the grammatical structure of the sentence, not on length, even with children as young as three years. The correlation between sentence length and repetition of correct order was only .03. If the sentences were presented in reverse order, however, the correlation was .87. When word order is reversed, the sentences become strings of words with no grammatical structure and consequently the major basis for chunking is not available. Further, Menyuk states that even her three-year-olds were repeating nine-word sentences. Compare this performance with the

---

[1] In some cases this relationship may be weak, as in psychological experiments involving strings of digits. In this case the only relationship available may be contiguity. The items can be grouped according to the order in which they are received.

norms for digit span (episodic memory for individual digits) presented in Table 1. The average digit span for college students is only eight. Clearly, STM for digits is not the same as that for sentence repetition. The difference would appear to be related to the fact that sentences embody meaningful relations, both in grammatical structure and in the conceptual rules they represent.

This type of research has direct relevance to clinical work. A child's auditory memory span for unrelated words is not the same as that for sentences, because of the chunking inherent in sentence structure. It follows that in language training, auditory memory span is better approached through experiences that enhance the chunking potential of linguistic structure for the child, rather than through practice with longer and longer lists of unrelated words or items in episodic fashion. I have certainly known children whose utterance length was adequate but whose scores on sequencing tests were low. We will return to this matter in Chapter 3.

Mediation

Earlier I defined mnemonic device as a technique or aid an individual uses in the acquisition of information into memory. Mnemonics are examples of a more general memory process known as mediation. For example, if we're standing on a street corner and I ask you to remember the makes of the next five cars that drive past, you might name each car as it passes. You can then remember the names rather than the actual images of the cars. The names mediate or form a bridge between the task and its solution. Mature individuals use a wide range of

Table 1. Norms for Digit Span

Age in Years	Digits
2.5	2
3.0	3
4.5	4
7.0	5
10.0	6
College	8

From *Experimental Psychology, Revised Edition* by Robert S. Woodworth and Harold Schlosberg, p. 704. Copyright 1938, 1954 by Henry Holt and Company, Inc. Reprinted by permission of Holt, Rinehart and Winston. Quoted in Herbert Simon, "How big is a chunk?" *Science*, 183 (1974), p. 486. Copyright 1974 by the American Association for the Advancement of Science.

mediators in memory tasks, but language seems to be the most common mediator.

Mediational Deficiencies and Production Deficiencies

Flavell (1970) explored the development of mediated memory in children. Nonverbal tasks were used, such as remembering which pictures the experimenter identified from a larger group of pictures. He found that kindergartners tended not to use verbal mediators, that is, they did not name the items they were attempting to remember, but fifth graders did.[2] Concomitantly, the younger children's performance in remembering which items had been identified was not as good as that of the older children. It was consistently found, however, that if the younger children were induced to name these items, their memory for them improved. A striking finding was that, even

[2] In observing the children, he used a lip-reading procedure so that he could record covert naming—in which the children talked to themselves or mouthed the words silently—as well as overt naming.

after achieving successful memory performance when the examiner instructed them to
name the pictures to be remembered, the
majority of the younger children did not
spontaneously name pictures in later
memory tasks.

Flavell discusses these tasks in terms of
two types of memory deficiencies. The first
he calls a mediational deficiency. In this case
the mediator does not help memory. The
kindergartners did not demonstrate this kind
of deficiency because their performance did
improve when they were instructed to
mediate with words. The second type Flavell
refers to as a production deficiency. In this
case the child possesses effective mediators
but does not choose to produce them. The
kindergartners consistently demonstrated
this pattern. From the perspective presented
in the previous chapter, it can be seen that a
production deficiency is a difficulty with
metarules. The child has appropriate rules
relating mediators to their respective
"mediatees," but does not invoke (and
perhaps does not possess) the metarules concerning when to use such mediation. Further, Flavell sees mnemonic mediation as
related to problem solving. One learns to
choose mediators that will be effective in the
task at hand. Flavell refers to this activity as
"planfulness." With increasing maturity the
child learns to do something now (mediate)
that will aid performance in the future
(recall). We will return to the idea of planfulness in the section on cognitive strategies.

Short-Term Memory Strategies

Let us look briefly at another type of
research that has been conducted on STM
processes. It is well known that STM performance is reduced in retarded subjects. Belmont and Butterfield (1969; 1971; Butterfield and Belmont 1975; Butterfield,
Wambold, and Belmont 1973) have attempted to increase STM span in retarded
subjects through specific training procedures. They used an episodic visual
memory task in which subjects had to recall
the position in which a letter was exposed
relative to other letters in a sequence. The
letters were exposed one at a time. Subjects
controlled the rate at which the letters were
exposed by pressing a button whenever they
wanted to see the next letter. In this way the
investigators could follow each subject's acquisition and retrieval strategies separately.
By noting how long a subject paused before
exposing each new letter, the investigators
obtained information on how the subject acquired each sequence, or attempted to commit it to memory, without having to ask that
subject to recall it. In acquiring a sequence
of nine letters, for example, the normal
adults studied would be likely to expose
three letters fairly quickly, pause, expose the
next three with little delay between them,
pause again, and then finish quickly. After
this acquisition phase the experimenters exposed one letter from the sequence, but on a
different display panel, and the subject's
task was to indicate which position it had
been in the sequence. That is, the subject
had to retrieve that information from
memory. If the letter was in a position
following the second pause, subjects tended
to respond quickly. If it was earlier in the sequence, subjects tended to pause before indicating that letter's position.

On the basis of these observations, and
interviews with subjects, Belmont and Butterfield described the process as follows. A
subject would chunk the first three letters
and then rehearse that chunk; then the process would be repeated for the second three.
For the last three letters, the subject depended on an "echo response," perhaps
from sensory store. In the retrieval phase the

subject responded quickly if the letter was one that had been acquired through the echo response. If the letter was earlier in the list, the subject paused while running through the chunks that had been rehearsed. It should be noted that while this was the most typical pattern for normal adults, some subjects showed different patterns, such as cumulative rehearsal, in which the subject rehearses a continually longer list.

This two-pause pattern, then, was identified as a strategy that was effective in the task. The investigators then trained retarded subjects to follow the same pattern in the task. The results were remarkable in two ways. First, the "deficit" in STM that the retarded subjects had originally demonstrated was virtually eliminated. Second, there was little generalization of this strategy. On subsequent days the retarded subjects tended not to employ the strategy, although the investigators could reinstate it with further training. In Flavell's terms, the retarded subjects showed a production deficiency. Butterfield, Wambold, and Belmont (1973) conclude that their retarded subjects had the memory processes for successful participation in the task. What they lacked was the executive control to invoke and coordinate those processes. Again, the difficulty is in the acquisition of appropriate metarules.

Short-Term Memory and Language Disorders

This work by Flavell and by Belmont and Butterfield has important implications for work with language-disordered children. I interpret it to mean that deficiencies in STM, in both normal children and retarded individuals, are partially the result of difficulties in higher level processing skills rather than of any lack of basic capacities.

Simon (1974) interprets the growth of STM as represented in digit span (Table 1) the same way: the increase in digit span with age is due to improvement in chunking ability, which is a processing skill. Not all researchers agree with this position, however. Huttenlocher and Burke (1976) argued that the increase in digit span with age in normal children is not due to progression in cognitive strategies such as rehearsal and chunking. Rather, they suggest that this increase is due to development of the basic skills in identifying individual items and in retaining the order of those items. They note, for example, that auditory memory span is shorter for nonsense syllables than for familiar words, and that melodic contour can be an important aid in retaining auditory sequences.

There is considerable interest in the STM skills of language-disordered children, and a number of such children are described as deficient in STM. It seems reasonable that all the views discussed above will be relevant in this regard. That is, it appears unlikely that STM deficiencies are related to some basic capacity of memory. Rather, they represent difficulties in identifying or recognizing items, serial encoding, cognitive strategies, and problem solving. These areas, in turn, are related to meaningfulness, ecological validity, and motivation. The presence of this variety of variables in short-term memory span clearly implies a great deal of individual variation in this skill and in its relationship with language disorders.

Retention and Type of Processing

We consider now one more relation between language and retention: quality or type of processing. Craik and Lockhart (1972) proposed that the division of memory into separate short-term and long-term stores might not be the most appropriate metaphor for representing the fact that we retain some information permanently and other information only briefly. Rather, they suggest that there is but one memory. Information is retained according to how it is processed when it is acquired. Craik and Tulving (1975) explored this possibility with an incidental learning paradigm. In this procedure, printed words were presented briefly to a subject one word at a time. Each subject was instructed to respond to various words in ways that were devised to induce the subject to process the words differently. Instructions were of three kinds. First, the researchers might direct the subject to process the word according to its physical characteristics, such as, "Is it printed in lower case letters?" A second type of question was directed at phonemic processing, such as, "Does the word rhyme with bus?" The third type focused on semantic processing, such as, "Is it an animal word?" or "Would it fit in the following sentence: 'The boy ate the _____ .'?" These questions tended to orient the subject to process each word in a particular way. Subjects were not told to remember the words, but after a series of words the subjects were tested on their recall of those words.

Craik and Tulving (1975) report the results of ten experiments using varieties of this procedure. They found that quality of processing was highly related to retention of words. The words that were best retained were those with which the subjects were induced to do the most semantic elaboration, that is, think about the meaning of the word, associate it with other words, and in general relate it to semantic memory. This effect occurred in spite of variations in amount of effort, intent to learn, difficulty of orienting questions, response time, rehearsal time, and it occurred even when differential rewards were offered for words identified with the different processing levels.

This series of studies also has relevance to clinical work with language-disordered children. Retention of words is not based solely on the cognitive strategies and problem solving referred to above but also on semantic considerations. The more meaning a word has, and the more it relates to other words and ideas, the more it is likely to be retained.

Summary of Memory

In general, we code things in memory in two ways. Some information we retain in specific unitary form. Recall of that information might be called reproduction. We reproduce a relatively specific image, whether it be visual, auditory or whatever. Memory of this type is called episodic. One might analogize that we retain brief episodes of our lives in fairly complete detail as they occur. Other information is retained in generalized form. We retain the meaning of a sentence but not the specific wording. Recall of this information is reconstruction. We reconstruct the event rather than calling it back whole. Memory of this type is called semantic because of the importance of language in the process.

It seems that we are continually acquiring new information into semantic memory in automatic or involuntary fashion. If something is meaningful, we are likely to retain it. Retention of episodic information can occur automatically—for instance, remembering a face—but it may also be retained because we specifically attempt to commit it to memory. This intentional memory involves invoking metarules that specify and control the use of various mediational activities and cognitive strategies. These procedures involve time and effort.

Some information is retained only briefly while other information is retained relatively permanently. There is a limit on how much information can be retained in STM at one time, but we can beat this limit through chunking or by storing some information in LTM. Language and memory are inseparable companions. Language is, of course, impossible without memory, but, in turn, language plays an enormous role in memory, through its versatility in representation and mediation.

Finally, we reviewed three specific programs of research concerning the processes of remembering. In intentional memory tasks a child may possess a memory strategy but fail to produce it at appropriate times. Similarly, retarded individuals can be trained in the component strategies of a memory task and then perform with these strategies so that their "memory deficits" are virtually eliminated on that task, but again they do not utilize those strategies on their own. They have not learned the metarule at the top of the hierarchy. Finally, retention of words is related, not only to the strategies exercised, but to the degree to which the meaning of the word is considered and related to semantic memory. These research programs emphasize the importance of cognitive strategies and metarules, and we now turn to this last aspect of human information processing.

COGNITIVE STRATEGIES

It is apparent from the discussion of STM that we do not merely receive or register information. We actively process it. The methods we use to process information may be called "cognitive strategies." This idea owes much to computer simulation of intelligent behavior in which the computer program directs the activity of the computer. A cognitive strategy, then, gives organization to the way we process information. It controls behavior and thinking (Simon 1969). We have already encountered examples of these strategies. Chunking obviously organizes information. Mnemonic devices such as rehearsal similarly organize our activity. Cognitive strategies are learned and, of course, must themselves be stored in memory.

The Nature of Cognitive Strategies

The term cognitive strategy has been used in different ways by various authors. I take it to represent a continuum from very automatic activity that may occur almost completely without awareness, such as many of the processes used in reading by skilled readers, to very conscious, purposive activity, such as that employed in various types of problem solving. Cognitive strategies are involved in all intellectual activity.

From these considerations it follows that cognitive strategies must be hierarchical in nature (Miller, Galanter, and Pribram 1960). Thus, in carrying out some activity regulated by a particular strategy, various subroutines may be called up. The higher level strategies are sometimes referred to as executive functions. It should be clear that strategies in the executive functions may also be described as metarules. They determine the use of other strategies further down in the hierarchy. This is the "planfulness" mentioned by Flavell (1970).

As mentioned earlier, Flavell's production deficiencies and the lack of generalization Belmont and Butterfield encountered in training STM skills in retardates both involved difficulties with metarules (I will refrain from calling them "metastrategies") and problem solving. The subjects possessed cognitive strategies that would be useful in the tasks, but they did not call up those strategies on their own.

Current interpretations of the development of memory and other areas of information processing in children emphasize changes in cognitive strategies rather than changes in structural components (Hagen, Jongeward, and Kail 1975; Simon 1972). As Flavell (1970) and Brown (1975) point out in reference to memory development, wherever conscious cognitive strategies are involved, developmental progressions will be found. Language is critical in the development of cognitive strategies, both in activities such as mediation and because, by its very nature, language provides a means for organization. At the same time, language processing depends on various cognitive strategies. We see again the interplay between language and intellectual functioning discussed in Chapter 1.

Individual Differences

At a more general level, individuals have been described as manifesting different cognitive styles. Some children are reported to be impulsive, solving problems quickly, and often reported as making fairly high numbers of errors. In contrast, other children are described as reflective, solving problems at a slower rate and with fewer errors (Kagan 1965; Denney 1973; Messer 1976). Impulsive children have also been described as global in perceptual style; they are sensitive to the overall contour or gestalt of a stimulus. Reflectives, on the other hand, are described as analytical; they focus on perceptual attributes and details within a stimulus (Denney 1973; Zelniker and Jeffrey 1976). Thus, not only have particular

cognitive strategies been studied, but individuals have been described as showing differences in cognitive styles in which whole hierarchies of cognitive strategies are subsumed.

In spite of this research, cognitive strategies should not be construed as being uniform among groups of people. The bulk of the literature has not been concerned with this issue, but individual differences abound. In reference to the impulsive and reflective groups described in the preceding paragraph, a substantial group of children cannot be classified into either group. In the Zelniker and Jeffrey study, for example, one third of their sixty-one subjects were not classified into either group. Battig (1975) provided impressive evidence of individual differences in subjects' strategies in various experimental tasks. Not only do different subjects use different strategies on a task, but typically the same subject will use different strategies on the same task at different times. Denney's (1973) review also illustrates individual differences in the use of cognitive strategies. Similarly, Belmont and Butterfield found adults using different strategies in their STM task. It should be noted that this variation has been observed in the cognitive strategies over which the subjects have conscious control. It may be inferred, then, that much of this variation is associated with decision making and problem solving.

It follows that an equal amount of individual variation will be found in the cognitive strategies associated with children's language learning. Brown (1973) attests to the variation young children exhibit in structuring utterances, a variation he ascribes to the children's problem solving in developing those utterances. No one who has worked with language-disordered children can fail to be impressed with the individual differences among these children and within the same child across different situations.

CONCLUSIONS

I have described human information processing as having five aspects: sensory systems, attention, intermodal connections, memory, and cognitive strategies. All five appear to be indispensable in the use of language as well as in other activities. Perhaps the most important factor to stress is that all functions are highly interdependent and interrelated. The sensory systems are useless unless there is further processing of the information they receive. Attention selects information for further processing and egress to memory. At the same time, memory and cognitive strategies direct attention. Cognitive strategies are stored in memory and simultaneously they are very influential in determining what gets into memory. The picture of human information processing we end up with is one of a dynamic, multiply determined, adaptable system, responsive both to outside stimuli and to its own functions. People think, and they are flexible in how they go about it.

The Importance of Meaning in Language Learning

The relations between human information processing and the use of language have been discussed in previous sections. What general conclusions can we make? First, it seems to me that the key to language learning is meaning. The retention of language is a semantic memory function and it is primarily acquired through automatic memory, that is, through meaningful ex-

periences. I will define meaningful here as having import in the child's life, or being functional for the child, or possessing ecological validity for the child.

It may be argued that in the case of a language-disordered child, this primary avenue of language learning has failed to some degree and that it will have to be augmented with intentional learning. This argument has validity in many cases, but teaching language to young children through intentional memory carries with it two difficulties. First, the child may not possess or put into operation appropriate cognitive strategies. Second, intentional memory involves work. Children, like the rest of us, abhor work, particularly work that is not meaningful to them. As language is presented in ways that are truly meaningful, the stimuli become more salient and the probabilities increase that the child will learn the material automatically. Children can also be induced to work, of course, through contingency management. Finally, teaching language through episodic memory functions, as in repeating sentences, would seem less than ideal because it may not foster attention to the components of the sentence. Care must be taken that the child learn the reconstructive function that is characteristic of the generation of sentences. In short, the various views of memory lead me in the same direction. Whether the training is structured or unstructured, language must be presented to clinic children in ways that are meaningful for the child.

Metarules and Hierarchical Organization

A second general conclusion I would draw is, as pointed out in the first chapter, the importance of metarules and hierarchies of cognitive strategies. With reference to metarules, children not only have to know words and grammatical structures, they have to decide to use them in appropriate situations. Children who seem to comprehend well (although this is difficult to determine precisely) but whose expressive language is severely impaired may be described as having primarily production deficiencies. They "know" more language than they use. Surely this interpretation fits a child who typically produces a particular grammatical structure in errored form but occasionally produces that form correctly. That child does not need to learn that form; what is needed is the metarule concerning when to use it.

Metarules occur in association with cognitive strategies. Cognitive strategies, in turn, are the means of organizing and processing information as it is received as input and as it enters memory. Children have to learn these strategies, but the irony is that we do not know precisely what the "best" strategies are. We do know that young children have not yet developed a full armamentarium of cognitive strategies, or the metarules governing their use, and that individuals of all ages vary greatly in the strategies they employ. Because of the many unknowns involved, I would not advocate training clinic children in the use of particular cognitive strategies, although this is certainly a fruitful area for research. We can, however, be aware of a child's cognitive style as much as possible and adjust our training procedures accordingly. In addition, we can teach language to children in ways that may induce the development of cognitive strategies. One way to view this matter is to approach the use of language as a series of problem-solving tasks (Winitz 1973). From the preceding comments it will be seen that the problems to be solved will involve the meaningful use of language.

Language Processing

A third general conclusion I would make is that the psychological processes involved in using language are dependent on the general functions of our information-processing systems. Psycholinguistic skills such as those in the *Illinois Test of Psycholinguistic Abilities* (Kirk, McCarthy, and Kirk 1968) and other tests are based on the fundamental functions of sensory reception, attention, integration, memory, and cognitive strategies. Consider the *Peabody Picture Vocabulary Test* (Dunn 1965), for example. Performance on this test requires selecting, from an array of four pictures, the picture that best matches a word presented auditorily. Thus, both the visual and auditory sensory systems are required. The child must attend to both the pictures and the word and disattend other stimuli that may be present. Intermodal connections are required to match the auditory stimulus (the word spoken by the examiner) with the visual stimulus (pictures) and respond with either the motor gesture of pointing or a spoken response. STM is required to hold the word in mind while selecting a picture, and this selection, of course, depends on LTM. Cognitive strategies are present in ways such as following the directions and scanning all pictures before making a choice. Poor performance on the test could conceivably be due to difficulties with any one of these functions.

We see, then, that these information-processing functions have broad implications, both for assessment and in developing intervention strategies. They will help in understanding children's use of language and in providing some clues for making training more efficient. In addition, they provide a useful background for looking at auditory processing and the perception of language, the topics for the next chapter.

3

THE PERCEPTION
OF LANGUAGE

We have looked at concepts and rule hierarchies and how they are intimately related to language, and at five functions of human information processing that are at the very core of language use. This chapter will explore how we use this knowledge and these processes in the perception of language. Language learning depends on input, but making sense out of that input requires perception. I will begin with a discussion of what perception is and describe some general theories of perception. We will then look at the perception of language and then specifically at sentence perception. Finally, we will apply these perspectives on perception toward an understanding of the auditory processing factors that are often mentioned in conjunction with children's language disorders.

THEORIES OF PERCEPTION

Perception may be defined as the organization and interpretation of sensory input on the basis of past experience (Eisenson 1972). It involves discrimination, in that a stimulus must be differentiated from other stimuli, and categorization, in that the stimulus is recognized or given meaning. There is a fine line between perception and cognition. In Gallagher's (1975) view, perception is based on the surface characteristics of a stimulus and on relatively few associations, whereas cognition moves beyond surface characteristics to internal processing of information in memory. Perhaps the two are best seen on a continuum. It may be argued that a very young child's processing would be more toward the perceptual end of this continuum because young children have not accumulated much in memory. Thus, core concepts may be based largely on perceptual processing, but as children learn the associated words and more elaborate concepts their processing becomes more cognitive.

Current theorists stress that perception is an active process rather than a passive receiving of information. We are constantly selecting and analyzing sensory input. We direct attention to different stimuli and recognize or categorize various stimuli. Perception always involves interpretation. We attempt to assign meaning to the stimuli we attend to and in general try to make sense out of the input to the sensory systems.

Components of Perception

The first part of my discussion of perception is based largely on Lindsay and Norman (1972). Most of our knowledge of perception is based on research in the area of vision. We will consider four major factors that are involved in perception. The first is the stimulus itself, whatever it is that we are perceiving. The stimulus might be recognized by comparing it with a set of generalized images, one for each category we can perceive. Lindsay and Norman refer to this process as the template theory of perception: For each category there is a template; if an incoming stimulus matches a particular template, it is recognized as belonging to the category associated with that template. This theory has been discounted because of the tremendous variety of stimuli that often belong in one category. Consider the varieties of stimuli that would fit in the categories of "cup" or "person." They vary in shape, color, size, and many other details of appearance. Further, they can be seen in different positions, from different distances, and with different types of lighting. It is hard to imagine just what the template for one of these categories would be like. A second theory is based on perceptual attributes, which are analogous to the criterial attributes discussed in Chapter 1. An individual could identify cups and persons occurring in considerable variety according to their perceptual attributes. It has been proposed that speech sounds are identified in this way, although in phonological theory the perceptual attributes are usually referred to as distinctive features.

The Context

There are some situations, however, where the stimulus alone cannot provide the full basis for perception. Suppose you look down a line of telephone poles marching across the desert. The more distant poles appear smaller than the closer ones, but you perceive them as all the same size. The perceptual attributes of the phone poles don't help you with their size. A second factor is needed, namely, context. We perceive stimuli in relation to context. The context provides a frame of reference in which to interpret stimuli. You hear a sharp bang at a Fourth-of-July picnic, and you interpret it as a firecracker. You hear the same sound coming from a dark alley behind a bank . . .

Previous Experience

A third factor underlies the stimulus and the context, and that factor is previous experience. We interpret stimuli in terms of our experiences in the past. You have traveled along rows of poles at one time or another and you know that they don't get progressively smaller. You've had many other experiences with perspective and distance. Similarly, most people in our culture have experienced firecrackers on the Fourth, although most of our experiences with loud reports in dark alleys may be vicarious. Past experience contributes to

perception in two ways. It provides the input into memory upon which we base the identification and interpretation of various stimuli; we learn perceptual attributes, for example, through experience. The second contribution of past experience to perception is of particular importance in the perception of language: past experience leads us to expect certain types of stimuli in certain contexts.

Expectations

As Lindsay and Norman put it, we develop sets of rules that limit the possible alternatives in various contexts. These rules are based on past experiences with that context. Thus, the fourth factor in perception is that much of the interpretation of sensory input is based on what that input *must* be, rather than what is actually contained in that input. If you dial a phone number, your expectations of what the first thing the receiving party will say are limited to a relatively few possibilities. The same is true in many other situations.

Analysis-by-Synthesis

These four factors are the basis for another theory of perception, which is referred to as analysis-by-synthesis. According to this theory, we are constantly developing expectations and revising these expectations during the interpretation of a message (Lindsay and Norman 1972). We develop and revise these expectations according to the rules mentioned above. In other words, we anticipate what's coming on the basis of previous experience and the context. It seems to me that analysis-by-synthesis is remarkably well suited to understanding how we perceive sentences. We predict what's going to be said, and then we monitor our predictions. If the input is familiar and predictable, as in an exchange of greetings, we can monitor casually, sampling only enough to check that our predictions are accurate. On the other hand, if prediction is difficult or if our predictions prove to be in error, we follow the input very carefully. The great redundancy in language also contributes to the process. This redundancy makes prediction easier, permits some material to be monitored only at superficial levels, and provides additional opportunities for monitoring in material that must be processed thoroughly. Analysis-by-synthesis becomes highly developed in mature speakers. Some people get so proficient in their predictions that they finish your sentences for you!

The process of constantly predicting what's coming and continuously monitoring and altering these predictions greatly reduces the information load that we have to process in perceiving spoken language. When we are listening to other people talk, we simply don't have to attend to all the detail in their sentences.

Analysis-by-synthesis depends directly on the functions of the human information-processing system. As it involves prediction, it involves directing attention. As it involves comparing predictions with actual input, it involves STM functions. Previous experience, of course, is stored in LTM. Interpreting utterances in a context usually involves intermodal connections. Obviously, sensory systems are involved. The whole process of analysis-by-synthesis is a cognitive strategy, a learned routine for processing information. Prediction of grammatical structures enhances chunking. For example, when you hear a ''the'' you expect a noun to follow. You are prepared, because of previous knowledge of the grammar, to chunk the article, the noun, and anything between them.

It should be emphasized that we carry out analysis-by-synthesis operations extremely quickly. Prediction in this process does not involve long periods of thought. It occurs in real time as we listen to sentences. The process is generally carried out without any particular awareness or specific intention to do so by the listener, although, of course, it can be done consciously.

Very young children and children who are severely impaired in language probably employ a rudimentary form of analysis-by-synthesis. Due to limitations in STM and knowledge of language, they may be forced to listen for the most salient items in the utterances they hear and either ignore the rest or fill in from the context and what they have in LTM. The salient items for individual children may include words or constructions that are stressed, particularly those that are recognized and those that have particularly important meaning for the child. The result may be that the child appears to have better language comprehension than is actually the case. Suppose a parent says to a young language-disordered child, ''Suzie, if you want some ice cream, get in your high chair right now,'' a fairly complicated sentence and doubtless beyond a young child's STM span. The child goes right to her chair. All the child really needs to get from that sentence is ''ice cream,'' if she knows from previous experience that she has to sit in her high chair to eat it and, of course, assuming that she wants some ice cream. In addition, the parent may provide many cues in the context, such as pointing toward the chair, walking toward the freezer, or perhaps even getting out the ice cream. It is well known that hard-of-hearing children become masters at filling in from the context. Some language-impaired children may do as well.

In summary, analysis-by-synthesis illustrates the complexity of language comprehension and the intimate relationship between human information processing and language usage. Mature language users employ analysis-by-synthesis in very sophisticated fashion, but probably young children and language-disordered children interpret utterances with some form of the process. They use whatever information they can from the stimulus, the context, their previous experiences, and their expectations of what is coming.

LANGUAGE PERCEPTION

Now that we have had a brief look at theories of perception and how they relate to language, let us look at the perception of language more closely. It should be clear from the outset that there is no single, accepted index of when a sentence is perceived or comprehended. The problem is that comprehension is covert—whatever we do to measure it involves some response by the subject, some act beyond comprehension itself. Johnson-Laird (1974) suggests that when an individual can decide if a sentence is true, that sentence is probably understood. Glucksberg and Danks (1975) state that when a subject can make appropriate use of the information derived from a sentence, then that sentence must be understood. Both of these methods of investigating comprehension have been used in research and in clinical assessment.

An additional difficulty is that, so far, anyway, there is no effective way to separate sentence perception from comprehension or understanding. Rommetveit (1971) has suggested that the two are not necessarily the same. As he notes, you may recognize a word as being one you have heard before but still not know what it means. This experience always seems to happen to me at the worst time, such as when I'm trying to act knowledgeable about something in a conversation. Examples such as this illustrate processing at the perceptual end of the continuum, rather than the conceptual. Such occurrences may be frequent in the language-learning child, and could involve whole sentences as well as individual words. In any case, the terms perception, comprehension, recognition, and understanding are used almost interchangeably in the psycholinguistics literature in referring to sentence processing. I will not distinguish among them in the following discussion.

The Dual Nature of Language Perception

Fry (1970) states that language perception involves both acoustic and linguistic information. The acoustic information is the input signal. The linguistic information includes knowledge about linguistic structure, words, and statistical information about the nature of linguistic sequences. We will expand these notions shortly. The first point to note is that language comprehension is a twofold process (Fry 1970). That is, only the acoustic information is in the stimulus. The linguistic and statistical information are in the listener's mind. In general, these two aspects of language processing have been studied separately, the first as speech perception and the second as sentence comprehension. In fact, however, there is a complex interaction between the two in the comprehension of utterances.

Marslen-Wilson and Welsh (1978) employ

a useful terminology in discussing these two levels of language processing. They refer to "top-down" and "bottom-up" strategies for processing. In a top-down strategy the acoustic input is processed selectively according to high level constraints. The process is similar to the effects of previous knowledge and prediction in analysis-by-synthesis discussed earlier. We develop expectations of what a message must be, or, at least, we limit the number of alternatives for what that message might be. In a bottom-up strategy, on the other hand, the acoustic input itself plays the major role in determining what the message is. Both strategies are the same in that they function to develop interpretations for acoustic data; they derive meaning from sequences of sound. They differ in the direction in which this process occurs.

It does not seem, however, that we must choose one or the other. Marslen-Wilson and Welsh (1978) argue that both strategies are used together. Bottom-up strategies are important because we do indeed focus on what the speaker says, the acoustic signal. At the same time, top-down strategies are necessary to compensate for ambiguity, noise in the signal, and incomplete utterances. Marslen-Wilson and Welsh describe the two processes as occurring simultaneously. In parallel with our earlier discussion of analysis-by-synthesis, the balance between them depends on the situation. If the input is incomplete or obscured by noise, top-down processing will assume more importance. Similarly, if the input is simple or redundant, the listener will emphasize top-down strategies. If detailed processing is necessary on the other hand, then the acoustic signal will be emphasized through bottom-up processing. Doubtless there is much switching around in the balance between the two as a listener monitors con-

tinuous talking, such as in a conversation. We adjust this balance to make comprehension as efficient as possible. As Marslen-Wilson and Welsh put it, "Word recognition is . . . a self optimizing interactive process" (1978, p. 61). We see, then, that language comprehension is an integrated process that can vary with the situation and with the strategies a listener possesses. Before considering how such a phenomenon might be assessed, let us look more closely at what is involved in bottom-up and top-down strategies.

Bottom-Up Processing

Recognition is basic in language comprehension. That is, we assign the input to categories, such as different sounds and words. As Fry (1970) points out, one aspect of this recognition process is that an individual who knows a language knows what the categories are. That is, knowledge of one category presupposes knowledge of the others. The category /r/ only makes sense in relation to the other sound categories in the language. Speech recognition, then, is a decision-making process: The listener decides which sounds and words are in a stimulus. Recognition is consequently dependent on language learning. One cannot assign sounds to the categories unless one has already learned those categories.

Another phonemenon, called "categorial perception," also supports the importance of learning in the recognition of speech sounds. Categorial perception occurs primarily with stop consonants. In terms of acoustic properties there is a range of variation within what we perceive as a particular stop, as in the duration for which voicing precedes a vowel in a syllable such as /ga/. When this variation is carefully controlled through the use of specialized instrumentation such as a speech synthesizer, listeners will classify sounds within a certain range of variation as being the same, for example, as all representing the /g/ sound. Variation beyond this range, however, is perceived as representing a different stop. In other words, we are sensitive to variation between the stop consonant categories in our language but insensitive to variation within the category of a particular stop; hence the term "categorial perception." A parallel phenomenon is present in the difficulties a native English speaker has in discriminating sounds in other languages that do not match the sound patterns of English, such as the aspirated /t/'s in Chinese languages or the unaspirated /p/ in French. In addition to the learning components that seem to be involved in categorial perception, there is also the possibility of a neurological component. Categorial perception has been demonstrated in some babies at only a few months of age (Eimas 1974; Morse 1974).

Pattern Recognition and Parallel Transmission

Ultimately language perception depends heavily on pattern recognition. In bottom-up processing the patterns are in the arrangements of acoustic cues, namely frequency, intensity, periodicity, and time relationships (Fry 1970). The recognition of speech sounds is relative rather than absolute. For example, the acoustic characteristics of a particular speech sound will vary depending on whether that sound is produced by a young child, an adult female, or an adult male. We recognize that sound through its pattern of acoustic cues, not through specific values of each cue.

The pattern recognition in bottom-up speech perception, however, is not merely the recognition of a series of patterns in a row, one for each speech sound that we perceive. Rather, the perception of certain sounds (again, the stop consonants) is so linked to that of other sounds that there is nothing in the sound stream that can be isolated as representing those sounds. The patterns involve sequences that encompass more than one phoneme. Liberman (1970) has illustrated this phenomenon nicely. Using data from synthesized speech experiments, he showed, for example, that there are no separate segments in the sound stream that represent the two sounds in the syllable /di/. The vowel is represented by two formants, or areas of emphasis, in the sound spectrum, but these formants are also present during the consonant.[1] The consonant is represented by transitions, or abrupt changes, in these formants,[2] but when this transitional portion of the sound stream is played on the speech synthesizer by itself, it does not sound like a /d/ but like a chirp. Further, if a different vowel, such as /u/, is used with the same consonant, the frequency of the higher formant is changed for both the vowel and the consonant and the direction of its transition for the consonant is changed, but we still perceive a /d/. Thus,

[1] A formant has been defined as a resonance of the vocal tract (Denes and Pinson 1973) and as a band of acoustic energy (Liberman 1970). Any vowel or vowellike sound involves a range of frequencies or pitches occurring simultaneously, although we do not hear them as individual pitches but as one composite (vowel) sound. Certain groups of contiguous pitches are emphasized for each vowel, that is, they are produced at higher energy levels. These groups, or bands of energy, are called formants. They are different for each vowel because the position of the articulatory mechanism is different for each vowel.

[2] Ideally, in the production of a vowel the frequency area of each formant remains about the same for the duration of that vowel. A transition is a relatively brief change in the frequency of a formant, occurring either at the beginning or end of a vowel. Transitions are not perceived by the ear as changes in frequency but are interpreted according to the speech code.

one piece of acoustic information, the formant, is carrying information about more than one sound, and there is no sound segment that independently represents the consonant. Liberman concludes that there is no linear one-to-one relation between the sound stream and the sequence of phones. Rather, "Speech . . . transmits information about successive segments simultaneously, and on the same acoustic cue" (Liberman 1970, pp. 308–309). This phenomenon is referred to as "parallel transmission." Information about one phoneme is transmitted in parallel with that about other phonemes.

Segmenting the Stream of Speech

The overlapping of acoustic cues for individual phonemes illustrates another aspect of speech perception, which has been referred to as the segmentation problem (Glucksberg and Danks 1975). We perceive speech as a sequence of individual phonemes or segments, yet researchers have not been able to identify any such segments in the processing of speech. As we have just seen, these segments do not occur at the acoustic level of processing. Curtis (1970) pointed out that they have not been demonstrated at the physiological or neurological levels either. Parenthetically, I might mention that this problem of segmentation occurs in the study of other levels of communication as well. Palmer (1971) described the difficulties the linguist faces in rigorously attempting to segment utterances into words. There simply is no completely successful way to identify the words in a stream of speech. We are so brainwashed by print, where words are easily identified by spacing, that this problem does not often occur to us. At the same time, though, have you ever noticed that speakers of other languages always "run their words together"? This problem is one

reason that linguists focus on the morpheme. Condon and Ogston (1967) discussed the problems in attempting to isolate units at the level of nonverbal behavior, such as arm movements, body postures, and facial expressions. The problems of segmenting behavior into units are important also in Pike's (1967) work with the analysis of the structure of language and other forms of social behavior. It seems that behavior occurs in a constant stream at all levels. Attempts to identify units of behavior within this stream are difficult because much of the change occurs in overlapping gradations, rather than in abrupt contrasts.

A final irony with the segmentation problem is that T. C. Pits (The-Celebrated-Person-in-the-Street) has no difficulty with it. She or he can identify individual phonemes, words, gestures, and so on, whenever it seems necessary. This situation may lead the clinician to an oversimplification of the nature of perception in communication.

In reviewing this section the reader might argue that not all of the processes described here are truly bottom-up. If it's true that bottom-up and top-down processing are always interacting together, then it might well be impossible to isolate one from the other completely. In any case, I have focused on variables directly related to acoustic input. In summary, bottom-up processing involves pattern recognition, the patterns are relative rather than absolute, and they are often overlapping and interdependent.

Top-Down Processing

To me one of the most remarkable aspects of speech perception is in the following. Although it is difficult, we can follow speech at about twenty-five to thirty phones per second (Liberman 1970). Normal conversation contains around fifteen phones per second, but the temporal resolving power of the ear is only between seven and nine sounds per second (Lieberman 1975). This rate is the maximum at which we can distinguish between and identify different sounds one after another. Thus, we appear to be able to identify speech sounds that we are receiving at rates that surpass our resolving power. We can recognize speech sounds faster than we can recognize speech sounds! Enter top-down processing. The most reasonable way to explain this dilemma is through analysis-by-synthesis. We do not process every sound. We predict and fill in as we go. Let us look more closely at some of the factors involved.

One effect of the listener's previous knowledge in language comprehension is that it limits the possibilities for what a particular utterance might be and what it might mean. These limits are the high level constraints in top-down processing that Marslen-Wilson and Welsh (1978) describe. They are dependent on the listener's knowledge both of the world and of the rule system of language.

Sequential Dependencies

It was mentioned earlier that knowledge of language includes statistical information. This information may be described as sequential dependencies or conditional probabilities. The latter parts of a message are constrained by what precedes them (Fry 1970). The classic example is from information theory. If subjects are asked to guess what letter comes next in a printed sentence, the accuracy of their guesses improves as they get further and further through the sentence. On a more general level, several kinds of predictors have been proposed.

Lyons (1977) mentions positional and contextual factors. In addition, the listener is guided by general expectations of what the message might be. More specifically, Johnson-Laird (1970, 1974) discusses the importance of grammatical markers and the properties of certain lexical words. In general, then, we employ whatever information is most useful in applying top-down constraints, depending on what the situation is. These processes occur in all aspects of language, including the phonetic, morphological, syntactic, semantic, and discourse levels.

Top-Down and Bottom-Up Processes Combined

Consider a couple of examples of the interaction between top-down and bottom-up processing. Both my children used to have imaginary friends when they were preschoolers, and these friends would come and go. My son, however, had one such friend whom he kept mentioning for weeks. This imaginary friend's name was Chester Doors. It developed that Chester Doors was very helpful—he took care of my son's clothes and toys. After some time I asked if I could meet Chester Doors. "Sure," my son said. He took me into the bedroom and showed me his chest of drawers! Certainly errors in bottom-up processing were involved here, including both recognition of at least one sound (in "of") and the sequencing of the /r/'s. At the same time, these errors were not severe. Doubtless we said the "of" with minimal stress, perhaps as only a schwa, and he did get the correct number of /r/'s. Top-down processing was also operating, however. He took the acoustic signal as he perceived it and interpreted it in terms of words that were already in his lexicon, with a little playfulness thrown in.

Another example involves my daughter when she was in sixth grade. I recall finding her one evening rummaging through the atlas and encyclopedia, muttering to herself, obviously not finding what she wanted. After watching her for a while the teacher in me couldn't stand it any longer, and I asked her what she was looking for. "The Arch of Pelico," she answered. "Oh," I said, the teacher in me now prepared to retreat because I'd never heard of it. "What country is it located in?" "I don't know; there are several of them," she answered. We talked awhile longer and I finally realized that what she was looking for was "archipelago." Her teacher had said the word in class in conjunction with a geography lesson. Her bottom-up processing was fairly successful for that noisy environment. She had the melodic contour and accent pattern correct and all of the sounds except for a few unstressed consonants. She was missing a key element for top-down processing, though: She didn't know that vocabulary item. The result was that she made a "best guess" in the context of a geography lesson.

In both of these examples one can see how bottom-up and top-down processing combine in analysis-by-synthesis. The examples underscore two other points of major importance in language perception. First, it is indeed an active problem-solving process. We do not merely "register" acoustic stimuli. Children have to develop interpretations for the stimuli they receive. Perception involves cognitive strategies. Along this line, both Bever (1970) and Slobin (1973) have proposed various specific strategies that children might use in sentence perception.

Second, bottom-up and top-down processing are inseparable in the decision making children engage in during language comprehension. The child does not depend wholly on one or the other. As will be developed in the latter portions of this chapter, this view of language perception has important implications regarding what an auditory perceptual disorder might be.

SENTENCE COMPREHENSION

So far we have been looking at language comprehension in fairly general terms. However, many of the assessment and training procedures employed with language-disordered children center around the child's use of sentences. Therefore, it will be of value to explore the area of sentence comprehension in more detail. Researchers have explored the relative importance of three factors in sentence comprehension: linguistic structure, meaning, and cognitive processing. We will discuss each in turn.

Linguistic Structure

It seems obvious that linguistic structure plays a role in sentence comprehension, but it has proven remarkably difficult to tease out just what that role might be. The development of generative transformational grammar had a great impact on psycholinguistic studies of sentence perception. This theory assigns a very prominent role to linguistic structure in language. A number of studies have been carried out to explore this role in sentence comprehension. In this research the subject hears a recorded sentence. At the same time the subject hears a brief click sound. Through use of appropriate instrumentation the experimenter can position this click to occur precisely at any point during the sentence. The experimenter then asks the subject just where the click was located relative to the sentence.

In several studies, clicks were placed in

words that were near boundaries between syntactic constituents. For example, in the sentence *I saw the man who ate the last piece of cake,* the click might be placed either in *man* or in *who.* Subjects often report hearing such clicks as occurring between those two words, that is, they misplace the click to a position between the two clauses in the sentence. These results were interpreted as demonstrating that syntactic structure was primary in sentence perception. In subsequent research, however, it was demonstrated that other factors also influence how subjects misplace clicks. Stress and melodic contours are important. Further, if a click is presented during a period of noise, rather than during a sentence, subjects will still misplace that click toward the middle of the noise. Hence, the results of the click studies are equivocal. Further discussion of this work will be found in Fodor, Bever, and Garrett (1974), Glucksberg and Danks (1975), and Patel (1973).

Grammatical Chunks

In spite of the difficulties in interpreting this research, we do segment sentences in terms of their grammatical structure. As N. Johnson (1970) points out, we appear to register information in grammatical chunks. Johnson's research focused on sequential processing of sentences. A subject is asked to recall a sentence that was presented earlier. From many such trials with many subjects, Johnson calculated the probabilities that if a subject recalls a particular word correctly, the next word in the sentence will also be recalled correctly. The results indicate that subjects had more difficulty recalling the following word if there was a syntactic boundary between the two words. In the sentence mentioned above, *I saw the man who ate the last piece of cake,*

words like *saw* and *piece* would be recalled more accurately than a word like *who.* This research emphasizes sequential dependencies, but only within grammatical constituents.

Sequential dependencies related to grammatical sequences are not the only factors operating, however. If a subject is given a sentence and then one word is repeated from that sentence with the instruction that the subject give the first other word from that sentence that comes to mind, the subject will select a word on the basis of semantic associations, rather than associations related to serial order.

Weisberg (1969), quoted in Glucksberg and Danks (1975), presented subjects with sentences such as, *Slow children eat cold bread.* The sentences were constructed so that there were no close associations among the words they contained. The word *slow* elicited the word *children,* as we would expect from the sequential nature of the sentence, but *children* elicited *slow.* Thus, it seems that while sequential order has a role, meaning may be a more powerful factor in sentence processing.

Meaning

It has already been pointed out in Chapter 2 that what is remembered from a sentence is its gist or meaning, rather than its syntactic structure. Sentence recall depends largely on the reconstructive functions of semantic memory. The specifics of grammatical structure are lost quickly (Johnson-Laird 1970, 1974).

There is other evidence for the primacy of meaning over syntax in sentence comprehension. We attempt to comprehend anomalous sentences through meaning rather than through structure. In fact, if the semantics and the syntax of a sentence are contradictory, we will rely on the semantics in developing an interpretation of that sentence (Hunt 1971). If you doubt this statement, consider what you do in trying to understand young children whose grammatical skills are not yet fully developed, or language-disordered children: You focus on the meanings they are attempting to express. In a similar vein, Brown and Hanlon (1970) reported that the parents of the three young children they studied provided positive feedback to the children for utterances that were semantically appropriate, rather than syntactically correct.

Meaning has also been prominent in research in artificial intelligence. In experiments in which computers are programmed to process aspects of natural language, it has been found that the programs must be based on meaning and general knowledge, rather than syntax (Glucksberg and Danks 1975). On the basis of his work in this area, Hunt suggested that "The rules required for comprehension appear to be much simpler than the rules usually considered necessary to describe the grammar of a language" (1971, p. 83). We can relate this statement to an idea presented earlier in the section on analysis-by-synthesis. It was suggested that children may appear to comprehend more than they actually do through the process of analysis-by-synthesis and the problem solving related to it. In addition, following Hunt's suggestion, it may be that comprehension doesn't necessarily require complete linguistic processing, anyway, or at least that comprehension isn't as difficult as it appears to be in terms of syntactic processing. Admittedly these questions go far beyond the available data, but they are still relevant to clinical training, where the differences between

comprehension and expression take on special significance (Chapters 9 and 10).

In view of the importance of meaning in comprehension, one may ask what syntax does contribute to the process. First, in conjunction with stress and melodic contour, it helps identify grammatical units in sentences. These units, or chunks, are important in the processing of meaning. Second, syntax gives a variety of cues concerning the semantic relations in a sentence. Third, it provides one layer of redundancy in sentence comprehension. Much of the information that is represented syntactically is also represented lexically or in the context.

Cognitive Processing

As already mentioned, sentence perception or comprehension always involves choice or decision making. The listener must decide on an interpretation for each utterance that comes along. In many cases this decision is easy and straightforward because of the redundancy provided by previous utterances and the context. Further, in many situations it isn't terribly important that a precise interpretation of each utterance be accomplished—in casual talk about the weather, for instance. In other cases, however, one must work very hard to develop precise interpretations. Our whole legal system is based on careful interpretation of written language. Similarly, a student reviewing lecture notes for an exam is involved in interpreting the instructor's remarks. Quite different types of interpretation become important in reading poetry or in psychotherapy. I am reminded of the old joke in which two psychiatrists exchange casual greetings such as, "Hi," and "How ya doin'?" as they pass each other in a hallway. Each then goes on down the hall wondering what the other "really meant" by those remarks. Language comprehension involves problem solving of some sort. We think as we listen.

Variation in Language Processing

This view emphasizes the importance of cognitive strategies in language comprehension. Cognitive strategies, in turn, imply individual differences, as was discussed in Chapter 2. We don't all think the same. As Glucksberg and Danks put it, "There is no single way that people perceive, remember, or comprehend any given type of linguistic material" (1975, p. 85). I have already suggested this variety in terms of the flexibility inherent in analysis-by-synthesis and the interplay between top-down and bottom-up processing. In order to consider how a child might process sentences, however, we need to look at this variation in more detail. While there are many factors influencing how an individual will process a sentence, perhaps they can be organized into three major areas.

The Listener's Skill and Knowledge. First, the way an individual processes a sentence is dependent on the skills and knowledge that individual possesses. Here we go back to the five aspects of human information processing upon which perception is based. Children will vary in attention, memory, and so forth. As stressed in Chapter 2, different children will have at least somewhat different cognitive strategies available to them in approaching language comprehension. Also important is the child's knowledge of the language system and of the topic of discussion. It is hard to execute the top-down processing necessary for analysis-by-synthesis if you don't know what's going on.

The Listener's Purpose. A second area that influences sentence processing is the individual's purpose in dealing with a particular sentence. In performing on a test of auditory memory span, for example, the purpose is to recite back the stimuli just as they were presented: "six, three, seven, five, nine, four, eight." The task focuses on intentional memory of an episodic nature and evokes strategies we have available for that task. In contrast, consider a situation in which you are given directions on how to get to somebody's house. The task is still intentional, but its episodic quality may be diminished. Comprehension becomes dominant. What you need is to be able to reconstruct those directions as you're driving along. Alternately, imagine that you've just been told that you have been awarded a large cash bonus for good deeds. Your processing is likely to be quite different again. It may involve pinching yourself or leaping up and down. It's doubtful that you will need to invoke intentionally any particular strategies to retain this information. Many other examples could be given. The way we process a sentence depends very much on how we will use the information that sentence represents. As will be developed shortly, testing during language assessment may involve distinctly different purposes for a child than using language in more natural situations, and may thus elicit different processing strategies.

The Information in the Context. A third factor that influences sentence processing is the information available in the situation. As has been repeatedly emphasized, we use cues in the context and in previous utterances in interpreting an utterance, as well as the cues in the utterance itself. It is from the context and the preceding discourse that we develop many of the constraints that are central in top-down processing. Miller and his associates (Miller, Heise, and Lichten 1951; Miller and Isard 1963; both quoted in Fry 1970) concluded that the effects of context are to limit the number of choices or possible interpretations that a particular utterance might have, specifically a top-down function. This situation is particularly true with ambiguous sentences. Frequently a listener doesn't even detect ambiguity in a sentence when that sentence is encountered in an appropriate context. If you're on a hunting trip with friends and conversation develops about "the shooting of the hunters," you're very likely to know immediately whether to flee, duck, express sympathy, or listen for other hunters in the distance.

Ambiguity leads to another aspect of the relation between an utterance and its context. Johnson-Laird (1970) suggests that ambiguity or vagueness in a sentence directs the listener to relevant aspects of the context. If you're not sure how to interpret a sentence, one thing you do is to look for cues in the context. The nature of the vagueness or ambiguity, however, directs you to look for certain types of cues. If a child says, "Is it this one?" you look to see what item the child is indicating. To quote Johnson-Laird, "In this way a sentence defines its own context" (1970, p. 265). At the same time, if the nonlanguage aspects of a situation are ambiguous, we can look for appropriate cues to understanding the situation in the accompanying utterances. Thus, there is a reciprocal relation between a sentence and its context. A sentence is the context for its context. From the problem-solving point of view, a listener interprets a situation, not just an utterance. Let us explore the implications of this expanded view of sentence comprehension.

The Picture-Utterance Match Task

It could be said that there are three elements to sentence comprehension. There is the sentence itself, the context in which the sentence is heard, and there is the decision making or problem solving in which an interpretation for that sentence is developed or selected. In much mature conversation the relation between the utterances and the context may be extremely tenuous. Two adults can stand on a street corner and discuss many different topics, from lollipops to language. The context remains the same. For the situations we are interested in, though, the context is more directly relevant to the utterance. One of the most common procedures in psycholinguistic research and in the assessment and training of language-disordered children is to present utterances and pictures together. The subject's task, then, is to relate the picture and the utterance. In language assessment and comprehension training it often involves choosing one from a small set of pictures that best matches an utterance, such as in the *Peabody Picture Vocabulary Test* (Dunn 1965) described in the preceding chapter or the *Test for Auditory Comprehension of Language* (Carrow 1973). In expression training, a picture or series of pictures is often used to elicit an utterance that contains a particular grammatical structure from a child.

The Effects of the Task in Testing Comprehension

Glucksberg and Danks (1975) have reviewed the use of similar tasks in psycholinguistic research. A number of studies have attempted to determine whether or not certain sentence types are more difficult to process than others. For example, it appears to take longer to process passive sentences than active ones. This finding was the result of experiments employing varieties of the picture-utterance matching technique described above. The subject hears a sentence and sees a picture. The task is to decide whether or not the two match. For example, the picture might show a car hitting a truck. The utterance might be, "The car hits the truck," or, "The truck hits the car." While the details of this research are more complicated than I'm indicating, the point is that it takes subjects longer to decide if passive sentences such as "The truck was hit by the car" match the picture than it does for active ones such as those above.

Olson and Filby (1972) altered the task slightly. In essence, first they showed a picture of just a truck. Then they showed a picture of a car hitting the truck. Using this technique, passive sentences were processed more rapidly than active ones, a reversal of the previous pattern. The extra time required for processing passive sentences in the previous work, then, was not due to anything inherent in the passive construction, but rather was due to the particular task used in the experiment. As we will see in Chapter 7, Glucksberg, Trabasso, and Wald (1973) and Glucksberg and Danks (1975) have described other experiments which support the same general conclusion. The way a subject processes a sentence is dependent on the specific task the subject is asked to perform.

Clinical Implications

Now we come to a most interesting problem. As I pointed out, many of the assessment and training procedures used with language-disordered children employ variations of the same task that has led to

spurious results in psycholinguistic research: picture-utterance matching. The implication is that these tasks may elicit problem-solving strategies that are specific to the task, rather than representing "knowledge" or "use" that is typical of the child's language performance. There are some data supporting this *caveat*. Prutting, Gallagher, and Mulac (1975) compared children's responses on the expressive portion of *The Northwestern Syntax Screening Test* (Lee 1971) to their grammatical structures in language samples. In the expressive portion, the Lee test assesses particular syntactic structures through a picture-utterance matching task in which the child first notes matches between two pictures and two utterances produced by the clinician and then produces the matching utterance for each picture. It was found that with this procedure the children made errors in grammatical structures that they produced correctly in their spontaneous language samples. Similarly, Dever (1972) demonstrated that children's failures on another picture-utterance matching test of grammatical structures were not related to the same children's ability to use those structures in spontaneous talking. The task in this case was that used by Berko-Gleason (1958) in studying morphological development.

Clinicians and researchers have attempted to develop instruments for assessing children's skill with grammatical structures. As has been demonstrated, context greatly affects one's comprehension of language. This problem has been approached in test construction by minimizing the context, usually to a set of from two to four pictures. The effect is to restrict top-down processing. It is reasoned that the child is thus forced to attend to the grammatical construction of the utterance. The context cues simply aren't sufficient. Ironically, it's turned out that in these attempts to "isolate" language knowledge, a particular problem-solving task has also been isolated. Unfortunately this problem-solving task has problems of its own, as has been discussed above. A parallel dilemma exists in attempting to train specific grammatical structures through picture-utterance match tasks. I will deal with the clinical implications of these situations in later chapters. For now let me say simply that the teacher or clinician should be very cautious in interpreting picture-utterance match tasks as representing children's knowledge or skill with particular grammatical structures. A more extensive perspective will be required.

This discussion of cognitive strategies and the processing of language leads directly to the final topic of this chapter, auditory processing. With a background in human information processing and in language perception and its attendant cognitive processing, we are now in a position to consider auditory perceptual skills directly.

AUDITORY PERCEPTUAL PROCESSES

Our focus is restricted now to the processing of acoustic stimuli, particularly language, through the auditory channel. Many authors and clinicians in fields such as speech pathology, language pathology, and learning disabilities have characterized this processing in terms of a number of specific skills (e.g., Chalfant and Scheffelin 1969; Wiig and Semel 1976). Included are processes such as awareness of sound, awareness of speech, auditory localization, auditory figure-ground discrimination, auditory discrimination, auditory memory span, and auditory sequencing. These phenomena are often referred to as auditory perceptual

skills; they are assumed to underlie the perception of language.

There are two fundamental questions to ask about auditory perceptual skills such as those just listed. First, are they relatively unitary, independent phenomena? The implication in treating them as separate skills is that they are. Second, are they causative or symptomatic in relation to children's language disorders? The assumption frequently is that they are causative. If these skills underlie language perception, then problems with any of them could impair language learning and use. In response to these two questions, I would like to argue that auditory perceptual skills are highly interdependent and, in fact, are better understood in terms of the more general operations of human information processing than as unitary skills of and by themselves. In a sense, the second question then loses some of its potency. Be that as it may, Rees (1973), Sanders (1977), and Bloom and Lahey (1978) have all argued that there is very little convincing evidence that impairment in auditory perceptual skills functions is a source of language disorders in children.

Perspectives for Considering Auditory Processing

At this point our friend, T. C. Pits, would be quick to argue that auditory perceptual skills are very real. Indeed, some language-disordered children get their words out of order, or have difficulty discriminating between certain linguistic forms, or are impaired in their ability to repeat back utterances spoken by someone else, and so on. Further, several theoretical models of language processing provide formal support for these observations. These models represent language processing as a linear sequence of steps. In Nation and Aram's (1977) model, for example, language input goes through stages of sensation, then perception, and then comprehension. Other language models also hypothesize that language processing involves a series of stages or levels (Wiig and Semel 1976; Kirk and Kirk 1971; Wepman, Jones, Bock, and Van Pelt 1960; Cooper 1972; Chalfant and Scheffelin 1969). It is not my purpose to discuss the merits of these models. I merely wish to illustrate that if one thinks of language processing as a series of steps, then it makes sense to include auditory perception and the skills it entails as comprising one step.

These models may be contrasted with views of language processing as holistic (Sanders 1977) or simultaneous (Marslen-Wilson 1975; Marslen-Wilson and Welsh 1978). From this perspective language input does not go through a series of stages but rather is processed at a number of levels simultaneously. The ideas of top-down and bottom-up processing discussed earlier illustrate this perspective nicely. The linear sequential models put the emphasis on bottom-up processing: first sensation, then perception, then comprehension. Marslen-Wilson (1975), however, has demonstrated that we process phonetic, linguistic, and semantic information all at the same time. We can only accomplish this feat through the addition of top-down processing. Top-down processing, in turn, implies knowledge of the language system. Sanders states the matter succinctly: Auditory processing is part and parcel of language processing. "It does not seem to be the relatively independent function that some writers claim it to be" (1977, p. 193). Further, as I mentioned earlier, the idea that language is processed top-down and bottom-up simultaneously makes it difficult to conceive just what a level of auditory perception might be. Top-down processing is not specifically auditory,

so auditory processing must be bottom-up; but bottom-up processing is heavily influenced by its top-down counterpart and in addition does not seem to function as a series of stages.

Consider now the relation between auditory perception and the aspects of human information processing from Chapter 2. It should be immediately apparent that skills such as discrimination, memory span, and sequencing are heavily dependent on all five aspects of human information processing. In fact, auditory perceptual skills might better be seen as applications of these more general information-processing functions, rather than as a separate level of skills. Sequencing, for example, consists of processes in the sensory systems, attention, memory, and cognitive strategies such as chunking. Discrimination revolves around the same set of skills. Auditory memory was analyzed in just this way in the preceding chapter. Viewed in this way, the several skills involved lose their independence. All are overlapping manifestations of more general principles.

Implications for Intervention

I will save a thorough discussion of etiology for Chapter 6, but let me point out now that the causal relation between auditory perceptual skills and language disorders is at best circular. Because auditory processing is part of language use, rather than a separate level, one could imagine causation going in either direction, or perhaps being related to other factors. Thus, improving language skill might enhance sequencing or auditory memory span for language, rather than the other way around (Bloom and Lahey 1978). Similarly, a retarded child might show deficits in overall language skill and of auditory memory and sequencing of language stimuli as well.

T. C. Pits, however, refuses to go away: "What shall we do with children who have difficulties with auditory perceptual skills such as memory and sequencing in their use of language?" I answer in terms that are becoming familiar from previous chapters. Avoid excessive reification of auditory perceptual skills. That is, do not isolate those skills as independent entities. Rather, approach auditory processing as an aspect of language use. For example, the tasks for the child in the evaluation and training of auditory processing factors are typically far removed from how those factors are involved in the use of language in meaningful communication. Discrimination work often consists of listening to pairs of unrelated words in a nonmeaningful context, or even listening to bells and drums; sequencing work usually focuses on unrelated items. In both cases the child is denied the opportunity to develop or enhance relevant cognitive processing strategies because those strategies depend on the presence of meaningful language in a context. The strategies the child does develop, indeed, may not be directly applicable to processing language in normal contexts. Therefore, it would seem desirable to focus the assessment and training of auditory processing skills directly on how those skills are manifested in the child's use of language. If a child gets words out of order, approach this problem as a difficulty in that child's knowledge and use of language, rather than as a difficulty in auditory processing apart from language.

Perhaps I should add that I am certainly not suggesting that we abandon attention to auditory processing in language-disordered children. Rather, I want to recommend a richer perspective for auditory perception than is often applied, and I simply want to urge a little caution in an area that we don't understand well. An extensive discussion of auditory processing will be found in Sanders (1977).

CONCLUSIONS

First, let me comment further about reification. You may have noticed that while I have cautioned against the reification of constructs such as rules in Chapter 1 and auditory processes in this chapter, I have cheerfully reified other constructs myself, such as short-term memory in Chapter 2 and analysis-by-synthesis in this chapter. My first thought is that there are good reifications and not so good reifications, but that's not fair. It may well be that it is not possible for us to consider abstract human capacities such as information processing and language usage without at least some reification. Does language exist apart from our use of language? My point is that it's one thing to observe an abstract function, such as short-term memory or auditory discrimination, as it is manifested in a particular context, but it's quite another thing to consider that function as existing as an entity on its own. Some theorists may need to do the latter, but clinicians and teachers are perhaps better off concentrating on the former. Consider a child who produces sentences of appropriate length but who tests out below norms for digit span, or a child who articulates certain sounds correctly but misses those same sounds on an auditory discrimination test. We cannot make sense of these situations in terms of the generalized functions of short-term memory and auditory discrimination. My suggestion is that we consider these functions as embodied in the situations in which they occur, rather than as abstract skills. We can then approach them in terms of the problem solving the child must do in each situation.

Language Perception

Returning to the subject matter of this chapter, I began by looking at various theories of perception. I selected analysis-by-synthesis as the only one flexible enough to represent language perception. This theory emphasizes a view of perception as an active process. We predict what's coming, compare our predictions with the input, adjust and fill in as we go. Language perception seems to go in two directions at once. We take the acoustic input, recognize patterns, and assign meaning to them. The patterns are relative and overlapping, rather than discrete and linear. In addition to this bottom-up processing, we develop both general and specific expectations of what an utterance might be. These top-down constraints make language processing much more efficient. Both directions of processing occur simultaneously in analysis-by-synthesis. The balance between the two varies with the situation, including the type of information, the ease with which the signal can be heard, the listener's previous knowledge, the context, and other factors.

Perception, including both its bottom-up and top-down components, is based directly on the ideas presented in Chapters 1 and 2. It is dependent on previous knowledge, which consists of concepts and rules stored in long-term memory. It depends on input from the sensory systems. It requires attention and at the same time guides attention. It often involves material from more than one sensory channel. Perception itself can be viewed as an open set of cognitive strategies.

Selection among these strategies is governed by metarules that are invoked by past experience and the demands of the particular situation.

Within this general view sentence comprehension may be seen as related to three factors: linguistic structure, meaning, and cognitive strategies. It turns out that meaning is more important in this process than linguistic structure, an ironic conclusion in view of the intense interest in syntax that is current in the field of children's language disorders. In any case, sentence comprehension implies developing an interpretation for each sentence. This process, in turn, may be described as one of problem solving or decision making. We see again the active nature of language comprehension. In addition, the cognitive strategies through which these decisions are made vary greatly with the situation and the listener's purposes and skills.

Clinical Implications

These conclusions lead us to some views more directly related to language training. First, it is very difficult to assess language perception. This difficulty stems partly from the fact that comprehension is covert and partly from the fact that we do not comprehend only language, we comprehend situations in which language and the context are often inextricably woven together. In spite of this complexity, there are some hints that language comprehension may not be as difficult as it appears. All of these conclusions render the standard clinical approach to assessing language comprehension somewhat suspect. This approach, which is based on comparing pictures with utterances, may elicit problem-solving strategies that are very different from those the child needs to comprehend language in natural situations.

Finally, it seems that the auditory processing factors that are commonly invoked in attempting to understand language-disordered children may be of less substance than has often been thought. Auditory perceptual skills such as discrimination and sequencing are not independent entities that underlie the use of language. Rather, they are inseparable aspects of the process of using language itself. In assessment and intervention it may be more helpful to approach these factors directly in terms of how the child uses language, rather than isolating them for special consideration.

In consonance with the previous chapters, this chapter has emphasized the importance of meaning and active problem solving in language use. Further, it has underscored the flexibility with which human beings of all ages process language. With this background let us turn now to a more careful consideration of language itself.

4

LANGUAGE STRUCTURE AND FUNCTION

In the introduction to this book it was pointed out that language has both representational and communicative functions. Further, language was described as a system including a lexicon, or vocabulary, and a grammar, or set of rules for combining elements. Since then we have looked at concepts, rules, information processing, and the perception of language. With this background let us return for a closer consideration of language itself.

Language is often described in terms of five levels. Phonology is the study of the sound systems of languages. Morphology is concerned with minimal units of meaning and of grammatical pertinence and with word formation. Syntax involves the structure of phrases, clauses, and sentences. Semantics is the study of the relations between language and meaning. Finally, pragmatics focuses on language use. The term "grammar" is frequently used to refer to both morphology and syntax, and I will use it in that way. It has sometimes been thought that one could consider any one of these areas relatively independently of the others. It seems more realistic, however, to view each level as interacting with the others. As has been discussed earlier, language is structured in hierarchical fashion.

STRUCTURE AND FUNCTION

Perhaps the most general goal of linguistics is the rigorous description of language. This goal is pursued differently by various schools of thought in linguistics, but some generalizations can be made. At the very least a linguistic analysis of a language will have to include a description of the structures of that language and a statement about how those structures function. The linguist attempts to identify the regularities in a language. One way we can look at this process is as follows. Any language contains a great deal of variation. The problem for the linguist is to determine just which aspects of this variation are significant in the structure of the language under study. One could gather a corpus of utterances and describe all the variation in that corpus in exquisite detail. The result might be a listing of all the structures or components used in that corpus, with similar elements sorted into categories. Such an analysis would be purely descriptive. It would not necessarily provide any information about how those elements or categories function. It would be analogous to monitoring secret messages without knowing the code. We could describe all the characters in the code and their arrangements, but we still wouldn't have broken the code. Or, for another parallel, the situation is similar to that of an American baseball fan watching a cricket game for the first time. The players may do familiar things, such as throwing and hitting, but the baseball fan's knowledge of cricket is purely descriptive. It does not include the functions that underlie the activity on the field. In linguistic terms, the observer has not yet discovered the rule system associated with the game.

Pike (1967) has characterized this matter in terms of two levels of analysis. One is purely descriptive or observational with no interpretation, and the other focuses on those differences that are important, meaningful, and functional.[1] A descriptive analysis can be done from outside the system, but an analysis of function can only be done by getting inside the system. The difference between the two can be seen easily in phonology. Some speakers of

[1] Pike (1967) refers to these two levels as "etic" and "emic" respectively.

English pronounce *either* and *neither* with a long *i* and others with a long *e*. Or, one speaker might end the word, *cup,* with an aspirated /p/ and another without aspiration. An observer who knew no English would not know whether or not these variations are important. The best that person could do would be to list or describe these variants. An observer who comes from within the system, however (that is, a speaker of English), could tell that this variation is not significant in the language. This English speaker would also know that the variation between *cup* and *cub* is indeed functional or significant in the language.

In studying a language, then, a linguist needs descriptive or observational data. At the same time, in learning how to interpret these data, how the elements of the language function, the linguist moves inside the system to a large extent by learning as much of the language as possible and by consulting informants who are fluent in the language. The distinction between description and function in analysis is not restricted to language. Research in nonverbal behavior in humans is an example. There are plenty of descriptive data available; but there is considerable uncertainty concerning the interpretation of these data relative to the functions of nonverbal behavior. We will explore this matter in the next chapter. A similar situation exists in the study of interaction within the family unit. Pike (1967) presents a number of other examples.

RELATEDNESS

Virtually all authors emphasize the complexity of grammatical structure, and, indeed, the grammar of a language consists of a most complicated rule hierarchy. The fundamental principle behind grammar, however, is simple enough. Bolinger (1975) referred to this principle as "relatedness." Language expresses relations. The grammatical structure of a sentence indicates how the components of that sentence are related to each other. Recall from Chapter 1 that a rule is a relation between concepts and that a linguistic category such as a grammatical function may be considered a relational concept. The key element in this view is embodied in the term relations. Hence, in concert with Bolinger (1975), we can say that grammatical rules specify relations among linguistic categories or elements. In the sentence *Eddie kissed Edna,* there is nothing in the words themselves to indicate who was the kissee and who was the kisser. That relationship is represented by word order, which is a matter of grammatical rules. Similarly, in the sentence *The little tiny brown dog bit the great big black dog,* we know which dog was brown and which dog was black and which dog did the biting because those relationships are spelled out by the grammar. It is clear, too, that the relatedness in the grammar of these utterances parallels the relatedness in the realities to which they refer. In many sentences the relatedness may be more subtle than in these examples or more difficult to ferret out, as in the classic *Dogs dogs bite bite back.* These difficulties, however, should not detract from the point that the basic business of grammar is to spell out the relationships among the parts of the sentence.

Grammatical Operators

The relatedness of grammar is represented in several ways. First, it is expressed through word position, as in the preceding examples. Second, it can be represented by what Bolinger (1975) refers to as "grammatical operators" that function in the sentence to indicate grammatical relationships. Operators serve as organizers in the sentence. Through emphasis and phrasing, for example, one gives a listener cues about the organization of an utterance. Similarly, punctuation marks, by setting off segments of a sentence (such as I'm doing now), help the reader understand the organization of that sentence.

Grammatical Morphemes

In addition, certain morphemes function as operators. These morphemes are called "grammatical morphemes." Examples would include function words such as *such as, to, the, other,* and *and,* and inflectional suffixes such as, *-ing, -s,* and *-ed.* Through their grammatical functions these morphemes help indicate the organization of the relationships in the sentence. For instance, if a sentence begins, *Give me the . . . ,* we know to expect a noun phrase; if a word ends in *-ing,* our first guess is that it's a verb. These examples are related to the perceptual strategies discussed in the preceding chapter. Observe how much easier it is to process the *dog bite* sentence from above with the addition of some operators: *Dogs that are bitten by other dogs bite back.* Not Pulitzer quality perhaps, but the relationships are clearer now than in the original statement.

Lexical Morphemes

Morphemes may be either lexical or grammatical (Bolinger 1975). The emphasis in lexical morphemes is on content. Lexical morphemes represent the wide range of concepts we can express with words. Bolinger notes, on the other hand, that grammatical morphemes function in two ways. First, as already mentioned, they are grammatical operators. Second, they represent certain

aspects of meaning that are so basic to language that they recur constantly, such as plural, tense, possession, and the pronominal function of representing meanings already established in a discourse. The difference between these two roles of grammatical morphemes becomes blurred in actual use. The distinction between lexical morphemes and grammatical morphemes, however, is of considerable practical importance.

Clevenger and Matthews (1971) present an example that will be instructive in this regard. They analyzed a speech on elementary education by a college student. Table 2 lists the ten most commonly occurring words in the speech and the percentage of the total number of words in the speech that each of the ten words represents. Almost a quarter of the student's total output in this speech consists of only ten different words. Further, and to the point here, all of those ten words are grammatical morphemes. The eleventh word was *child* (1.5 percent) and

Table 2. Relative Frequencies of Occurrence of Ten Words in a Speech

Word	Percent
the	5.0
of	3.0
a	2.5
and	2.4
for	2.3
is	2.2
not	2.1
that	2.0
in	1.7
can	1.6
Total	24.8

From Theodore Clevenger, Jr. and Jack Matthews, *The Speech Communication Process,* p. 42. Copyright © 1971 by Scott, Foresman and Company. Reprinted by permission.

the thirteenth word was *education* (1.2 percent). One would expect these two lexical morphemes to be used frequently because they are so closely related to the topic of the speech.

The contrast between the two types of morphemes is striking. Grammatical morphemes form a rather small class, that is, they are relatively few in number, whereas lexical morphemes form a very large class. At the same time, grammatical morphemes occur much more frequently than do lexical morphemes. Each sentence needs its operators, drawn from the same relatively small pool, but the speaker can choose from a vast selection of lexical morphemes.

Grammatical Operators and Language Training

We can say that lexical morphemes belong primarily to the semantic or referential system of language, whereas grammatical morphemes, as the name suggests, are part of the grammatical system. The difference between the two is important in language training. A lexical morpheme is typically taught as a concrete concept. We show a child a shoe or pictures of shoes and teach the word. A grammatical morpheme, in contrast, is a relational concept and can only be taught in the context of the relationship it represents. While one can teach a word such as *car* by associating it with cars the child sees, one cannot teach *is* by associating it with examples of *ises* the child sees. *Is* represents a relationship between other words, for example, *The ball is green,* and can only be taught in its relational (i.e., grammatical) context.

In addition to strategies for training, grammatical morphemes raise other questions of clinical interest. As has already been stressed, they form a relatively small class

but they occur very frequently. At the same time, language-disordered children frequently have difficulty with these morphemes. If utterance length is limited, a child may employ few grammatical morphemes or none at all. A child with longer utterances but difficulties in the area of syntax will also show errors in the use of grammatical morphemes, for example, in verb constructions. Other things being equal, one might hypothesize that it would make sense to focus training on these morphemes because overall level of language use would improve more from incorporating some grammatical morphemes than from acquiring an equal number of lexical morphemes. "Other things being equal" here would include at least that the child already has enough lexical morphemes to have something to talk about and that the child is combining words. The irony is that grammatical morphemes are difficult to teach because of their abstract, relational nature.

Summarizing this chapter so far, a linguistic analysis must both describe the elements of a language and specify the functions of those elements. The core of a linguistic analysis is a set of rules that specify the relations among the elements, to show how various items in the language are related to each other. Relatedness, then, is the basic concept behind linguistic rules. Relatedness is indicated in various ways, such as grammatical morphemes, vocal inflection, and word position. Grammatical morphemes, in turn, are of particular interest in language training.

STRUCTURAL LINGUISTICS

Various schools of thought have developed within the field of linguistics. The ideas presented above are characteristic of one of those schools, which is called structural or descriptive linguistics. Structuralism is an eminently practical endeavor. The goal is to analyze and make a permanent written record of many different languages as efficiently as possible. The motivation for this goal developed partly out of a concern among anthropologists to preserve the languages of many native cultures that were literally dying out. Certain religious groups with extensive missionary programs had a similar need for efficient procedures for analyzing languages, as did the world powers, especially during World War II, when they came in contact with many different language groups. All of these motivations were applied and practical in nature. Another factor influencing structuralism was the Watsonian emphasis on behaviorism in psychology during the twenties and thirties.

The result of all these factors was a focus in linguistics on developing techniques for analyzing languages utilizing objective data and methods. The function of meaning in language was deemphasized because of its subjective nature. Meaning could often be reduced to judgments about whether two utterances had the same meaning or not, a process directly paralleled in our use of same-different judgments in auditory discrimination testing. The focus was on developing "discovery procedures" for identifying linguistic structures. The use of minimal pairs in isolating phonemes is an example. Two words are chosen which differ in only one sound contrast. If the two words do not mean the same thing, then the two sounds in contrast must be separate phonemes. Thus /tin/ and /din/ do not mean the same thing, and so /t/ and /d/ must be different phonemes. On the other hand /lip/ and /lip^h/ do mean the same thing and consequently /p/ and /p^h/ are not separate phonemes. No analysis of meaning is necessary beyond the same-different distinction. Hence a minimum amount of interpretation beyond descriptive statements is needed for linguistic analysis.

Function, Class, and Position

Meaning, however, refuses to go away. In particular, it is difficult to identify grammatical functions without additional reference to meaning. One approach to this problem was that developed by Pike (1967). His approach to language emphasizes three interrelated concepts: function, class, and position.[2] Function refers to grammatical function, class to the group of items that represent that function, and position refers to where an item from that group can occur in a sentence. A nongrammatical example will help in understanding these terms. Consider positive reinforcement. The function of positive reinforcement is to increase the frequency of occurrence of the event that immediately precedes the reinforcer. The class of phenomena that can represent or implement that function is large, including praise, food, money, tokens, and affection. Finally, the reinforcer must occur in a certain temporal position relative to the other events in the situation. It is important to note that each of these three concepts is interdependent with the others. The function (reinforcement) doesn't get far unless it can be manifested or represented somehow. It becomes manifested through one of the members of the class of events that can be identified as positive reinforcers. At the same time, that group of events is identified as a class because each can function in the

[2] Readers familiar with Pike's work will note that this section is based on tagmemics. I am avoiding his technical terms, such as tagmeme and slot, for ease of exposition.

same way; in the context of this discussion the members of the class are interchangeable. The function is the basis for identifying the class; the class in turn represents the function. Finally, that class does not appear willy-nilly. It must appear in a particular position in the temporal sequence.

A similar analysis is applied to various aspects of language. For example, there is a class of words in English called articles. These articles have certain functions in sentences. The same reciprocal relationship as in the previous example holds between the class and the function. The function of articles can be determined by observing how that class of words behaves. Conversely, the group of words called articles form a class because they all function in the same way. Finally, that class has a distribution in sentences, that is, articles occur in certain positions only.

It may be argued that the definitions of these terms are circular, in that function and class are each defined in terms of the other, but this argument misses the point. What is important is the relationship between them. Pike (1967) talks about a grammatical category as a correlation between a class and a function. The two are inseparable. In analyzing the grammar of a language, classes, functions, and positions are identified by juggling around among the three, but this situation occurs only during the process of analysis. After the analysis is finished class and function form one unit, which occurs in certain positions.

The Pivot-Open Construction

A similar analysis can be performed when the functions of the classes are not clear. In this case the classes are defined only in terms of the positions in which they occur. A relevant example is the "pivot-open" construc-

tion in young children's early word combinations. In earlier studies it was found that some children were using two word classes. The pivot class contained a relatively small number of words. The open class, on the other hand, contained a larger number of words and seemed to acquire new words frequently. In any individual child's utterances, some pivot-class words tended to precede an open-class word in two-word combinations, and some followed open-class words. In the terms developed above, we now have classes and positions. Some researchers stated their analyses in this fashion, with the minimal attention to meaning that is characteristic of structuralists, as was discussed earlier. This is sometimes referred to as an "item and arrangement analysis."

Other researchers, however, looked at the words in each class and attempted to define what their function might be. The terms pivot and open represent a very conservative move in this direction. These words were chosen partially because they are not the names of any word classes in adult English. The open class was so named because new members are easily added to this class. The term pivot connotes some sort of link with the open class without specifying what that relationship might be. More precise labels for these classes were also proposed. The open class typically identifies the topic of the utterance, while the pivot seems to provide additional information about that topic. Hence, the terms "topic" and "modifier" were proposed. One can see that considerable interpretation is involved in applying these terms. In effect, we are guessing that the two classes of words function differently for the child and guessing what those functions might be. Later analyses of this type of construction included the context in which the child's utterance was made and therefore permitted more precise interpretations of what the child's utterances might mean (Bloom 1970). These interpretations suggest that the child who uses two-word combinations has a richer command of language than the analysis into two classes would imply.

Clinical Implications

The relationships among function, class, and position are of considerable power in viewing linguistic rules. No matter what kind of structure appears in a child's utterance, it can be analyzed from this perspective. Applying these concepts in teaching grammatical structures gives us a relatively concrete way to approach grammatical rules, making those rules less abstract to deal with. That is, to teach a child a grammatical structure or rule, all three components will have to be dealt with. Consider some examples. If a clinician elects to teach a telegraphic talker to use *the,* the focus is on a class (albeit a class of one) and a position, but not on a function. If a teacher attempts to teach a child to express wants with words rather than gestures, the focus is on function, with the class not clearly specified. It seems artificial to separate the aspects of grammatical categories in this fashion. One cannot teach the function of expressing needs verbally unless the child has a class of at least a few words to use in this capacity. Similarly, if *the* is taught as a filler for a particular position, why should the child use it? It has no function. We will return to this matter later in the chapter.

As implied by the example on positive reinforcement, Pike has suggested that the same type of function-class-position analysis can be applied to areas of human behavior other than language. As examples he presents analyses of football, church services, and even breakfast. Each of these events includes various functions that are represented by classes of behavior and that occur in some sort of sequence. This type of application, in principle at least, suggests the possibility of analyzing verbal and nonverbal behavior together. For example, a child may have the communicative function of denial but express it with a class of gestures rather than words. Or a child may express wants by pointing and whining rather than with words, or with one-word expressions accompanied by gestures. As we will see in the next chapter, however, there are problems in pushing this type of analysis too far. At least some nonverbal communication is qualitatively different from language.

Summary

This section has introduced additional concepts of structural linguistics, with the focus on objective, observable data. We have seen, however, that structuralists vary considerably within this focus. In earlier work dependence on the subjective area of meaning was minimized. In more current structuralist work meaning is employed in determining the function of grammatical categories. Pike's (1967) view of grammatical categories as relations among function, class, and position illustrates that view. Our understanding of the nature of linguistic rules is enriched by these ideas. Grammatical categories are relational concepts, embodying relations among functions, classes, and positions. Grammatical rules indicate relations among grammatical categories. Description and function are thus inseparable. As has been illustrated, this view of grammatical rules has important implications for clinical training. I shall expand on this topic later on.

The relationship between objective data and subjective interpretation in linguistic analysis, as illustrated in the discussion of the pivot-open construction, is a central problem in linguistic theory. How much should linguistic analysis be based on an objective analysis of observed data, and how much should it be based on interpretation and theoretical or mental constructs? At this point we will consider generative transformational grammar.

GENERATIVE TRANSFORMATIONAL GRAMMAR

Transformational grammar[3] developed from structuralism but with a very different focus. Transformationalists feel that the insistence on only certain kinds of objective data is too limiting. Central to transformational grammar is the idea of mentalism. Mental activity is carried out in the mind; it is not observable. Mentalism in transformational linguistics means that the informant's mental activity (concerning language) is an acceptable type of datum. Thus, the transformationalist is interested, not only in utterances, but in the speaker's ideas about those utterances. This perspective has been very useful in approaching certain areas that had been problematical in structuralism, such as the relationships between certain sentence variations. The transformationalists' wholehearted endorsement of mentalism has also allowed, perhaps encouraged, linguistic analysis to be based on theoretical

[3] For our purposes generative grammar, transformational grammar, and generative transformational grammar all mean the same thing.

(mental) constructs in addition to observable data.

Deep and Surface Structures

Consider the difference between active and passive sentences, as in *Eddie ate the cheese* and *The cheese was eaten by Eddie*. We know (mentalism) that these sentences mean approximately the same thing, a fact that structuralism was unable to deal with in any elegant fashion. Transformationalists, on the other hand, proposed that the two sentences were the same at some underlying, deep level. Thus, sentences could be described in terms of two levels. The deep structure, a theoretical construct, is the meaning level or the abstract structure of the sentence. The surface structure, also a theoretical construct, is the string of words that directly parallels the actual utterance. (This string still must go through a set of phonological rules before the utterance itself is realized.) The two sentences about Eddie, then, would be described as two different surface structures with the same deep structure. A statement such as one often sees at highway construction sites, *SLOW MEN AT WORK*, on the other hand, is associated with at least two deep structures. This two-level analysis has permitted many insightful observations about sentence structure and the relationships between sentences.

Transformations

Another theoretical construct employed by generative grammarians is the "transformation." This device was originally used as a way to show relations between sets of sentences, such as, *Eddie ate the cheese, Eddie didn't eat the cheese, The cheese was eaten by Eddie,* and, *Did Eddie eat the cheese?* Each of these sentences can be related to the others through a process of transformation; each can be transformed into the others through certain changes in word order and the addition or deletion of various elements. Transformations, however, were soon employed more extensively as the links between deep and surface structure. The abstract form of a sentence and the actual string of words uttered are viewed as being connected through a series of transformations. As languages were studied by transformationalists, specific transformations were hypothesized in relation to various types of surface structures. In English, for example, there are the "wh-question transformation," the "passive transformation," the "noun complement transformation," and so on. Each relates to a particular type of (surface structure) linguistic form and specifies the relation between that surface structure and its corresponding deep structure. While many authors refer to various transformations by name as if they were entities, it is to be emphasized that these transformations do not exist except in the form of consensus among transformationalists to use those names to represent certain theoretical constructs. In the terms I have been using they are reified abstractions.

Competence and Performance

As has been stated, transformationalists emphasize the speaker's ideas and knowledge about language and the abstract structures underlying utterances, rather than the utterances themselves. In line with this orientation, transformationalists have attempted to describe language structure in its pure form, rather than in some form contaminated by all the vagaries of actual talk-

ing by human speakers. This goal has been described in terms of the distinction between "competence" and "performance." Competence refers to everything one knows about one's language. As you might predict from the discussion of the psychological reality of rules in Chapter 1, much of this information appears to exist without any particular awareness by the speaker. Consideration of competence would not be possible were it not for mentalism. Performance, on the other hand, is what one can actually do with language; it is the sentences one can actually comprehend and produce. Performance, then, is subject to all the complications and limitations of the human information-processing system, while competence is not.

An analogy may be helpful. In playing cards there are various levels of rules as illustrated in Chapter 1. Competence is analogous to a player's knowledge of the rules of the game and of various moves and strategies to win. Performance, in contrast, is what that player actually does while playing. For example, I often forget what cards have already been played and occasionally even who's turn it is. These are problems with my performance. They do not reflect my competence, or knowledge of the game in the abstract. Similarly, the generative grammarian is interested in the ideal speaker-listener, who is not subject to performance limitations such as memory, attention, and shifts in purpose.

Transformational Grammar and Language Training

Through the writings of Chomsky (1957, 1965, 1972a, 1972b) and his colleagues, transformational grammar has assumed a position of great importance in current linguistic work. The emphasis has been more on developing a theory of language than on analyzing many different languages, as in the applied approach of the structuralists. The basic tenets of the theory, such as deep and surface structure and transformations, have been modified and enriched in various ways. The theory has had an impact in other disciplines interested in language, such as the study of children's language acquisition and psycholinguistics.

Ironically, language clinicians currently face a surfeit of linguistic theory. There is vigorous debate among schools of thought in linguistics. Transformational grammar has divided into more than one camp. Theoretical developments have been coming along so quickly that one year's accepted dogma rapidly becomes old hat and in need of revision. While this tempo of change is exciting and stimulating, it does not provide the stable framework necessary to develop and evaluate intervention strategies for language-disordered children. Such program development takes years to complete.

There is a central fact, however, that ultimately may dictate the paths we will follow. Language clinicians and teachers, by definition, must focus on performance. We deal with children in the here and now of real behavioral contexts, subject to all the nonlinguistic factors of human information processing and of human relations. Rather than deny or ignore performance limitations, we must seek them out and attempt to explicate them. If a child is found to have a deficit in sensory input, attention, memory, or the like, the clinician must deal with that performance deficit in approaching that child. If a child does not use language in some situation, we must focus on the exigencies of that situation, regardless of how much language competence we judge the child to have. In short, we are interested in the words children demonstrate they can actually comprehend and the utterances that they produce. Such an orientation does not reduce our focus to some sort of bare bones behaviorism at all. It merely asserts that our primary concern is with the child as a language user.

Transformational grammarians are attempting to develop competence models of language. What is meant by a competence model is a representation of the knowledge that an individual must possess in order to use language. This goal is legitimate and of interest in children's language disorders as well as other fields. At the same time, there is no claim that such a competence model actually represents the form in which language users possess or apply that knowledge. Thus, the majority of transformationalists do not mean to imply that we "really use" transformations as they have been described. Rather, as language users, we must carry out some sort of processing operations to realize those aspects of language represented by transformations and, for that matter, all other linguistic rules as well. As in previous chapters, we use metaphor to discuss complex human processes such as cognition and language.

Transformational grammar, as its name suggests, has focused primarily on the level of grammar. At the same time, through the door of mentalism, it has spawned new approaches to the relationship between semantics and grammar. Recent developments in theory, such as generative semantics and case grammar, may be described as attempts to make meaning more central in grammatical analysis. This effort has had considerable impact on the study of children's language acquisition and language disorders.

SEMANTICALLY BASED GRAMMARS

The essential tenet of a semantically based grammar, such as generative semantics or case grammar, is that there are a number of semantic roles or functions that are fundamental in sentence structure. These semantic roles underlie the surface structure of sentences and are not to be confused with traditional grammatical cases (at a surface level), such as subject, verb, and object (Fillmore 1968). One can say, for example, *I broke the lock with a rock,* or, *I used a rock to break the lock,* or *A rock was used to break the lock,* or simply, *A rock broke the lock.* In each sentence the semantic role of the rock is the same: It is the instrument involved in breaking the lock. This role remains the same in spite of the fact that the grammatical case of *rock* varies from object of a preposition, to object of a verb, to subject of the sentence.

Consider some other examples. In *The summers are hot in Tucson* and *Tucson is hot during the summer,* the semantic role of *Tucson* is the same, namely, to specify a location. Similarly, *summer* makes the same temporal reference in both sentences. As with the rock and lock sentences above, however, the grammatical cases of these words vary in the two sentences. The same observations may be made about *Jake* in *Jake found the snake, It was Jake who found the snake,* and *The snake was found by Jake.*

Semantic Functions Underlying Sentence Structure

These examples illustrate what is meant by a semantic role or semantic case. Both Fillmore (1968) and Chafe (1970) have developed tentative lists of semantic roles. Chafe,

for example, begins by making a distinction between the area of the noun and the area of the verb and then proposing cases for each area. Some of the cases within the area of the verb are as follows.

State. A verb of this type specifies that something represented by a noun is in a certain state or condition, as in *The pudding is cold* or *The work is finished.* The nouns in these sentences are represented as being in the states of being cold or being finished, respectively.

Process. Process verbs specify that something represented by a noun changes from one state to another. The sentences *The milk was spilled* or *The wind died down* represent changes in state. The milk changed from unspilled to spilled and the wind from blowing to calm.

Action. This category is not related to states, but to the idea of action, that something gets done, as in *Sarah walked all night* and *The horse began to buck.* Both of these sentences include the idea of "doing."

The area of the noun includes roles such as these:

Patient. A patient is something that is specified as being in a particular state or that changes from one state to another. In the above examples, pudding, work, milk, and wind are all patients. Patients are sometimes described as logical objects, as opposed to grammatical objects (Glucksberg and Danks, 1975).

Agent. An agent is able to initiate and perform an action, such as Sarah and the horse above.

Instrument. An instrument is something that effects a change in state but that is not an agent. Typically, an instrument is an inanimate object that is used by an agent, as with *bat* in, *Betty hit the ball with a bat.*

Location. This semantic case identifies

the location of a particular state, process, or action, as in, *Alfred went outside* or *It's windy in San Francisco.*

Experiencer. An experiencer is an animate being who is mentally disposed in some way. Examples here would include *Susan wants her dessert* and *Charlie hates football. Susan* and *Charlie* are neither agents nor patients, but they can be described as being in certain mental dispositions.

Complement. A complement is something that comes into being as the result of an action. In *Picasso painted the picture,* the *picture* comes into being through the action of painting. Similarly, *hymn* is a complement in *The choir sang a hymn.*

Chafe (1970) describes some other cases but the total list is small. Fillmore's list is even smaller. It seems that there are a relatively small number of basic semantic functions underlying sentences. It is important to remember that they may be represented in various ways in actual utterances. They are not literally to be taken as nouns and verbs in the surface structure. Rather, they are abstract semantic functions.

The importance of semantic roles in sentence structure rests in how they are combined. Thus, *The men boiled the soup* contains an agent (*the men*) and a patient (*the soup*). The verb is both a process (changing from unboiled to boiled) and action (the men did it). Of primary importance is the relation between semantic roles from the area of the verb and those from the area of the noun (Chafe 1970). It turns out that there are various restrictions on which "noun" cases can occur with which "verb" cases.

One can see a certain amount of parallel between the description earlier of grammatical categories in terms of function, class, and position, and the present discus-

sion of semantic roles: Both revolve around function. In addition, these functions must be represented somehow in utterances. The two views, however, differ in the mechanisms of this representation. The grammatical categories discussed earlier are components of surface structure and are realized directly through the classes associated with them. Semantic roles or cases, on the other hand, are posited as a deeper, semantic, level and are realized indirectly through a series of transformational processes similar to those in transformational grammar. Nevertheless, both approaches might posit some of the same functions in the grammar of a language, such as instrument and location, although they would vary in their handling of grammatical relations such as subject and verb.

Clinical Implications

The relevance of semantic roles to children's language disorders may be developed as follows. Considerable research has been done on young children's early word combinations in normal language acquisition. Brown (1973) has pointed out that some investigators, particularly Bloom (1970), Schlesinger (1971), and Brown himself, have characterized these early word combinations in terms strikingly similar to those of case grammar. These utterances can be interpreted as expressing relations between a small number of semantic roles. Thus, *Daddy go* expresses an agent-action relation, *Milk all gone* represents a patient-state relation, and *Toy got broke* represents a patient-process relation. Brown (1973) has argued extensively for the importance of such semantic role relationships in children's early word combinations.

Following these analyses, some language clinicians have adopted semantic roles as a basis for early language training (Mac-Donald and Blott 1974; Miller and Yoder 1974). As we will see in later chapters, the logic for this strategy is compelling. Children are likely to be aware of these relations because they are central to human experience at all ages. As Brown (1973) points out, they are based on sensorimotor learning and do not depend directly on language. At the same time, they form a core of language and communicative skills that will be relevant to the child immediately and can be elaborated in later language development. We will consider this matter in more detail in Chapter 8. The focus on semantic roles leads us now to a more general consideration of meaning in language.

SEMANTICS

Meaning can be viewed in many ways. The first part of my discussion will be based largely on Lyons (1977). We will begin by exploring three fundamental terms in semantics. These terms indicate different aspects of word meaning.

Reference

"Reference" is the process of identifying what is being talked about (the referent). Thus, reference applies in specific instances only. Words in the abstract do not have reference. It is only when they are used in particular contexts that they can refer. As Lyons says, words can't refer; only speakers can refer. If I say, *These kumquats are good,* and there is a basket of kumquats present, my utterance has a referential function. Similarly, I may look in a store window and say, *That's a beautiful coat,* while admiring a particular coat. Note that I could then enter the store and tell the clerk, *I'll*

take that one, while gesturing at the same coat. This utterance is referential although it does not contain the name of the intended referent. Most vocabulary training with language-disordered children is referential. We identify particular items or pictures of items, and the child learns the word as it refers to those referents. The more severely the child is impaired, the more the vocabulary training will be referential, because any other method of training would involve abstraction that might be difficult for the child.

Denotation

Many people argue, however, that words have meaning beyond reference. A word stands for a whole class of items. This usage is called "denotative" meaning. An important point about denotation is that word meaning comes from outside the language system. Segments of reality are denoted by words, but those segments are not part of language itself. It is in denotation, perhaps, that word meanings are most closely associated with concepts. I can use the words *kumquat* or *coat* to discuss all kumquats or coats as classes, without referring to any particular exemplars of those classes at all. It can be seen that this statement is parallel to saying that those two words symbolize their respective concepts.

There is some debate about whether one should simply say that a word represents a class or say that a word represents the concept which in turn represents the class (Lyons 1977). Part of the reason for this debate is that the term "concept" has been defined differently by different authors. If it is argued that possessing a concept merely means being able to classify objects in terms of whether or not they are represented by a particular word, one might take the former view. If, on the other hand, possessing a concept means more than that, as I have suggested in Chapter 1, the second alternative might be more appropriate. In the typical child, words and concepts develop together. Given the variation and flexibility in cognitive development referred to in Chapter 2, it seems probable that both views might apply to a particular child during the development of various words and concepts.

In summary, there are two important aspects to denotative meaning. First, in contrast to reference, a word denotes a whole class of items, or a concept, rather than being tied to individual acts of reference in particular contexts. Second, in parallel with reference, a denotative meaning comes from outside the language system.

Sense

The third type of meaning is called "sense." This term has been used in two ways. It is often used synonymously with meaning in general. Some semantic theorists, however, have used it in a more restricted fashion (Lyons 1977; Olson 1970b). For these authors the sense of a word is its meaning in terms of its relations with other words. In contrast to denotation, sense is the meaning of a word from within the language system. There are a number of sense relations among words. Two common ones are synonymy, as in *shout* and *yell* or *fast* and *swift,* and antonymy, as in *hot* and *cold* or *up* and *down.* Sense relations between words of the same class are called paradigmatic relations. Examples would include relations between one noun and other nouns or one verb and other verbs. In contrast to sense relations of this type, there are syntagmatic relations, or the relations between words of different classes, such as nouns and verbs or nouns and adjectives.

Some further examples will be instructive at this point. Consider the word *spoon.* In terms of reference this word would be used to identify or refer to a particular spoon in an actual utterance. Its denotation would be more general, including the whole class of spoons, or perhaps the core and concrete concepts of *spoon.* Its sense would include paradigmatic relations with words such as *fork, knife, soup, dinner,* and syntagmatic relations with words such as *eat* and *serve.* As a second example, take the word *teacher.* In reference it would be used by a speaker on a specific occasion to refer to a particular teacher. Its denotation would include the whole class of teachers, in this case a relational concept. With regard to sense it would be related paradigmatically to words such as *student, class, school* and *education,* and syntagmatically with words such as *learn* and *teach.*

Reference, Denotation, and Sense in Language Training

It is fruitless to attempt to decide which type of meaning is most important or closest to reality. All play a part, and all are relevant to language training. As has already been pointed out, vocabulary training usually revolves around reference. We teach the child to associate a word with particular referents, and often very few of them at that. Countless clinical and classroom hours have been spent holding toy cars in front of children and saying, "car," holding blocks and saying, "block," and so forth. But we are not happy if children can only name a few exemplars of a concept. We want to teach the child the concept that accompanies the word, or, stated differently, we want the child to generalize. In present terms, this goal means a shift from reference to denotation. We want the child to be able to use a word for the whole class of items it symbolizes. Finally, we want the child to use the word in sentences. This type of usage requires sense relations. A clinician may ask a child to make up sentences with the word *spoon* in them. Normally you would accept *I want a spoon to eat my lunch* but not *I'll eat my spoon for lunch.* Further, there are some words that have no capacity for reference and very little denotation. They are the grammatical operators, discussed earlier, whose meaning is primarily in the area of sense relations. It would be difficult to specify denotations for words like *if, and,* and *whether,* but they do signify important sense relations.

Word meaning, in the abstract, involves both denotation and sense. Word usage in utterances involves both of these plus reference, to varying degrees. What is important in clinical work is that, while they overlap and interact, they are not identical with each other, and training one type of meaning does not necessarily imply that the others are learned as well.

Utterance Meaning as Differentiation Among Alternatives

Given this state of affairs, how can we develop a perspective on word meaning that will be directly useful in language training? Lyons (1977) has emphasized that the use of language to communicate information implies choice, or selection among alternatives. As was spelled out in the preceding chapter, comprehension involves choice in that the listener must decide on an interpretation for each sentence. Choice is also central to the speaker's task. One must decide what to say and how to say it.

Along these lines, Olson (1970b) has proposed a referential theory of meaning.

He is looking at meaning in utterances, in the actual use of language, rather than in the abstract as it has often been considered by semanticists (for example, Katz and Fodor 1964). Olson suggests that the meaning of an utterance is in how that utterance differentiates among the alternatives in the situation. An utterance, then, specifies one alternative from those available in a contrast set. Suppose you are buying ice cream for a child. The child's desires will be expressed with different words, depending on what the alternatives are. You say, *What do you want, Billy?* He answers, *A cone,* the contrast set consisting of items such as a bar or a cup. Or he might say, *Ice cream,* in contrast with sherbet. Again, he may say, *A triple-double,* the alternatives now being lesser-sized servings. Finally, he will probably specify a flavor, *Pistachio,* from the contrast set of flavors available. You and Billy may have to run through all these sets of alternatives before a decision is made.

It is noteworthy that Billy's intended referent is the same for each utterance—he knows what kind of confection he wants—but the utterance varies with different sets of alternatives. Obviously, he could combine all the above information into one utterance if he wished and had the skills to do so: *A triple-double pistachio ice-cream cone,* but that does not detract from the point. The meaning of an actual utterance lies, not in abstract considerations of denotation and sense, but in how that utterance differentiates among the alternatives available.

The preceding statement requires some explanation. First, notice that I said the meaning of an utterance, not of a word. In the abstract, word meaning can be described in terms of sense and denotation, but Olson's is a theory of use, of how words in actual utterances represent meaning. Second, the alternatives in a communicative situation do not have to be physically observable in all cases (Olson 1970b). They can be present or implied. One can talk about ice cream whether or not there is any available at the moment. The contrast with other goodies is implicit in using the term ice cream. Similarly, we can discuss communism, Roman civilization, or Smokey the Bear. Third, the above statement is not intended as a God's Ultimate Truth pronouncement about meaning. It does not deny the existence of denotation and sense. Rather, it provides an approach to meaning that is less abstract and consequently more amenable to use in clinical training. In large measure, the teacher can determine which alternatives will be available in training children to use particular words. Further, Olson's theory helps relate the choice of words to particular utterances, that is, different words are used with a specific referent, depending on which alternatives are important. Finally, this theory lends itself to the problem-solving theme that I am developing as an approach to working with language-disordered children.

As was mentioned, the element of choice discussed by Lyons (1977) is present for both speaker and listener. The speaker's choices are concerned with the intent of the message and how to represent that intent relative to the contrast sets involved. As we will see later in this chapter, the speaker's choices are also based on guesses or assumptions about what contrast sets the listener may have in mind and other factors about that individual. The listener's choices center on identifying what the speaker has in mind, given the alternatives in the situation. As suggested in the chapter on perception, the listener attempts to comprehend the situation, including both the utterance and the context. We now see that the context can be further described as a set of alternatives.

Over time, a child will experience a word in various contexts. That is, the word will be used in relation to different contrast sets. Concomitantly with these occurrences, the word directs the child's perceptions in different ways. Consider the word *apple*. On one occasion the contrast may involve oranges; another time bananas or other fruit; again, the contrast may be with a decorative wax apple or with a ball. The use of the word in a variety of contexts will direct the child's perceptions to the contrasts in each of those situations. As in Chapter 3, the various alternatives are contexts for utterances containing the word *apple,* but those utterances are also contexts for those sets of alternatives. Through this reciprocal process the child develops the general command of the word that has been described as denotation and sense. The child's concept of apples also becomes enriched. In general, the child's knowledge of a word develops through experience with that word in various referential contexts.

Implications for Language Training

Olson's (1970b) theory is rich in implications for language intervention. It focuses on actual utterances in use. Such utterances are the core of language training. The theory is concerned with reference, which is how we teach words. In this regard, recall Lyons's (1977) remark that language doesn't refer, people do. Further, reference is conceived in a way that implies more than merely associating a word with an object. Rather, through the problem solving involved in selecting among alternatives, it develops an approach to reference that enhances cognitive activity and provides a link between specific referential uses of words and the more general development of word meaning.

Grammar as Options-to-Mean

The idea of choices among alternatives has also been used to look at language in broader scope. Halliday (1973) has developed a useful perspective in this regard. He begins with what he calls a behavior potential. A potential is a set of options. A behavior potential, then, is a set of options for how one can behave, or choices in what one can do. Behavior potentials are culturally and socially determined. That is, the choices you have for your behavior are heavily influenced by the situation you're in; the things you can do while in an elevator are different from what you can do in a classroom or at a picnic or on a public sidewalk. The culture provides a set of metarules that put limits on the behavior potentials available to you in different settings.

Language is one set of options in the behavior potential. Halliday (1973) describes language as a meaning potential. It is a set of options-to-mean. The focus in Olson's (1970b) view is on the function of language in relation to alternatives outside of the language system. Halliday is concerned with alternatives within the language system. Thus, the semantic roles presented above are options that one can mean when using language. That is, one can express meanings such as agent or action. The grammatical categories discussed earlier in association with Pike's (1967) theory may also be interpreted in this perspective. That is, functions and classes are similarly options to mean. For example, as Lyons (1977) mentions, verb tense depends on oppositions of temporal reference. Similarly, the choice between *the* and *a* depends on whether or not the accompanying noun is singled out in some way. In general, as Halliday puts it, "The options in the grammatical system are realized as structure and vocabulary . . ." (1975, p. 249). In addition, it should be clear that speakers and listeners share roughly the same sets of options.

Implications for Language Training

In parallel with Olson's theory, Halliday's view of grammar as options-to-mean has considerable clinical appeal in the perspective I am developing. First, it approaches grammar through meaning. When we look at language samples in Chapter 8, we can ask what a particular child can mean, rather than merely what grammatical structures are present. We can identify the options-to-mean that the child actually demonstrates in the sample. Second, it relates grammar and meaning to cognitive processes. If using utterances involves choosing among options, this process can profitably be viewed as a series of problem-solving tasks. In both comprehension and expression, the child is constantly making decisions.

Another facet of Halliday's work is relevant to clinical concerns. Certain grammatical options are related to the interpersonal situation in which a person is functioning. Consider sentence structure. An independent clause may be either imperative or indicative; if it is indicative, it may be either declarative or interrogative; if it is interrogative, it may be either of the yes/no form or the wh- form. As Halliday points out (1973, p. 56), these forms indicate that the speaker is taking on the various social roles associated with each form and assigning the complementary roles to the listener. In effect, by using a certain form of statement, you are establishing a certain kind of human relationship, at least for the moment. For example, in using an imperative, you set yourself up as one who can give commands and your listener as one who should receive commands. It is a moot point whether the form of statement actually influences the relationship or the relationship influences the form of statement. Each occurs in the context of the other and each reinforces the other. The point is that the use of language is inseparable from participation in human relationships. Talking and responding to talk are ways of behaving toward other people. We will explore human relationships more thoroughly in the next chapter.

The Social Code

Extending this view even further, ultimately a language user develops not only a linguistic code but a social code as well (Krauss and Glucksberg 1977). Not only must a child learn language, but the child must also learn to use language to communicate with other people. Typically, there is more than one option-to-mean available in a communicative situation. The semantic role of "agent," for example, can be expressed in many ways; so can the social role of "one who can give commands." The child learns to select options that will function in the interpersonal context of the moment. This is Krauss and Glucksberg's social code. These selections depend partly on the speaker's assessment of the human relationships involved and partly on an assessment of the listener's background and skills as they interact with the referential alternatives available in the situation. The more delicate semantic choices, as Lyons (1977) says, are often determined by the environment.

Consider an example. Suppose you lose a fifty-cent piece. There is a young child present who can help you look for it. The referential alternatives include that coin and a contrast set of other things one could look for, such as buttons, pennies, pebbles, and other objects. The options that you select in describing the coin will reflect your opinion of how best to differentiate the coin from the contrast set in terms the child will understand. For example, you might decide not to name the coin but to describe some of its most salient perceptual attributes, such as roundness and shininess. The options you choose in enlisting the child's aid in the first place depend on your view of your relationship with that child. You may utter a command or request the child to help or attempt to intrigue the child into helping, depending on such factors as how well you and the child know each other and what you know about how the child responds to those various approaches. Thus, language, meaning, and human relations are all tied together.

Summary

We have explored a number of views of meaning in this section. First, the general distinctions between reference, denotation, and sense were considered. In order to develop a more direct clinical perspective, however, we related language and meaning to choice. Language is used to differentiate among alternatives, to specify one alternative from a contrast set in specific instances of communication. More generally, language can be seen as a set of options-to-mean. Grammar is thus viewed as a set of ways to mean, rather than as simply a set of rules. These options-to-mean include both ways to represent alternatives relative to a contrast set and ways to communicate one's intended meaning to particular listeners.

This perspective on meaning will be useful in devising clinical interventions for two reasons. It permits us to view language use in terms of problem solving and therefore to focus on some of the cognitive activity accompanying talking and comprehending. At the same time, language is seen as a way to deal with other people, thus emphasizing the relationship aspects of language use.

CONCLUSIONS

This chapter has been a most eclectic discussion of linguistics and language. I have been searching for ideas that will be useful in approaching language training. A problem that linguists of all persuasions have faced is the relationship between description and interpretation, between form and function. We have seen that we will need to be concerned with both in working with language-disordered children. One approach to this problem is through Pike's ideas of the interrelatedness of function, class, and position. The teaching of any grammatical structure must involve all three components. This view allows us to go beyond merely asking what grammatical structures a child uses.

We still need a way to focus these ideas directly on the child's using language to communicate. Halliday's (1973, 1975) ideas provide one way to bridge this gap. Language consists of sets of options-to-mean. Function, then, can be taught in terms of what the child can mean, and thus grammar is directly related to communication. Options-to-mean range from the general semantic functions of the semantically based grammars, such as agent, action, process, and patient, to the more delineated semantic functions of particular grammatical morphemes, such as plural and past tense. In training, all of these options-to-mean will be represented by certain classes of utterances, such as words or phrases. In addition, these classes will occur in larger utterances in specified positions or orders.

I am particularly intrigued with Halliday's (1973, 1975) description of grammar as options-to-mean, rather than as options-to-express-meaning. Meaning is thus seen as embodied in what people do with language, rather than being reified as existing in language itself. This view dovetails nicely with my theme that we do not teach children language, we teach children to use language in communicative situations. A store of options-to-mean, then, is essential both to comprehension and expression.

Olson's (1970b) theory presents additional perspective on how utterances can mean. The meaning of an utterance resides in how that utterance differentiates among the alternatives in a situation. This view emphasizes referential meaning, which again suggests language in use. In addition, it carries the potential for developing an empirical approach to teaching children language. Utterances can be related to the alternatives available in the teaching environment.

While there is sharp debate among various schools of thought in linguistics, work with language-disordered children can benefit from ideas from various sources. The clinician needs the structuralist emphasis on empirical analysis of actual utterances in assessing language samples and formulating certain kinds of training goals. At the same time, the interpretation of how language means for a particular child will certainly be mentalistic at times.

The emphasis on alternatives and choice as discussed by Halliday, Olson, and Lyons relates language use to problem solving and decision making. This perspective provides a direct link between language use and cognitive processing, which we will be able to exploit in developing approaches to clinical management. At the same time, the structure of utterances is related to the social context in which they are employed. An imperative is an interpersonal as well as a grammatical statement. Language is as heavily influenced by the social context of its use as it is by conceptual, cognitive-processing, and linguistic factors. In the next chapter we will explore human relationships as they relate to communication and language use.

5

COMMUNICATION AND
HUMAN RELATIONSHIPS

Human relationships develop and are maintained through communication. At the same time, communication is only possible in the context of human relationships. When individuals communicate, by definition they form relationships. In this chapter we will be concerned with the nature of communication and human relationships and with the reciprocity between these two phenomena. Because language is a means of communication, the use of language cannot be separated from participation in human relationships. This view was brought out in the latter portions of Chapter 4. For example, Halliday (1973) noted that the choice of a particular form of statement assigns social roles to both speaker and listener. In asking a question the speaker takes on the role of "person who can ask questions" and assigns to the listener the role of "person who will answer questions." Further, as noted by Krauss and Glucksberg (1977), one structures utterances with a listener and a situation in mind, not merely on the basis of a set of linguistic rules. Thus, in this chapter we will look at the interplay between language and human relationships. In approaching this goal we will also consider some comparisons between language and other forms of communication.

A DEFINITION OF COMMUNICATION

We may begin with a definition of communication. Following Watzlawick, Beavin, and Jackson (1967), I define communication simply as transfer of information. As these authors suggest, all behavior has message character. Not only language, but facial expression, posture, gesture, tone of voice, choice of clothing, and myriad other activities all transmit information of some

sort. One can say, "Hello" with words or with a flick of the eyebrows. A person can say, "Take me seriously," through dress, tone of voice, and facial expression as well as with words. One sends the message "I am in a hurry" simply by being in a hurry, whether or not one talks about it. In fact, it can be seen that it is impossible not to communicate (Watzlawick, Beavin, and Jackson 1967). Imagine yourself seated on a bus after a hard day's work. Someone sits down next to you and attempts to strike up a conversation. Because of your mood at the moment, you simply ignore that person. Clearly even a "refusal to communicate," as in this case, can communicate a powerful message. The relationship between meaning and choice discussed in the previous chapter now takes on an added dimension: One cannot choose not to behave. In Goffman's (1967) terms, we exude information. We cannot avoid producing messages.

This view of communication carries several implications. First, as mentioned above, no intent to communicate is necessary. An individual who is frying an egg is communicating, just as a lecturer or newscaster is. Behavior transmits information whether or not we wish to communicate, as in the example of "refusing to communicate" cited above. Second, this definition does not require that all communication be complete or true, or even that it be understood. Messages that are vague or contain outright lies still involve information exchange and are thus instances of communication. Similarly, if information has been received, then communication has occurred, even if the receiver is not sure what that information means. Third, a receiver must be present to perceive whatever information is entailed in someone's activity, whether it be through physical presence, telephone connection, reading the printed word, or other means of contact. Messages must be apprehended for communication to occur. Finally, in face-to-face encounters, transmission and reception of messages occur continuously and simultaneously. As I talk to other people, they receive my words and note my other activity. Their behavior in listening and watching is itself information, which I monitor even as I continue to talk. At the same time, they are watching me watch them . . .

As was just mentioned, receiving a message is an act of perception. As with all perception, we interpret the information we receive from the various sensory channels. This reception and interpretation occurs through the information-processing functions and conceptual networks discussed in previous chapters. We continually attempt to extract meaning from the activity of others. As emphasized in previous chapters, this attempt is a continual process of choice and decision making. The interpretation of behavior, or the extraction of meaning, is central to all communication, from the hand holding of a boy and a girl, to conversations between business associates, to election campaigning, to the deployment of weapons systems by various nations. It is the quintessence of clinical work. A child wonders what we're up to at the same time that we attempt to understand that child.

DIMENSIONS OF THE COMMUNICATION PROCESS

There are three dimensions of communication that are fundamental in the process of sending and interpreting messages. They are concerned with how information is coded, whom it has meaning for, and what type of information is involved. We will consider each of these dimensions separately.

Discrete and Continuous Communication Systems

We use symbols to represent concepts. A number of different types of symbols occur. One dimension along which symbols vary is that between "discrete" and "continuous" symbol systems (Chafe 1970). In a discrete symbol system each symbol is separate and distinct from each other symbol. In a continuous symbol system there is constant variation between symbols, with each symbol grading into the next. An analogy will help in seeing the difference between the two. Assume that the lines in Figure 1 represent two paths up a hill. The one on the left has steps cut into it. The one on the right ascends the hill at a constant rate. The line on the left is analogous to a discrete symbol system. Each step is distinct from each other step. It is not possible to stand between steps, so you can tell where you are on the hill by noting which step you're on. The line on the right, on the other hand, is analogous to a continuous system. There are no separate steps, but rather, each point on the line grades into the next.

We communicate with both types of communication systems. Consider facial expressions. Everyone can recognize smiles and frowns, but suppose someone starts with a big smile and then slowly diminishes that

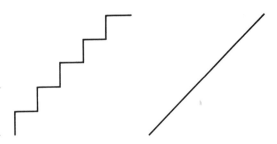

Figure 1.   Discrete and Continuous System

smile until there is no smile at all, but just a "straight face." At precisely what point did the person stop smiling? You cannot tell, because facial expression is a continuous system. The same is true of tone of voice, posture, and other means of nonverbal communication. On the other hand, consider the Morse code. Each letter in the alphabet is represented by a distinct combination of dots and dashes—a discrete system. Language is a fairly discrete communication system because we have no difficulty recognizing words as separate and distinct from each other, although, of course, the meanings they represent may not be entirely discrete.

Discursive and Nondiscursive Communication

A second dimension in which communication varies is the continuum between "discursive" and "nondiscursive" messages (Szasz 1961). As Szasz uses the term, discursiveness refers to communication in which the meanings of the symbols are shared knowledge among the communicators. The Morse code is discursive because each user of the code knows the proper combination of dots and dashes for each letter. Street signals are discursive because all drivers know what red, yellow, and green lights mean. A phone book is discursive because each name has a specific number, and anyone can look it up. To the extent that we agree on word meanings, language is discursive. Because of its shared meanings, discursive communication permits the exchange of knowledge.

In nondiscursive communication, on the other hand, the symbols do not have shared meanings among the communicators. They are idiosyncratic or presentational (Szasz 1961). There is no conventional agreement

about what the signs or symbols mean. Abstract art is a good example of nondiscursive communication. It has meaning, yes, but the meaning is specific to the painter and to each individual who views the work. Autistic behavior is often highly nondiscursive. It is idiosyncratic to the particular child. Words and gestures may be used, but not with their conventional communicative functions.

Discursive and nondiscursive communication are best seen on a continuum with most messages falling somewhere in between. Much communication with language is relatively discursive. When we attempt to make verbal communication precise, we are attempting to make it as discursive as possible. The General Semantics movement (Korzybski 1948; Johnson 1946; Hayakawa 1949) represents this goal nicely. On the other hand, language can be very nondiscursive, as in the work of certain poets. Similarly, nonverbal communication varies from discursive, as in the gestures of a policeman directing traffic, to nondiscursive, as in the movements of a modern dancer.

Linear Knowledge and Intuitive Information

The third dimension in communication is concerned with the types of information that may be communicated. Szasz (1961) makes a distinction between "knowledge" and "information." In his terms, knowledge can be presented by conventional, discursive symbols and is therefore publicly accessible. Information, on the other hand, cannot be represented directly with discursive symbols and consequently may not have this quality of public accessibility. Thus, for Szasz an abstract painting may be said to contain information but not knowledge. Its meaning cannot be represented adequately with discursive symbols such as words. Ornstein (1972) has made a similar distinction using terms such as linear, rational, and verbal-intellectual to describe knowledge, and intuitive, holistic, and arational to describe information. Examples of linear knowledge abound. The entire scientific and technological enterprise of our society depends on linear knowledge. Perhaps the best example of intuitive information, on the other hand, is meditational states. Typically, individuals who experience these states are literally unable to describe them with words and thus end up with nondescriptive statements such as "being at one with the universe."

Because the behavioral sciences have developed within our cultural emphasis on linear knowledge, they approach human behavior in just that way. The discussions of concepts and information processing in this book are good examples of this orientation. The essence of human relationships, however, is more likely to be intuitive than linear. A woman may say to a child, "I am your mother." This statement specifies their relationship in terms of linear knowledge. At a deeper level, however, their relationship contains fundamental aspects that cannot be adequately described with words because they are intuitive in nature. We cannot understand such a relationship entirely in linear terms, much as we would like to. Similarly, our experience of emotions is primarily intuitive rather than linear. Researchers attempt to understand emotions through linear means such as physiological studies of the organism during various emotional states and social learning theories. The actual experience of emotion, though, is more often described by poets.

You may have difficulty with the idea of intuitive information at first, because I have to present it linearly but you have to intuit it! Think of what it means to be close to a loved one or to experience a profound work of art or a strong emotion. These experiences are real and meaningful, but they cannot quite be put into words. They are examples of the intuitive side of consciousness. Notice also that the experience of intuitive information is not reserved for a few people with Great Powers. Rather, we all deal with intuitive information regularly, although this type of consciousness is not emphasized in our culture.

Summary

Let us review briefly. The three dimensions of communication may be represented as planes in a cube, as in Figure 2. Each dimension can vary somewhat from the others, although they're not entirely independent of one another. The interior of the cube may be seen as some sort of "message space." All human communication involves all three dimensions, so that any message can be placed somewhere in that space with respect to each dimension. A newspaper, for example, is discrete, discursive, and linear. A touch of hands between lovers is con-

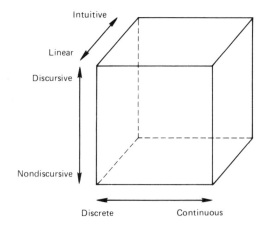

Figure 2.   Dimensions of Communication

tinuous, nondiscursive, and intuitive. Much communicative behavior contains complicated mixes among the three dimensions. An angry scolding delivered to a young child by a parent may be discrete in the words used but continuous in tone of voice, posture, and facial expression, with both verbal and nonverbal aspects of the message being fairly discursive and linear to the child. At the same time, the meaning of the incident in the relationship between parent and child may have both linear and intuitive elements.

An understanding of these three dimensions enlarges our perspective in approaching the language-disordered child. I began this chapter with the assertion that all behavior has message character. Now we have a better idea of what kinds of messages there are and why some messages are more difficult to understand than others. Halliday's (1973) behavior potential, mentioned in the preceding chapter, begins to take on shape. Our options for behaving vary along these same dimensions. Similarly, there is convergence among other ideas from previous chapters. Language is a set of options-to-mean (Halliday 1973). The meaning of an utterance rests in how it differentiates among the alternatives in the situation (Olson 1970b). The comprehension of language involves choosing among alternative interpretations for an utterance in a context. All of these factors operate together. The success of these processes in language use is largely dependent on the fact that language is discrete, discursive, and linear to a high degree. Further, in clinical work our major concern is communication. These three dimensions provide a structure for interpreting all behavior in terms of its message character so that we can focus on the communicative import of behavior in attempting to understand the language-disordered child as a communicator. I will return to this matter later in this chapter and elsewhere in this book.

NONVERBAL COMMUNICATION

In typical face-to-face communication, verbal language is not separate from nonverbal communication. The previous discussion provided some hints on the differences between verbal and nonverbal communication. Verbal language tends to be relatively discrete, discursive, and linear, while nonverbal communication is likely to be more continuous, nondiscursive, and intuitive. Both of these characterizations oversimplify and hence are not to be taken too literally. As Lyons (1977) states, there is no sharp distinction between verbal and nonverbal communication.

Levels of Nonverbal Communication

Let us now take a more explicit look at nonverbal communication. I will take nonverbal communication to mean both kinesics, that is, body movement, facial expression and posture, and what is sometimes referred to as paralanguage, that is, tone of voice, sighs, cries, laughs, and other productions of the vocal mechanism that are not specifically linguistic. Nonverbal communication ranges across all three of the dimensions described above, as does language, but its most frequent communicative functions are different from those of language. I will describe four categories of nonverbal communication, each shading into the next.

Conventional Gestures

All nonverbal behavior has a continuous quality to it. Nevertheless, some conventional gestures are so culturally stylized that they are recognized as representing discrete messages. In this category of nonverbal communication the messages are discursive and linear. In our culture, for example, we recognize the palm vertical, arm outstretched signal for "stop," the military salute, the child's wave "bye-bye," and other gestures. Similarly manual communication codes for the hearing impaired, such as American Sign Language and Exact English, are discrete, discursive, and linear. Indeed, they are designed specifically to function as languages.

Nonverbal Communication Accompanying Language

A second category of nonverbal communication is that which directly accompanies spoken language. Included here are gestures, vocal emphases, head nods, facial expressions, and the like. These behaviors appear to have two functions. First, they modify, amplify, and in other ways comment on the verbal message. Thus, important words are identified with tone of voice and gesture. The mood of an utterance is amplified with vocal quality, rate of speech, facial expression, and posture. Typically, these nonverbal messages do not contribute additional linear knowledge to that in the verbal message. Rather, they supply information about how to interpret the verbal message.

Scheflen (1974) has described additional types of nonverbal behavior that accompany verbal communication. Through body motions and shifts in posture we punctuate our discourse, marking when we have made a point and when we have finished a "paragraph." Again, the function is to comment on and structure the verbal message.

A second function of the behaviors in this category seems to be a "tuning in" between communicators. Condon and Ogston (1967) have shown that speakers coordinate small behaviors such as eye blinks precisely with their talking. It is striking that they found that listeners coordinate their eye blinks in the same way. That is, a listener blinks in exact coordination with the speaker's stream of speech. While such behavior is connected to language, it also has a relationship quality to it in a subtle identification with the speaker that is more intuitive in nature. Condon and Sander (1974) have demonstrated that even young babies coordinate their movements with the speech of their caretakers, demonstrating this same type of identification.

The behaviors in this second category, those that accompany spoken language, tend to be less discrete, discursive, and linear than those in the first category of conventional, culturally defined behaviors. In general, behavior in the second category aids in the interpretation of verbal messages. At times, however, it may lead to confusion about what was meant by a particular tone of voice or gesture. It may be added that it is impossible not to communicate in this way during verbal interaction. One must have some tone of voice, facial expression, and posture.

Nonverbal Communication Regulating Social Interaction

Scheflen (1972) also described a third category of nonverbal communication. This type of nonverbal communication is not directly related to verbal language. In interpersonal groupings people consistently use a set of gestures and postures to regulate their social interaction. By nonverbal means we include or exclude certain individuals from a conversation, censure an individual who has committed some sort of transgression, demonstrate alliances, and in other ways regulate the behavior of the people in a group. Thus, we orient our bodies toward each other, turn away from certain individuals, direct eye contact at various individuals, gesture toward each other, and so forth. Similarly, we hold young children's hands, help them with their clothing, point things out to them, and carry them around. Nonverbal signs in this category, then, function as messages about the relationships among the people in the interaction. It is, again, impossible not to transmit these signs. They are obviously continuous rather than discrete. It is difficult to assess the degree of discursiveness in these signs. Most people in a culture appear to use them in the same ways, which suggests a degree of discursiveness, but they are often used beyond awareness, or at least are not consciously thought of as messages, which gives them a nondiscursive quality. We tend to think of such behavior as related to each individual's internal state rather than as relationship communication. Finally, because of their relationship character, these messages tend to be more intuitive than linear.

Iconic Signs. Szasz (1961) has termed such nonverbal messages "iconic signs." The relationship between an iconic sign and what it refers to is one of similarity. That is, an iconic sign is somehow similar to what it means. Thus, if one is dejected, the shoulders sag, the face droops, and the tone of voice drops. These behaviors are similar to the state of being dejected and therefore are iconic signs. We indicate interest in other people at gatherings by such behaviors as

talking to them, orienting the body toward them, and looking and nodding at them. Again, the relationship between these behaviors and what they refer to is one of similarity and in this way they function as iconic signs. An iconic sign is different from a word because a word is a conventional symbol. The relationship between a word or conventional symbol and what it represents is purely arbitrary. There is nothing similar between the word *affection* and the state of receiving or giving affection. A hug, on the other hand, is somehow similar to affection and is thus an iconic sign.

As another illustration, recall the core concepts and their attendant functional relations discussed in Chapter 1. A child demonstrates functional relations by using objects appropriately. This behavior is interpreted as indicating that the child possesses the corresponding core concept. We can now see that we interpret such behavior as iconic signs of the core concept. Pouring with a pitcher is similar to the core concept of pitcher, whereas the association between the word *pitcher* and the concept is an arbitrary relationship. In the interpretation of core concepts, one might say that the clinician, rather than the child, is assigning meaning to the iconic sign. That is, the child may not be attempting to communicate, but the clinician is attempting to understand.

In addition, however, severely language-delayed children may rely primarily on iconic signs in their communicative efforts. I recall a boy, for example, who used to kiss everything he liked, such as favorite clinic materials, the clinician, candy, objects from home, and pictures of his family. A little girl I knew used to sit in the living room and whine repeatedly while pointing in a general direction. Her mother would try to guess what she wanted. While this child used iconic signs to get things, it is clear that relationship communication was involved as well. The child initiated and the mother complied.

To the extent that language-delayed children employ iconic signs in their attempts at communication, that communication may be qualitatively different from that involving language *per se*. They are using an iconic representational system rather than the arbitrary symbol system of language. Communication is likely to be difficult for them because of the nondiscursiveness of many of their iconic signs. Further, iconic signs do not lend themselves to the type of abstraction inherent in language.

Idiosyncratic Nonverbal Communication

Finally, Szasz (1961) has described a fourth category of nonverbal communication, which is related to emotional disturbance. He discusses psychiatric symptoms such as hysterical paralysis. In this situation there is paralysis without any apparent organic cause. Szasz interprets this type of behavior as communication using iconic signs, but these signs are exceedingly idiosyncratic and specific to the individual involved. Accordingly, they are not only intuitive but extremely nondiscursive as well. It is therefore impossible to interpret such messages through the linear logic of conventional symbols. Exactly the same difficulty occurs in attempting to understand autistic behaviors such as repetitive movements or self-destructive activity. Such iconic signs are truly nondiscursive.

Similarly, many of the behaviors exhibited by language-impaired children may be interpreted as iconic signs. Activities such as crying, laughing, resisting direction, throwing tantrums, smiling, and touching may be viewed in this way. The message character of such iconic signs is likely to be nondiscursive and intuitive. As we will see, it is often useful to interpret these signs as bearing information concerning the relationship between the child and the clinician or teacher.

Summary

Summarizing, I have built a case for viewing nonverbal behavior as communication about the content of linguistic utterances and about human relationships. The child's options-to-mean (Halliday 1973) range far beyond the use of language itself. This observation does not mean, however, that there is one monolithic communication system available to the child. I have argued that, in general, nonverbal communication is qualitatively different from linguistic communication. Language tends to be discrete and linear. Nonverbal communication is primarily continuous and intuitive. When the totality of human interactive behavior is viewed, discrete, linear, nonverbal communication such as conventional gestures and specific manual communication systems is the exception rather than the rule. While both linguistic and nonverbal communication vary in discursiveness, language is likely to be more discursive because of its linear, logical nature, while nonverbal communication is less likely to be discursive because of the emphasis on relationships and iconic signs. In the terms of the preceding chapter, the communicative functions and the classes of behavior that represent those functions are likely to be less precisely defined than the functions and classes of language itself. In short, language and nonverbal communication complement each other, but they do not parallel each other.

MULTIPLE-LEVEL COMMUNICATION

I have mentioned several times the intimate connection between communication and human relationships. Watzlawick, Beavin, and Jackson (1967) have asserted that communication defines relationships. The thrust of their argument is as follows. When you behave toward someone in some way (i.e., communicate) you are doing two things. First, you are transmitting whatever message your behavior might indicate, such as, "Hello," "I am your friend," "What time is it?" "May I have that?" and so on. Second, you are communicating the message that it is permissible to behave in that way (generate that kind of message) in the particular relationship involved. This second message is often implicit. For example, in lecturing to a class, I will sometimes make wisecracks. By making such remarks, and by laughing when class members make similar remarks, I send the message that it is acceptable to joke in that class. The class members send a similar message to me with their jokes and laughter. Through this behavior we determine that the relationship we have in the classroom is one that permits joking, but we never talk about joking. The example is trivial (unless the jokes are bad) but the point has far-reaching implications. Entailed in exchanging messages about any topic is communication about what is permissible in the particular relationship involved. We structure or define our relationships through communication. In fact, a relationship between individuals consists of the total communicative exchanges that have occurred between those individuals.

Content and Relationship Communication

In accordance with this view, Watzlawick, Beavin, and Jackson (1967) have posited two levels of communication. The content level contains what we would normally think of as the message: the meaning of the utterance. The relationship level contains a message about the relationship between the communicators. For example, in an exchange between Sara and Susie, Sara may say, "Don't bounce that ball." The content message of this communication is in the semantic meaning of the sentence. The relationship messages are in what that sentence implies about the relationship between Sara and Susie, in this case that commands and denial are permissible in their relationship and that Sara can be in charge. Susie will respond in some way. She might say, "All right," indicating that she accepts Sara's definition of the relationship. On the other hand, she might say, "I like to bounce this ball," in which case she indicates that she does not accept Sara's relationship message and thus proposes a different type of relationship.

Let us explore this example in more depth. First, content and relationship messages need not be the same. In the example the content message deals with bouncing a ball, but the relationship messages are concerned with what kinds of statements can be made and ultimately with who's in charge. Further, no intention to convey a relationship message need be present. The relationship message is inherent in the act of communicating. In addition, both children's nonverbal communication adds further information to the exchange in ways such as emphasizing particular words and indicating how strongly they feel about what they are saying. These iconic signs may add further relationship messages of their own.

Another area of consideration from the above example is that the definition of a relationship is reciprocal. Neither Sara nor Susie alone can specify their relationship. They each contribute equally to defining how they will behave toward each other. This reciprocity is always present in relationships, even in situations where a very "dominant" individual bullies a very "weak" individual. If the second individual does not submit, the relationship will be different. We are often unaware of this reciprocity because we tend to feel that we cause events to occur rather than seeing events as multiply determined. Teachers and clinicians may become aware of the reciprocity of relationships when they work with children who insist on doing things their own way.

Finally, relationships are defined over time. The relationship between Sara and Susie is not established in the above exchange. It is still being negotiated, particularly if Susie does not comply with Sara's directive. Relationships become established through many communicative exchanges. In addition, relationships must be defined in many different contexts. What Sara and Susie work out concerning ball playing may not apply at all when their parents are present or in other activities such as playing tag.

In terms of our earlier discussion, content messages tend to be discrete, linear, and discursive. We generate such communication specifically to transmit some message. Relationship communication, on the other hand, seems primarily continuous, intuitive, and iconic. We "act out" how we think a

relationship should be, partly through what is implied in the content message about the relationship, and partly through the iconic signs of nonverbal behavior. Obviously, relationship messages can be linear and discursive: *I am your president.* Here the topic of discourse is the relationship. Even in communication of this type, however, there are intuitive aspects accompanied by nonverbal iconic signs. Is the speaker telling the truth? Teasing? Asserting superior status over us?

The Believability of Relationship Communication

We come now to another difference between the content and relationship levels of communication. There is no truth or falsity to relationship messages in the way that there is in content messages. In principle at least, the premise of a content message may be determined to be true or false because of the discursiveness and linear logic of such messages. In relationship communication, however, the issue is not the degree of truth in the message but whether or not the recipient of the message believes that message (Szasz 1961). Suppose two people are in an interaction. The behavior of one person defines their relationship in a certain way. That definition cannot be evaluated in terms of any truth or falsity it contains, because it is not based on linear logic. Rather, it is based on the intuitive logic of human relations. The other person in the interaction can either accept or reject that definition.

Imagine a situation in which a small boy is disobeying his mother. She tells him to do things and he not only doesn't comply but also says, "Why should I?" The mother replies, "Because I'm your mother," using a forceful tone and generally acting sternly to place the child in a subordinate position under her authority. The veracity of her content message can be verified because it is based on linear logic, which in turn can be referred to biological fact. She is indeed his mother. Her relationship message is roughly, *I am one-up and you are one-down.* There is no truth inherent in this message itself. The child either accepts or does not accept the position of one-down. Anyone who works with children has encountered similar situations. I still sometimes fall into the trap of setting myself up as the one in charge, only to find that the children don't see me that way at all and in fact are going their merry ways without me. Trotting out my linear list of degrees doesn't help, either, because that kind of truth is irrelevant in this particular relationship. All that matters is whether or not the child is willing to let me be one-up. Most of this communication is iconic.

Interpreting Nonverbal Communication

Viewing relationship communication in this way provides a powerful means for interpreting certain kinds of behavior. Szasz (1961) suggests that behavior such as hysterical paralysis may be approached in terms of its relationship character rather than as being symptomatic of emotional disorder. Similarly, behavior in language-disordered children such as frequent crying, inattention, resisting direction, and in certain cases language delay itself may be viewed as relationship communication through iconic signs. Jackson (1967) has suggested that such behaviors may represent "real" states or feelings within the individual, or they may be relationship tactics. These two possibilities are present whether or not these behaviors are produced with conscious intent. Be it real or tactical,

however, an iconic sign such as crying always carries a relationship message. The clinician may interpret such behavior by attempting to determine what it means or how it functions in the relationship between client and clinician, rather than taking it as representing some internal state or emotion in the child.

Interpreting children's behavior in this way is appealing to me for three reasons. First, it keeps the focus on communication, which is our area of professional expertise. Second, all clinical work and teaching take place through human relationships. An understanding of the child's relationship communication should be helpful in this connection. Third, using language is itself a relationship act. It is helpful to view the child's language functioning in conjunction with other relationship communication. I do not wish to imply that interpreting behavior in terms of iconic signs and relationship functions will always be easy. It can be very difficult because of the nondiscursive iconic signs and intuitive information involved. Further, it may be argued that such interpretation is not necessary because we can focus directly on behavior *qua* behavior. In my opinion, however, meaning is at the heart of language and communication. Working with communication disorders without coming to grips with meaning in some way is similar to trying to fix a car without looking at the motor. As we will see in Chapter 11, looking at behavior in terms of its relationship functions permits one to verify one's interpretations to a fair degree and thus removes some of the onus of interpretation, as opposed to observation and description, of behavior. Suppose a child cries frequently during training sessions. The clinician might interpret this crying as a relationship message meaning that the child would like things done differently: Perhaps the child wants fewer direct demands to respond or would prefer a different type of activity. Either of these involve a change in the relationship between child and clinician. The clinician can verify this interpretation by altering the demands placed on the child and observing if there is a concomitant change in the crying. Again, the point is that the child's behavior is interpreted in terms of its communicative or interpersonal functions.[1]

Examples of Relationship Communication

Consider some other examples. A child is asked to do something but responds with "No!" Another child responds by crawling under the table. A third participates in the activity but with extremely fleeting attention span. We are used to thinking of these messages as representing the child's attitudes and skills: The child is unwilling or unable to participate in the activity. All three responses, however, can also be viewed as iconic relationship messages: The child wants a change in how the relationship is structured. It is noteworthy that the clinician's responses to these behaviors are likely to effect changes in the relationship, even though the clinician may be thinking only of dealing with the child's behavior. On a broad scale, the clinician has two choices. One is to make the activity more enticing, give the child a break, offer a distraction, or in some other way mollify the child's

resistance. All of these options may also be seen as relationship messages. Their effect is to change the relationship in the direction of allowing the child more control over what occurs. The clinician's other choice is to get the child to participate in the activity by getting tougher and more demanding, or getting out the heavy consequences. In this case the balance of the relationship has again changed; the clinician asserts more control than ever. In general, the relationship level of communication is always present, whether we take note of it or not.

Iconic relationship communication is not always as straightforward as in the above examples. I recall one child, a four-year-old boy with severe language delay. Our clinic included a group program for language-delayed youngsters that was conducted in a large nursery school room. The little boy in question would make use of the various play equipment in the room but usually independently of whatever the other children were doing. If the group was in the story corner, he would be off somewhere else. I found that I could move him around the room simply by changing my own position in the room. As soon as I got within about five feet of him, he would move. I could literally control him in the same way a cow pony runs a steer. If he moved in one direction, I could "head him off" or encourage him in that direction according to how I moved. I should note also that we were doing all this while sitting on the floor. Thus, if I wanted him to join the group of children at the story circle, I could get him there, but it took a few minutes. In effect, we did an almost dancelike series of movements around the room, all in slow motion, and always about five feet apart. I do not offer this example as a demonstration of how to manage children, and there was more to our clinical intervention than I have described. I

[1] The preceding example has much in common with contingency management. From my point of view contingency management is a particular type of communication that leads to a very structured and predictable relationship. It defines relationships in terms that are highly discrete, discursive, and directly based on linear logic. The uncertainties of interpreting relationships on an intuitive basis are minimized at least for the clinician. One can see obvious appeal in such an approach.

merely wish to illustrate the nebulous character of some relationship communication. Both my behavior and that of the child were extremely nondiscursive. Meaning there was, but of an intuitive nature that I never did comprehend. The child continued this type of performance for about the first month that he was in the group. He then became more social in his activity and never exhibited the behavior again.

Personality

Participation in relationships suggests the importance of personality. Following Ruesch and Bateson (1951), I will view personality as inseparable from communication. Ruesch (1951) provides an analogy that will be useful in this regard. Consider the relationship between a river and its banks. Through its constant flow the river forms its banks. But the banks channel the direction of flow. One literally cannot come into being or change without the other. So it is with personality and communication. Because the focus of this book is on language disorders and communication, I will view personality from its communicative side or its interpersonal aspects, rather than in terms of its characteristics within the person. Because of the possibility of verification mentioned above, and because of the influence of the relationship context on behavior, I will approach behavior as communication rather than as representing internal states. It has been argued by Ruesch and Bateson (1951) and Bateson (1972) that human behavior can only be understood by viewing it in context.

ONGOING RELATIONSHIPS

As mentioned earlier, a relationship becomes established through many exchanges in different situations. The result is the development of a set of metarules that govern what can occur in that relationship. These metarules develop through both explicit and implicit or iconic communication at the relationship level. It is a truism that we know such rules, but we may not be consciously aware of them unless they are violated. Consider the rules in American culture for riding on crowded elevators. First, stretch up, not out; don't touch your fellow elevator riders. Second, be careful where you place your eyes; watch either the neck in front of you or the lighted numbers above the door. Third, engage only in the most superficial conversation; stick to the weather or the latest sports event. You comply with these rules, but you aren't particularly aware of them unless someone leans on you or stares at you or asks you a personal question.

It must be stressed again that metarules about behavior in relationships develop as a result of reciprocal exchanges between the participants in a relationship. While there may be cultural determinants, such as those governing behavior in public places, ultimately the parties to a relationship develop their own set of metarules by living that relationship.

Metacommunication

Bateson (1972), Haley (1963), and Watzlawick, Beavin, and Jackson (1967) have referred to the process of establishing metarules through relationship messages as metacommunication, which means communication about communication. Since relationship messages establish what behavior can occur in a relationship, that is, what can be communicated, they are indeed communication about communication. The concept of metacommunication sets some messages at a higher level than other messages, just as in our discussion of metarules in Chapter 1. Grinder and Bandler (1976) have argued that there is no way to tell *a priori* which messages are meta to other messages. For example, suppose an adult says, *I hate you*, but with voice and expression marked with warmth and affection. The metamessage is concerned with the relationship. Which one is it? We encounter the same situation with a small child who expresses intense anger at an adult but does not break away from a hug by that adult. Grinder and Bandler conclude that examples such as this vitiate the power of the concept of metacommunication. As I see it, the difficulty here is with the meaning of relationship messages. As stated in the previous section, they are not true or false. Their meaning is in how they function in the relationship. Consequently, the question of which message is the metamessage becomes irrelevant. In situations such as the preceding examples, in which there are contradictory messages present, the receiver has a number of options, including accepting either message, neither message, or responding with another double message.[2] The important point is that whatever confusion may exist concerning which messages are meta to which other messages, relationship communication is certainly present in any exchange, albeit not always easy to interpret. Normally, any such confusions that are important are clarified by the communicators as the interaction continues.

Patterns of Relating

Over time, then, the participants in a relationship develop consistent patterns of behavior toward each other. We may think

[2] The idea of simultaneous messages that are either contradictory or even paradoxical is related to the double bind theory of disturbed communication. (Bateson 1972; Sluzki and Verón 1971).

of these patterns as a set of metarules that evolve from the continuing metacommunication that is inherent in interaction. Some examples will be helpful. Some children in clinic demonstrate what is often referred to as "separation anxiety." They become very upset when taken into a room away from their parents. A common behavioral treatment for this situation is to apply a form of extinction. Keep the child in the room, crying and all. After a few sessions the crying will extinguish and the child will participate in clinical activities. Typically, very appealing activities are offered concurrently with the extinction procedure. I used this approach with one three-year-old language-delayed girl, but with little success. She would hang on the doorknob and cry for sixty minutes straight. When I left the room (there were other clinicians present) to talk to her mother, the mother was visibly upset, hands shaking like the proverbial leaf. Who had the separation anxiety? One can argue that the mother was upset just because the child was upset, but that's just the point. Over time and through many different types of communication, they had developed an intense closeness in their relationship, which our clinical procedure had abruptly violated. When they were reunited, each comforted the other through various iconic relationship messages such as hugging and patting.

Another child in a similar situation cried so violently that we decided to forgo the extinction procedure and permit the mother in the clinic room. This was the nursery school room mentioned earlier. The child, this one a five-year-old boy, would participate in any activity we offered, but only if his mother remained within two or three feet of him. He would turn frequently to his mother and smile or gesture at her. She would respond warmly, running her fingers through his hair and making other affectionate gestures.

Again, this pattern of "bonding" through iconic messages had a long history, resulting in a shared metarule that made separation very difficult for them.

Ultimately, an individual's behavior is often predictable in terms of the relationship roles that are being played. Consider your own behavior at a social gathering. Your options are largely spelled out for you by the metarules for that type of situation, and you will behave in predictable ways regardless of personality factors and your wishes of the moment. Communicative behavior is a product not only of the individual's internal states, it is heavily influenced by the social networks in which that individual functions as well. This point is often overlooked in considering language-disordered children, particularly those with language delay. As has been illustrated, a richer understanding of such children can be obtained by viewing them as participants in the social networks of their families.

The Family System

The family system is an example of enduring relationships in which a complicated and extremely subtle set of metarules develops. As with other relationships, family members are consciously aware of some of these metarules, such as "Don't shout at the dinner table." Other metarules, and the patterns they represent, seem to function beyond the awareness of the family members. Families develop styles of relating, including language use. Some areas are discussed openly, others are broached only implicitly. Family members develop systematic ways of influencing each other. Many patterns of family interaction have been described by scholars in fields such as behavior modification, anthropology, and general systems theory. Again, these patterns are not possible without the compliance and participation, whether consciously or not, of all family members involved. We will explore the area of family interaction in Chapter 12. For the present, the point is that each family operates in ways that can be described with a set of rule hierarchies. Indeed, the consistency of family relationships is so fundamental that it is the cornerstone of most work in family theory and therapy. Child development, including language development, cannot be separated from the family system.

Mechanisms of Change

I have been emphasizing the consistency and self-maintaining qualities of relationships. In view of the strong tendencies in these directions, one may wonder how change can occur at all. We can view participation in relationships as another class of problem-solving tasks. Consequently, one typically has several options for behavior in a relationship, some specified by the metarules of that relationship and others outside or counter to those metarules. Thus, one always has the potential of behaving in ways that will produce change. Hence, change may stem from individual problem solving and decision making, although it has relationship consequences. Children may be seen effecting such change as they explore the options available to them in the family. Further change in the child occurs through maturation and the development of new skills and orientations.

Change in an individual may also occur through relationship processes. As has already been discussed, relationships are mutually determined. If one participant in a relationship changes, others are likely to change, too, because the relationship is now different. Consequently, changing the behavior of a parent of a language-disordered child may be as effective as working directly with the child in some cases. Similarly, the clinician may establish a relationship with a child that is different from the child's other relationships, thus causing the child to behave differently. Further, any individual is involved in a network of relationships, many of them interlocking and overlapping. This situation increases the behavioral options available to the individual.

Thus, a person may change through individual problem solving or maturation or as a result of change in other individuals. Two points are important here. First, the tendency in human relationships is toward consistency rather than frequent change. In fact, parties to a relationship may well resist change in that relationship (Haley 1963). Second, change in an individual always affects that person's network of relationships. As children mature, for example, they are treated differently. In other words, the family changes, too, and consequently the stimuli the child now receives from the family are different from those received previously. Because of this reciprocity, questions of the direction of influence in a relationship often become moot. Is the child influencing the parents or are the parents influencing the child? As we will see in the next chapter, the answer to both questions is yes.

Summary

Summarizing this section, human relationships are reciprocal and self-maintaining. Through communicative exchanges, participants in a relationship develop a set of metarules that governs their behavior in that relationship. These metarules can become remarkably subtle and powerful in enduring relationships, such as those in families. Change in a child's behavior, including use of language, is always related to change in that child's relationships. The variety of possibilities for change discussed above expands and enriches the clinician's options for intervention. At the same time, the tendency toward consistency suggests that change in relationships is not always easily obtained.

THE LARGER SOCIAL SYSTEM

Human relationships are also defined and maintained at larger levels in the social system. Every culture works out consistent ways for people to interact with each other. There are accepted conventions for approaching the young and the elderly, minority groups, powerful individuals, disabled individuals, and so on, as well as ways to deal with other people in general. All of these conventions have relationship aspects to them. Some are formally specified in a culture, as in traffic regulations, social legislation, and procedures for selecting political leaders. Many are informal, such as conventions governing interpersonal behavior in social gatherings.

Within a society, subcultures are also defined in terms of consistent aspects of their behavior. While all share many features of the dominant culture, each differs from the others in special ways. Indeed, it is on the basis of these differences that groups are defined as subcultures. Such groups may have a common identity related to ethnic background, religion, geography, or other factors. As with interpersonal relations, each group is maintained through reciprocal influences among its members.

Language use, along with other behavior, is regulated by these cultural processes. At the same time, language is a major means of social identification. There is a reciprocal relation between language and culture, then. A cultural group dictates specific aspects of language use; conversely, individuals are identified as members of that group because they demonstrate those aspects of language (and other characteristics as well). The resultant picture is one of language variation governed by relationship factors, including relations within and between social groups.

Dale (1976) describes two general kinds of language variation. First, there is variation in association with cultural identity. Members of a social group tend to talk alike. Important here are both dialect and bilingualism. Second, there is variation related to specific talking situations, usually referred to as style. Thus, we shift back and forth between formal and informal styles, depending on what is appropriate at the moment. The social code decisions discussed in the preceding chapter exemplify this level of variation.

Dialect

A distinction is often made between dialects based on social stratification or identification and those associated with geographical areas. (Williams and Wolfram 1977; Dale 1976). Bolinger (1975), however, begins with the more general notion of a speech community. Whenever a group of people have some basis for common identity, they form a speech community. That basis may be geographical, as in the dialects of New England or east Texas, or it may be based on social and ethnic identification, as with the English spoken by ghetto blacks. Other speech communities center around less global aspects of people's lives, such as membership in a particular occupation or special-interest group. Individuals shift their styles of talking as they interact inside and outside these groups during their daily lives. Thus, variation in language use ranges from large scale social patterns, such as southern dialect, to specialized instances, such as the professional vocabulary of physicians. The difference between dialect and style is a matter of degree, but generally a dialect marks a person's life in more pervasive fashion than does a particular style. There are many people who speak only one dialect, but as Labov (1972b) notes, there are no single-style speakers.

Returning to social relationships, some aspects of linguistic variation are more acceptable in our culture than others. Moulton (1970) cites several examples. We can accept either different vowels or the same vowel in contrasts such as *Mary/merry/marry, either/either, cot/caught,* or *pin/pen.* On the other hand, we do not accept alternations such as *tank* for *thank* or *den* for *then.* Similarly, many people will accept alternations such as *I shall/I will* or *It is I/It is me,* but not such variants as *he done it* or *it don't matter.*

Members of the dominant culture in the United States tend to agree on such judgments. The result is a prestige dialect of American English. As McDavid puts it, "[there is] . . . widespread acceptance of the assumption that there is a standard variety of the language which for various reasons has become a model of usage" (1970, p. 85). This dialect takes on prestige because it is used by the more influential members of our culture, those who are better educated or more affluent. It is used in writing and in the broadcast media and is taught in the schools. Williams and Wolfram (1977) point out that all cultures recognize prestige dialects. The problem is that in comparison to the standard, other dialects are viewed as less acceptable. This lack of acceptance is not merely linguistic; it is related to value judgments about ethnicity, social class, educational level, and so forth. Just as in interpersonal relations, language is part and parcel of the relations among larger social groups.

Some writers suggest that Standard English is understood by all speakers of American English (Bolinger 1975; K. Johnson 1970). In a general way this notion is probably true, given the amorphous nature of comprehension as described in Chapter 3. As we will see in Chapter 9, however, expression requires much more precise control of all levels of language; thus, most people are fluent speakers of only one dialect of English. Regardless of their understanding, then, people are marked by the dialect through which they express themselves.

Bilingualism

Bilingualism means the use of more than one language in an individual's daily living. An American who studies German for four years but never lives in Germany would be considered as knowing a foreign language. A bilingual, on the other hand, functions regularly in the speech communities of both languages. Each language allows that individual to participate in certain types of cultural relationships, although, of course, those cultures may overlap. Just as with dialects, bilingualism is a social phenomenon, not merely a linguistic matter. Further, bilinguals are subject to the same judgments that nonstandard dialect speakers are in relation to ethnicity and social class.

There are many factors involved in bilingualism. First, there is the degree of skill in each language a speaker may have. These skills might be different for comprehension and expression. Second, there is the degree of similarity or contrast between the lan-

guages. Third, different bilinguals will demonstrate different patterns of use: One language may be used at home, the other at school; one language may be used in relaxed conversation, the other during emotional exchanges (Turner 1973). Again, both languages may be mixed in conversations and even in individual sentences (Gonzales 1975). Further, in some cases a "pidgin," or "mixed language" develops, incorporating aspects of both languages. Finally, there are the values that individuals hold about bilingualism and about the two languages involved in any particular case. These values may vary for children, parents, teachers, language clinicians, whole communities, and even governments.

There has been considerable research into the cognitive strategies employed by bilinguals and heated debate about whether bilingualism is an advantage or a disadvantage for schoolchildren. Given the individual differences in cognitive strategies illustrated in Chapters 2 and 3, and the complexities of bilingualism listed above, there does not appear to be a single answer to this question. Rather, we will have to approach each bilingual child separately.

The Peer Group

All the language variation discussed above, both dialectal and bilingual, has a common core in human relationships. There is a reciprocity between the metarules for a social group or speech community and each individual's tendency to behave in ways that evidence identification with that group. Language and culture go hand in hand. This situation has important implications for language acquisition and for intervention with language-impaired children. Children begin learning language in the family, but in almost every detail they end up using the dialect of their peers rather than that of their parents. Labov (1969) suggests that the native dialect develops roughly between four and thirteen years of age. A first grader has not yet fully developed the native dialect. It is particularly in the fourth and fifth grades that the peer group becomes the major influence in teaching and enforcing the native dialect. Indeed, ". . . the most consistent and regular linguistic system of a speech community is that of the basic vernacular learned before puberty" (Labov 1969, p. 35).

Going a step further, schoolchildren may be seen as a subculture of their own. From this point of view, Opie and Opie (1959) emphasized the fundamental importance of language in children's peer relations. Not only are there word games and favored vocabulary items, but children organize their social relationships through what Opie and Opie call oral legislation. Ownership, taking turns, fighting, winning and losing, trust, and friendship itself are regulated through expressions that are accepted and standardized in the oral tradition of each group of children. Younger children define aspects of relationships through utterances such as *Cross my heart and hope to die, Eeny meeny miny moe, Say "Uncle,"* and *Finders keepers, losers weepers.* Older children use more sophisticated combinations of word games and relationship negotiation such as the banter of black teenagers described by Labov (1972a). Truly, the talking of schoolchildren is a speech community of its own. It is inseparable from the subculture of childhood.

Socioeconomic Factors

Numerous studies have demonstrated that socioeconomic status affects child development. Many of these studies focused on academic skills. In general, children from lower economic groups have been found to have more difficulty with academic learning than children from the middle class. Much of this work emphasizes language. It has been hypothesized, for example, that lower-class individuals emphasize a restricted form of communication that does not encourage the elaboration of thought so important in the classroom (Bernstein 1973). A number of studies have focused on the language skills of lower-class black children. While some studies suggested that these children demonstrate poor language skills (for example, Raph 1965; Deutsch 1965), other authors argue vigorously that these findings result from subcultural differences in language use, rather than from any deficiencies in the area of language (Baratz 1968; Labov 1969, 1972a). I will not review this extensive literature other than to make two general conclusions. First, there is ample evidence that children from economically deprived backgrounds tend to do poorly in schoolwork, including language-related skills. Second, there is also convincing evidence that many children, especially those talking in nonstandard ways, evidence quite different language skills outside of school than they do in the classroom.

Summary

We have looked at different kinds of cultural variation. Bilingualism and dialect are associated with various subcultures within American society. Childhood is a subculture that crosses with these other subcultures. Poverty interacts with all three. The result is extremely complicated patterns of language use in the United States, including its public schools. Dialect and bilingualism are inseparable from cultural identities and values. At the level of culture as well as that of individual interactions, language use involves relationship factors.

Selection of a dialect or language, then, is likely to be more intuitive than linear.

Let me finish this section with three general conclusions. First, work with bilingual and nonstandard dialectal children will have to be based on something other than the perspective of language disorders. Dialects and bilingualism are not pathologies to cure. Second, in cases where language disorders are suspected, there are special challenges in the assessment of culturally different children. One must be sure that the children's skills are being sampled fairly and, especially, one must be able to sort difference from disorder. Third, attempts to change language patterns related to cultural differences in children are likely to be difficult. These patterns are maintained by reciprocal patterns of relationships. Further, these relationship patterns are primarily based on intuitive values and identifications, while our interventions are based on linear logic. Finally, we will be trying to alter children's language habits at precisely the time when peer pressure and identification are building to a peak. We will have to surmount some mighty metarules to change these habits. I will return to these matters in succeeding chapters.

CONCLUSIONS

In the view I have developed in this chapter, the behavior of each individual in a relationship is determined by a set of metarules that govern that relationship. Talking and responding to other people's talking are obviously examples of behavior. Therefore, language use is determined partially by the metarules of relationships, as well as by cognitive and linguistic factors. At the same time, language and other forms of communication are the means by which relation-ships are established and maintained. Hence, use of language and participation in human relationships are reciprocal and inseparable. A family with a two-year-old child establishes a relationship in which the child is learning language and consequently will make errors, and the older members of the family will accommodate those errors and help the child. If the child is language-delayed, that relationship will be one in which the child does little talking, but the family still communicates. Similarly, a child who talks more in some situations than in others usually does so for relationship rather than linguistic or cognitive reasons. The metarules in all of these relationships are established over time through various means of communication.

In addition, a major portion of the ecological validity that language has for children and adults rests in its use in human relationships. I would argue, then, that the most powerful intervention strategies for working with language-disordered children will be those that help the child develop language in relationship contexts, rather than as a purely linguistic skill. Consideration of how a child functions in relationships with the clinician and certain other individuals, such as family members or peers, is important because the child can only learn language and generalize from that learning in the context of those relationships. Consequently, I will touch on this topic at various places in the book and present an extended discussion in Chapters 11 and 12.

Nonverbal communication is relevant in this perspective because of its function in relationship communication. In conjunction with aspects of the clinician's behavior, the child's behavior is instrumental in structuring the clinical relationship in various ways. This relationship communication will include both verbal and nonverbal messages, but the assumption is that much of it will involve nonverbal behavior. It may be difficult to assign meanings to such behaviors because of their iconic nature and because much relationship communication is implicit rather than explicit. The clinician can, however, study the effects of the child's behavior in the relationship and thus attempt to determine its relationship function. This information can be used in developing intervention strategies and in working with parents. We expand our understanding of the child by interpreting all behavior as having communicative import.

Finally, all that has been said about individual relationships has parallels at higher cultural levels. Bilingualism and the use of nonstandard dialects are social phenomena,

not merely linguistic patterns. Similarly, as we approach school-aged children, we must remember that their communicative behavior is heavily influenced by the peer culture.

In the first five chapters of this book we have been concerned with a number of factors that are of importance in language use. We have looked at concepts and rules, information processing and perception, language structure and meaning, and communication and human relationships. While each area is significant in its own right, we have seen that language development depends on the relationships among these areas. With this view as a background, let us move now to a more direct consideration of the causal factors in children's language disorders.

6

CAUSATION AND CHILDREN'S LANGUAGE DISORDERS

If something goes wrong, it's natural to ask why. If the car won't start, you start looking for causes. Out of gas? Battery dead? If a child develops red blotches and a high fever, the physician likewise looks for causes. Similarly, if a child demonstrates impairments in the use of language, we wonder why. If we could understand the cause, we would be closer to understanding the child and the disorder. At the same time, the search for causal factors in children's language disorders has been frustratingly difficult. Generally speaking, these factors have proven to be extremely illusive. Further, this search has generated some controversy. Some feel that identification of etiology or at least the development of reasonable hypotheses about etiology must guide work with any individual child. Others are of the opinion that etiological information is largely irrelevant; what matters is dealing with the child in the here and now.

We will begin our search for causal factors by looking at how the question of causation has been studied. We will encounter some possible causal factors along the way. We will then consider some theoretical models of causation in developmental disorders, with an eye toward establishing a useful framework for our search. We will see that causation doesn't derive only from a set of factors; it is a complex process. From this perspective we will explore the matter of causation in children's language disorders, and make some conclusions about the relations between causation and intervention.

STUDYING CAUSATION IN DEVELOPMENTAL DISORDERS

Two major experimental designs have been employed in the search for etiological factors related to children's language disorders and many other conditions appearing in childhood. We will consider each of these designs separately. My discussion is based on the work of Sameroff and Chandler (1975). They did not focus specifically on children's language disorders, but rather on the causation of developmental pathology in more general terms.

Retrospective Studies

One approach to studying the causation of developmental disorders is through retrospective studies (Sameroff and Chandler 1975). In these studies children who demonstrate various developmental pathologies are identified. The researcher then examines these children's early medical records for information about pregnancy, birth conditions, and other factors. The studies are thus retrospective in that they look backward in time. The child now has a disability; what early factors could have caused it?

Through many studies of this type, four general factors have been identified (Sameroff and Chandler 1975). The first is anoxia, in which the infant is deprived of oxygen for a period of time. For example, an infant may not spontaneously begin to breathe at birth. The second is prematurity, in which the birth occurs before full term. Prematurity is often associated with low birth weight as well. The third is delivery complications, such as the use of instruments. The fourth factor is social conditions, such as the socioeconomic and ethnic status of the parents.

Each of these four factors has been considered as putting the baby at risk of suffering a developmental disorder of some sort. Again, they were identified by searching the early records of numbers of children with developmental impairments. Thus, the studies concentrate on disordered children. One could also concentrate on the high-risk conditions themselves, asking whether all babies whose births are associated with these conditions eventually demonstrate developmental disabilities. Research of this nature falls into the second type of experimental design used in studying the causation of developmental disorders.

Prospective Studies

In a prospective study infants demonstrating some high-risk factor are followed over time to see if, indeed, any developmental pathology does appear. These studies are difficult to do because the children must be followed for a number of years, say, up to age seven or ten. Some studies are done in just this way, by identifying children at birth and then evaluating them periodically for a number of years. In other studies birth records from a certain year in the past are screened. High-risk children are identified on the basis of these records. The children are then tracked down across the intervening years and their current status is assessed. A prospective study is thus a predictive one: Does the presence of a high-risk factor at birth predict later pathology?

Sameroff and Chandler's conclusion is significant: None of the four high-risk factors identified through retrospective studies functions as an efficient predictor in prospective studies. The presence of a high-risk factor during pregnancy or birth does not necessarily mean that the child will end up developmentally disabled. Consider longitudinal studies of anoxic infants. These babies do poorly on newborn measures. They still show effects at age three, but by seven years of age they show few differences from normal children in control groups. Similarly, prematurity and birth complications do not predict developmental disorders, although a number of studies have found that children with histories of low birth weight tend to be slightly depressed in IQ. They are still within the normal range, however.

There are contradictions in the literature on this subject. Some follow-up studies of children born with high-risk conditions report significant differences between those children and normal controls. Others report no such differences. Taub, Goldstein, and Caputo (1977) suggest a useful perspective on this problem. In studying children who were born prematurely, they found that these children did not catch up completely with normal children, but they did perform within normal limits for their age groups. Whether they were "different" from normal children, then, depends on how you interpret the data. Using statistical tests with groups of children, one could demonstrate significant differences. On the other hand, the at-risk children were performing within the normal range.

Of the four high-risk factors, the most powerful predictor (but still not a truly efficient predictor) is social conditions. Pasamanick, Knobloch, and Lilienfeld (1956) found that the percentages of babies having some birth complication varied dramatically with socioeconomic and ethnic status. Five percent of the babies of white upper-class parents demonstrated a complication at birth. For white lower-class parents it was 15 percent. For all nonwhites, 51 percent.

Other studies also emphasize the importance of environmental factors. One of the most illuminating is that of Werner, Bierman, and French (1971). These authors studied all the children born during one year on the island of Kauai in Hawaii. These children came from a wide mix of ethnic and socioeconomic groups. The results of the study indicated that complications at birth were not related to later developmental problems unless they were associated with poor environmental conditions. Further, when good prenatal care was available, the effects of socioeconomic differences decreased markedly.

The point here has not been to argue that there are no precipitating factors for developmental disorders. Rather, I wish to illustrate that the causation of these disorders is complex. Sameroff and Chandler conclude that, in large groups of children, the high-risk factors are generally not associated with incidences of developmental disorders very different from those in the normal population. When the factors identified as high risk in retrospective studies are tested through prospective studies, they lose their potency. Further, these factors may interact with each other, as found in the Hawaii study, in which certain medical factors were only important in conjunction with certain social factors. Of the four factors the social environment holds the most power as a predictor. With this information as background, let us now consider some theoretical models of causation.

MODELS OF CAUSATION

The conclusion from the previous sections is as follows: If you investigate the early history of a language-disordered child, you may be able to identify factors that could have caused the disorder, but if you follow up on children who show those factors as babies, they may not develop language disorders. How can we deal with this seeming contradiction? One thing we can do is to back off a bit and look at the whole idea of causation. What do we mean by cause? How does an etiological factor operate? Sameroff (1975; Sameroff and Chandler 1975) de-

scribed three different views of the process of causation.

The Linear Cause-and-Effect Model

In this model there is a direct, one-to-one relationship between cause and effect. For each effect there is a cause; for each cause there is a resulting effect. The logic is straightforward and appealing, and indeed very useful. If you have a flat tire (effect), you look for a puncture or other source of air leakage (cause). The term "linear" emphasizes the direct connection between cause and effect.

In the behavioral disciplines this view is often called the medical model, because it is an approach to cause-and-effect relationships that underlies a great deal of work in medicine. In diagnosis the physician deduces from the effects, that is, the patient's symptoms, just what disease condition has caused those effects. This model has been very successful in medicine in such great discoveries as that a particular mosquito carries malaria and that typhus is carried by bacteria in water. The linear cause-and-effect model is also important in the physician's daily activity in identifying everything from measles to ulcers.

In describing the linear cause-and-effect model, Sameroff (1975) illustrates another distinction in thinking about causation. This distinction has been with us for centuries. It concerns the relative importance of nature and nurture. The question is of great importance in considering developmental disorders and human behavior in general. How much of each individual's functioning can be explained in terms of neurophysical makeup and genetic endowment, and how much in terms of environmental influences and learning? The linear cause-and-effect model can be applied either way. Let us look at each of these possibilities briefly.

Causation within the Child

Figure 3 diagrams a linear cause-and-effect model that places the causes within the individual's constitution. We will use the term "constitution" here to refer to the child's neurophysical makeup and genetic endowment. The words "good" and "bad" inside the boxes refer to predicted outcomes. Note that the outcome reflects the status of the child's constitution, regardless of the environment.

We can think of causal factors in the child's constitution at two levels. The first comprises those constitutional processes that lead to developmental disorder in the first place. Heredity is important here. There are a number of genetic disorders that can affect language development, particularly as they relate to sensory and intellectual development. Reed (1975) gives an excellent discussion of genetic factors in developmental disorders. Mysak (1976) presents descriptions of many such syndromes. In addition to genetic factors, various disease conditions such as meningitis, may have significant constitutional effects. Also included at this level of constitutional processes would be the first three high-risk factors described earlier. In fact, the search for such factors is in large measure inseparable from the linear cause-and-effect model.

A second level of constitutional factors would include the conditions and syndromes that are associated with the first level. Important here are sensory disorders such as hearing and visual impairments, and cerebral disorders such as retardation and brain damage. These two levels are often considered together, as in a preschooler with poor language skill that is related to a hearing impairment caused by a genetic defect. Again, a child in first grade may have a language disorder associated with an aphasic condition resulting from traumatic injury to the brain. One sees the aptness of the term medical model in viewing the causation of disorders such as these. Indeed, it is well established that various genetic and medical factors are associated with language impairments. Let us now consider a second view of the linear cause-and-effect model, this time emphasizing the environment.

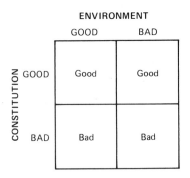

ENVIRONMENT

Figure 3. Linear cause-and-effect model emphasizing constitutional factors.
(Adapted from Arnold Sameroff, Early influences on development: fact or fancy? *Merrill-Palmer Quarterly*, 21 (1975), p. 282.)

Causation in the Environment

From a nurturist point of view, the linear cause-and-effect model would appear as in Figure 4. Notice that the outcome now depends on the quality of the environment, whatever the child's constitution might be. The assumption that environmental factors can influence children's language development is central, although often implicit, in clinical work and teaching. Any intervention is a change in the child's environment. Just as cases of severe retardation due to genetic anomalies support a constitutional view of cause and effect, so dramatic cases of en-

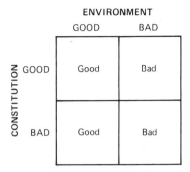

ENVIRONMENT

	GOOD	BAD
GOOD	Good	Bad
BAD	Good	Bad

CONSTITUTION

Figure 4. Linear cause-and-effect model emphasizing environmental factors. (Adapted from Arnold Sameroff, Early influences on development: fact or fancy? *Merrill-Palmer Quarterly,* 21 (1975), p. 282.)

vironmental deprivation support an environmental view. A girl named Genie (Curtiss 1977) is a case in point. Until the age of thirteen this child was confined to a small room with minimal human contact, and much of that apparently punitive. When the child was discovered, she was severely impaired in all areas of development, including language. It can be seen that the fourth high-risk factor, social conditions, fits well with an environmental view of linear cause and effect. The social environment can be characterized in various ways. We will concentrate on relatively large social environments first and then turn to the family environment.

The Sociocultural Environment. Bronfenbrenner (1975) presented some remarkable data on the effects of the community in which a child is raised. His technique was to compare the IQs of identical twins who were raised in separate environments. Because of the genetic similarity of identical twins, it would be expected that their IQs would remain similar, even when raised in different communities. Indeed, Bronfenbrenner notes that the IQs of identical twins who are raised in separate environments are more highly

correlated than those of fraternal twins who are raised in the same home. Let us look, however, at what happens when identical twins are separated and raised in different environments.

One group of thirty-five pairs of separated twins was tested with the Stanford-Binet, an IQ test that emphasizes language skill. The correlation of the IQs of twins who were separated but raised in the same town was .83. For those twins who grew up in different towns it was .67. Another group contained thirty-eight pairs of identical twins. Their IQ testing included both verbal and nonverbal performance. The correlation between the IQs of separated twins who were attending the same school was .87. With the twins brought up in different towns it was .66. Bronfenbrenner then reanalyzed the data on this second group according to the type of community in which each child was raised. Communities were classified according to size and economic base, such as industrial, agricultural, or mining. The correlation was .86 between the IQs of twins who were separated but living in similar communities. The correlation between those being raised in communities that differed from each other was only .26! Clearly, the environment has differential effects on the development of intelligence, even in identical twins. This finding is important in its own right but is also noteworthy because of the close relationship in our culture between measures of intelligence and language skill.

The Caretaking Environment. Perhaps the most dramatic demonstration of the power of the caretaking environment is in the work of Skeels (Skeels, Updegraff, Wellman, and Williams 1938; Skeels and Dye 1939; Skeels 1966). In the late thirties Skeels began a study of a group of twenty-six retarded children in a state orphanage.

The average IQ of the children and of their mothers was about 70. When the children were two, he placed thirteen of them in another state institution, in a ward of retarded women. The women acted as surrogate mothers for the children. In addition, nursery school facilities were provided for the children. About a year and a half later, these children's IQs had increased by an average of 28 points, while the children remaining in the orphanage had suffered a decrease averaging 26 points. The children who had received surrogate mothering had improved enough to be eligible for adoption, and all were placed in adoptive homes. During the sixties, Skeels (1966) tracked down each of the twenty-six children. Of those who had remained in the orphanage, all were still institutionalized except one who had died. In the adopted group every one was now self-supporting. Most had finished high school and four had attended some college.

We may have some reservations about Bronfenbrenner's findings and Skeels's early results. These results are based on IQ scores, which may be somewhat superficial at any age, but in particular are not valid with very young children (Lewis and McGurk 1972). The later outcomes of the Skeels study, however, are not open to such question. Through the surrogate mothering the children did become competent enough for adoption and, in their adoptive families, they ultimately became productive adults.

So far I have selected examples in which environmental influences were fairly dramatic. I will conclude this section with a different type of study, illustrating that relatively small changes in the environment can also have significant effects on child development. Whitehurst, Novak, and Zorn (1972) observed a language-delayed boy and his mother together and then altered the mother's behavior. The child had some comprehension but virtually no expressive language. These investigators found that small changes in how the mother talked resulted in large increases in the number of words the child used expressively. An increase in prompts (models of utterances for the child to say) from 1 percent to 7 percent of the mother's interaction with the child was accompanied by the use of roughly three new words by the child during each observation period. An increase in general conversational remarks from 45 percent to 61 percent achieved a similar result in the child's talking. These relatively small changes in the mother's behavior altered the child's behavior from using virtually no expressive language to uttering many dozens of words.

In conclusion, the environment is indeed a powerful influence on children's development at all levels, from social status and communities, to caretaking arrangements, to individual families and parenting styles. We will make considerable use of this fact as we go along.

Summary

Summarizing so far, I have illustrated two applications of the linear cause-and-effect model, one emphasizing the child's constitution and the other the environment. With either view I do not mean to suggest that people consciously adopt this model and then set about explaining various human conditions with it. Rather, the model is simply an abstraction to represent one way to view causation, and a very common one at that. Many people tend to think this way. I have encountered numerous parents who are looking for *the cause* for their child's difficulty with language. Similarly, many professionals concentrate on specific etiologies, both in research and in intervention.

A moment's thought reveals a severe shortcoming in either view of the linear cause-and-effect model, however. The locus of causation for any one child is neither in constitutional factors nor in the environment. It seems more reasonable to say that children's development depends on both. We move now to Sameroff's second model of causation.

The Interactional Model

Figure 5 illustrates the interactional model of causation. Observe that the outcome is now influenced by both sets of factors. The child's development results from the interaction between constitution and environment, as the name of the model suggests. This model makes more sense than the linear cause-and-effect model because it is more comprehensive. It explains the findings of the Hawaii study mentioned earlier, in which complications at birth were only predictive of developmental disorder when accompanied by certain socioeconomic variables. A child who is premature and then does not receive adequate medical care because the family is both rural and poor is at a higher risk than a child suffering only one of those conditions.

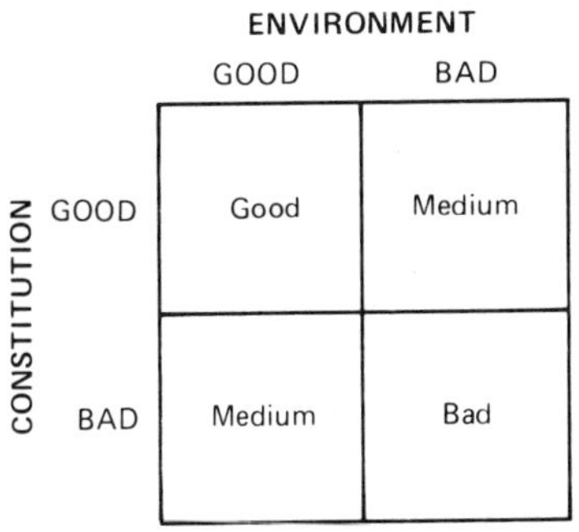
ENVIRONMENT
GOOD
BAD
CONSTITUTION
GOOD
BAD
Good
Medium
Medium
Bad

Figure 5. Interactional model of causation. (Adapted from Arnold Sameroff, Early influences on development: fact or fancy? *Merrill-Palmer Quarterly*, 21 (1975), p. 282.)

The interactional model, then, permits a richer account of causation. At the same time, this enrichment is bought at the price of increased complexity. No longer can we look for a single cause. A child with a genetic form of retardation communicates in a particular way, not only because of the degree of retardation, but also because of the type of environment in which that child is being raised.

Sameroff (1975) argues, however, that the interactional model is still an oversimplification. There are two interrelated problems. First, it assumes that constitution and environment do not change. The outcome for a child is the product of a particular combination of specific constitutional and environmental factors. Whatever the child's situation is, so it is likely to remain. Second, it assumes that the child and the environment do not affect each other. The interactional model is really a combination of both views of the linear cause-and-effect model. Consequently, causation is still unidirectional. The environment affects the child's development; similarly, the constitution has effects on the child's development; but the model does not include the possibility of constitution and environment affecting each other. Recall from Chapter 5 that relationships are reciprocal. Lines of influence run in both directions. Enter Sameroff's third model of causation.

The Transactional Model

The transactional model is qualitatively different from the previous models. It includes change over time and emphasizes the reciprocal influences between child and environment. Look at Figure 6. This diagram is different from the preceding ones. First, time is represented; both child and environment change over time. The "outcome" may be different at varying times in the child's life. Second, there are no boxes, but lines, suggesting again that conditions are not static and permanent. Third, there are arrows indicating that causation goes in both directions.

The model works as follows. At any point in time the child's constitution is in a certain state, indicated by C_1. In parallel fashion, the environment is also in a certain state at that same time, indicated by E_1. Both child and environment respond to each other, and thus change each other and are themselves changed. Consequently, at a later time (indicated by C_2 and E_2), each is now different. They are still influencing each other, so that at a still later time, both are different again. The process continues throughout life. Thus, environments influence children, but at the same time children influence environments. The net result is that children alter the environments that affect them and vice versa, in continuing reciprocal fashion.

An Example. Of the three models, the transactional model best explains the apparent contradictions between the retrospective and prospective studies mentioned earlier. Not only are there many factors influencing outcome, but the factors influence each other. Consider a hypothetical example. A child is born prematurely. Because of low birth weight, the infant spends its first weeks in the hospital. The mother is allowed limited contact with the child, and the father almost none. The parents worry a great deal, first, that they may lose the baby and then, as the infant gains strength, that the child may have difficulty in development. When the baby is allowed to go home, the parents become quite naturally oversolicitous. They feel lucky that the baby survived at all. As time wears on, they feel fatigue and a little resentment at the amount of work and lost sleep involved in caring for this delicate child. At the same time, the baby is fretful, cries much of the time, sleeps irregularly, and is difficult to feed. As the months pass, the parents become concerned that the baby is not developing at a normal rate, so they begin to provide as much stimulation as possible and push toward new

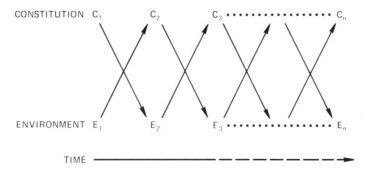

CONSTITUTION C_1 C_2 C_3 •••••••••••••••• C_n

ENVIRONMENT E_1 E_2 E_3 ••••••••••••••• E_n

TIME

Figure 6. Transactional model of causation. (Adapted from Arnold Sameroff, Early influences on development: fact or fancy? *Merrill-Palmer Quarterly*, 21 (1975), p. 282.)

achievements. The child does not respond well to these overtures, perhaps in part because of maturational lags associated with low birth weight. The parents push harder, at the same time feeling some guilt that perhaps they were too lenient during the child's early months. The child reacts to the pressure with increased resistance and the beginnings of tantrums. By now the parents are feeling combinations of desperation, guilt, and anger, but they continue to try. The child becomes increasingly uncommunicative and difficult to manage. At five the child is severely language delayed and is considered too immature and too much of a behavior problem for placement in regular kindergarten.

How do we identify etiology in a case like this? We can't lay it to the prematurity, because the child may have responded very differently to a different sequence of parenting styles. At the same time, we can't blame it on the parents, because another baby might have responded beautifully to them. It's important to notice, also, that the parents acted in reasonable fashion. They responded to the child's moods as best they could. They were not abusive or neglectful, but positively motivated and working for the child's betterment. If there had been severe pathology in either child or parents, the outcome might have been quite different. One can only understand causation in such situations in terms of the evolving transactions between parents and child.

Genetics and Neurophysiology

It may be argued that the genetic transmission of constitutional disorders contradicts the transactional model. A genetically caused hearing loss is a genetically caused hearing loss, period. Retardation due to Down's syndrome is genetic retardation, no matter what the environment. Many current writers in genetics do not make these absolute statements, however. As Scarr-Salapatek says, "It is not correct . . . to say that heredity sets the limits on development while environment determines the extent of development. Both are half-truths because they ignore the constant transaction between [genetic makeup] and environment during development" (1975, p. 15). Other writers also emphasize the importance of transactions between genetic and environmental factors (Reed 1975; Elias 1973). It is to be understood that, for these authors, environment includes not only the child's familial and sociocultural surroundings, but also conditions in utero from the moment of conception. Finally, Scarr-Salapatek (1975) discusses the reaction range, which is the variation in development that can occur from one genetic makeup, given different environments. It would appear, then, that genetics alone does not necessarily dictate precise outcome.

Again, it is not my purpose to denigrate the importance of genetic and neurophysical factors in child development. Rather, I wish to guard against simplistic and reductionist causal explanations on the basis of these factors. In fact, the medical profession is also expanding beyond the linear cause-and-effect model (for example, Minuchin, Rosman, and Baker 1978). Similarly, the behavioral sciences in general are moving away from the idea of specific etiology (Dumont 1968; Bronfenbrenner 1979). Especially with a multiply determined phenomenon such as language development, it is highly unlikely that a linear cause-and-effect explanation is going to tell the whole story. Even more important, it may not provide much directly useful information toward developing an appropriate intervention.

Parent-Child Interaction

For specialists working with language-disordered children, the practical focus of the transactional model is on the social exchanges between child and environment. It is through these exchanges that language literally comes to life. They form the communicative foundation for language and ultimately they are the embodiment of language use. In addition, as already mentioned, we target our interventions at the child's social transactions. It is important to my argument, then, to demonstrate evidence of mutual influence between child and environment in this area.

There is no doubt that the family influences the young child's language development. No matter what view one takes of the process of language acquisition, the fact remains that the family provides the model of language that the child will acquire, at least in the early stages. In the case of an only child, the parents provide this model. In multiple-child families other siblings are also involved. Moerk (1976) provided an interesting description of some of the teaching techniques that parents use in helping their offspring learn language. In addition to modeling the language, parents ask questions, elicit responses, provide feedback on the adequacy of the child's utterances, repeat utterances, and provide direct help in language learning in a variety of other ways.

In the past the influence of the parent on the child was the major focus of research in parent-child relations. Currently this emphasis is changing to a view of the parent and child as an interactive system (Martin 1975). Many studies now concentrate on the effects of the child's behavior on the parents. As indicated earlier, studies focusing on language have demonstrated that the parents' language use is heavily influenced by

the child's language functioning. Parents use increasingly shorter and simpler utterances as they interact with other adults, elementary school–aged children, and pre-schoolers (Broen 1972). At the same time, the parents' care in avoiding grammatical errors, pauses that interrupt grammatical constituents, and general linguistic sloppiness increases with younger children. Snow (1972) and Phillips (1973) have presented similar evidence of parental adjustments in language use according to the age of the child.

The age of the child is not the only controlling factor, however, and perhaps not the dominant one. Along these lines, Siegel (1963a, 1963b; Siegel and Harkins 1963) studied verbal interactions between adults and retarded individuals. The language levels of the retardates had been previously determined. Siegel found that the adults used shorter utterances and more redundancy when interacting with low-language-level rather than high-language-level individuals. This effect occurred even when the adults were misinformed about the retardates' language levels. For example, adults might be told they were going to interact with retarded individuals with high language levels, when in fact those individuals were low in language skill. More recent studies (Marshall, Hegrenes, and Goldstein 1973; Buium, Rynders, and Turnure 1974; Guralnick and Paul-Brown 1977) point in the same direction. Further, Snow (1972) found that mothers simplified their language more when talking to a child who was actually present than when asked to talk to a child who was not present.

While the child's output must be an important variable in these studies, Bohannon and Marquis (1977) have presented evidence that the child's indications of comprehension are a major factor in influencing the mother's language use. Mothers adjust their levels of talking according to their children's feedback concerning comprehension of what has been said.

Conclusion

In sum, we have a lot of evidence that we can put together in support of the transactional model in relation to language development. We know that parents influence children. We know that children influence parents. Further, we know that parents and children change over time, both through experience and through growth and maturational processes. Thus, we have all the components of the transactional model. Indeed, people develop throughout life in a never-ending series of transactions with the environment.

The transactional model carries with it a problem, however. This view of causation makes the identification of specific etiologies difficult. The direct connections of the linear cause-and-effect model become tenuous and illusive. Even if a clear-cut etiological factor is present, such as the presence of congenital retardation, that does not explain why the child communicates in certain ways at six or twelve years of age. It is only part of the equation.

In spite of this apparent drawback, the transactional model has a number of virtues. First, at least in my mind, it is more realistic. It takes into account the complexity of children's language disorders and their histories. Second, and perhaps most important, it offers the potential of intervention in whatever transactions are occurring when the clinician encounters the situation (Sameroff 1975). We can't change the past, but we can always work in the present. In addition, the transactional model frequently offers the clinician several avenues for intervention. More than one aspect of the child's transactions with the environment might have the potential for producing change. Third, at a more general level, this model puts the emphasis on communication, which is, of course, precisely what we want to focus on. Indeed, the transactions between child and environment are a series of communications of various sorts.

A Second Example. Let us consider an example at this point. Alison was referred to the speech clinic at the age of three years and two months. She had a history of one convulsion at about twelve months of age. She was small for her age and had not yet been successfully toilet trained. The referring agency suggested the possibility of mild retardation. Her expressive language was almost entirely limited to one word, *This.* She used it both in response to questions by the clinician and as a way to elicit remarks from whoever was present. Her mother reported that she used a few other words at home. She did not respond well to formal tests or directions, so her comprehension could not be assessed with confidence. She did, however, demonstrate appropriate play for her age level and would sometimes respond appropriately to suggestions given by the clinician during the course of play. Her hearing, assessed through play audiometry, appeared to be adequate for language development. She had an older sister in elementary school who was developing normally. Her father worked different shifts and had little contact with the clinic. Altogether, not an uncommon set of characteristics for a language-delayed child.

We enrolled Alison in the clinic, partly because her ability to communicate through language was truly impaired, and partly because the mother was deeply concerned. Through working with both child and parent, we hoped to understand the child's situation better, and explore possible interventions. We immediately became aware of a second level of this child's situation. Alison and her mother were intensely bound to each other. This is the child I mentioned in an earlier chapter who hung on the doorknob and cried for sixty minutes when her mother was out of the room. Her mother was equally upset. Over time, we were able to help them decrease their overinvolvement with each other, so that the child could function independently in the clinic room. The mother described the child as "very stubborn," and thought that perhaps her language delay was at least in part a refusal to cooperate. Similarly, Alison appeared to know what the toilet was for and how to use it, but training had not been successful. One can certainly imagine a transactional link between the lack of progress in maturation in different areas of the child's behavior and the intense parenting and concern supplied by her mother.

After a period of time Alison was demonstrating much more independent and mature behavior in the clinic and good comprehension, but she still did not talk. Two further events occurred that were important in understanding this child's communicative pattern. Both were learned of indirectly through parental report; we did not witness them. First, Alison talked on the telephone. She only talked to certain relatives, and then only when no one else was in the room. Apparently she would use multiple-word utterances in answer to queries about such things as what she was doing and where her mother was. The clincher came when the family went on vacation to another state to visit the child's uncle. Upon their return Alison's mother reported that the child had talked a great deal while at the uncle's house but had stopped talking during the return trip when they crossed the state line! While

one might want to take the state line element with a grain of salt, I believe the general substance of the mother's report. In line with these discoveries, our intervention focused increasingly on the relationship aspects of Alison's communicative behavior.

This example illustrates the transactional model of causation nicely. Whatever the original causal factors might have been, and there is a hint of maturational lag possibly connected with the convulsion, it's a far cry from the relationship game Alison was later playing with her mother and uncle. At the same time, both of these situations developed in the context of transactions between the child and her environment. The immaturity may have elicited overly solicitous parenting from the mother, but such parenting is likely to encourage immaturity. Again, Alison's minimal talking to her mother (and to her clinicians!) while talking to her uncle represents a transaction of a very different type. The meanings of these transactions are intuitive and nondiscursive in nature, but they had effects on the linear and discursive use of language in communication. In addition, while there were mild hints of constitutional dysfunction, our only reasonable interventions were through environmental changes. Finally, as we became aware of different aspects of Alison's transactions with her environment, we were able to intervene differently in each of these transactions. We diminished the intensity of the bond between mother and child, so that each could function more independently. We focused on Alison's language comprehension, so that we knew she had something to say. Finally, we focused directly on Alison's refusal to talk as a relationship tactic in her transactions with various individuals in the environment. I certainly would not claim that our understanding of this child was complete, but through the transactional model we achieved a more powerful perspective than we would have obtained by describing the situation as "language delay associated with developmental lag," or "language delay associated with overprotective mother," or even by combining both of those explanations.

General Systems Theory

At various places in this book I have emphasized reciprocal relations and interacting systems of relationships. These ideas are particularly apparent in the transactional model. It will be useful at this time to sketch this systems perspective in more formal terms. In association with cybernetics there has been an attempt to develop a set of principles that apply to any kind of system, be it mechanical, biological, or social. This set of principles is frequently referred to as general systems theory (Bertalanffy 1968). A system is a group of entities and the relations among them. We have looked at the human information-processing system, in which the entities include the five senses, attention, memory, and so forth. The relations among them reflect the idea that each is interdependent with the others. For another example, the entities in interpersonal communication are the context and the individuals in the interaction. The relations were described in terms of hierarchies of rules and metarules. Several characteristics of systems are important in understanding the causation of children's language disorders and in designing interventions. The first three of these principles are taken from Hall and Fagin (1956).

Closed Systems and Open Systems

A closed system is one that functions without influence from outside the system. A chemical reaction in a bottle is the classic example. Human beings are associated with open systems, which interact with, and are affected by, outside factors. A family is an example of an open system. It is a unit on its own, but it is influenced by cultural factors, from worldwide economic trends to the opinions of neighbors. The language-disordered child is similarly an open system. It is this fact that makes the transactional model viable. The child's functioning may be consistent or "rule governed," but it is influenced by the caretaking environment. That environment, usually a family, is another open system, which is changed by the child. At a higher level, this whole pattern of transactions related to the child's language disorder is itself another open system that we hope to change through intervention. It is the open-system nature of human beings and social groups that makes intervention possible.

Wholeness

This idea has already been mentioned but needs stronger emphasis. Wholeness means that all parts of the system are related and, more important, that change in one part of the system causes change in others. If you fill a balloon half-full of air and then squeeze one part of it, other parts will puff out accordingly. The idea of wholeness argues against the linear cause-and-effect model. Causation is multifaceted. Recall again from Chapter 5 that human relationships are always reciprocal. One person can't be dominant unless the "dominees" permit that domination. It is because of wholeness that it becomes possible to work with the parents of a young language-delayed child in order to increase the child's use of language. By changing the parents we change the transactional system and thus encourage change in the child. As we will see when we discuss punctuation, wholeness is perhaps the most easily overlooked principle of general systems theory.

Equifinality

The principle of "equifinality" holds that, in a system, similar initial conditions can yield different outcomes and that similar outcomes can result from different initial conditions. Equifinality explains why the retrospective studies discussed earlier were not supported by later prospective studies. The relations among the entities in a system also influence outcome. Consequently, high-risk factors by themselves are not good predictors. It can be seen that equifinality is at the very heart of the transactional model. The status of any individual at any point in life is the result of initial conditions plus that individual's whole history of transactions with various environments. No wonder we're all different.

Morphostatic and Morphogenic Processes

A major emphasis in general systems theory is on the relations within the system. Sometimes the effect of these relations is to maintain the system in a particular state and sometimes it is to induce change in the system. Hall and Fagin (1956) discuss these processes in terms of feedback mechanisms. Buckley (1967) delineated these mechanisms more specifically. Some types of feedback tend to maintain the system as it is. He refers to such feedback as "morphostatic" processes. It is these processes that allow a family to endure for decades. Morphostatic processes are also involved in the transactional model. For example, they would be important in any situation in which a child remains at an inappropriately immature

level. A four-year-old may not talk but may use nonverbal communication effectively. At the same time, the parents don't press for talking and become skilled in anticipating the child's needs and in reading those nonverbal messages. Thus, the family functions satisfactorily although the child does not develop expressive language. Morphostatic processes, such as those involved in the successful communication and the parents' view of their child's development, maintain the situation. Morphostatic mechanisms are extremely pervasive and often very powerful. Think a moment about what life would be like if there were no such processes.

On the other hand, people do change. Buckley (1967) refers to the mechanisms of change in a system as "morphogenic" processes. The fact that children grow and develop is a morphogenic process that causes other changes in the family. You do not act toward a two-year-old the same way you do toward a nine-year-old, much less a sixteen-year-old. Morphogenic processes also come from outside the family system, as in job changes and influences from the larger social system, such as education. In relation to causation, changes in transactional patterns result from morphogenic processes and, in turn, are morphogenic processes for further change. If we attempt to intervene in the transactional patterns associated with a particular child, that intervention is also a morphogenic process.

Toward the end of Chapter 5 I discussed the self-maintaining and reciprocal qualities of human relationships. In that context I emphasized the importance of metarules and rule hierarchies in relationships. It can now be seen that these rules are ways to describe the morphostatic processes in those relationships. I also explored the question of how change can occur in the presence of these system-maintaining morphostatic processes. It is worth noting that most of the morphogenic processes I suggested at that time take advantage of the fact that human relationships are open systems. Human behavior, both in and out of clinic, is the result of a subtle mixture of morphostatic and morphogenic processes.

Punctuation

Now we have an idea of some of the formal properties of the social systems in which children learn and use language. The ideas of mutual influence and multiple causation have been stressed. There is one further point that is relevant at this time. People frequently do not perceive the interrelatedness and mutuality of causation. We see ourselves as responding to some events and initiating other events. Our tendency to see life in this way has been called "punctuation" by Watzlawick, Beavin, and Jackson (1967). The ebb and flow of events go on, but we "punctuate" that constant stream into sequences of cause and effect, just as I punctuate this book into sentences, paragraphs, and chapters.

Consider an example. An eight-year-old girl doesn't talk much in class. She doesn't like the way she sounds and, indeed, her expressive language contains many errors in both grammar and articulation. Her teacher tries to "bring her out," by asking her questions during class discussions and having her recite before the class in other ways. The behavior of the child and the teacher can be described as a continuously repeating cycle. The child withdraws; she looks out the window or reads and does not participate in discussion. The teacher calls on her. She declines to respond. The teacher presses, and finally she responds in minimal fashion, in which, ironically, she does not display what language skill she does possess. In addition, there is some resentment in her manner. The teacher continues the discussion, eliciting comments from other students. Our language-disordered child withdraws again. Before long, the teacher calls on her again. A new cycle of the same pattern begins.

We talk to the child. She says she doesn't participate because the teacher picks on her and embarrasses her. (Punctuation: She is only responding to what the teacher is doing.) We talk to the teacher. He says he is just trying to encourage her to talk and get more involved in the topics of class discussion. (Punctuation: He is only responding to what the child is doing.) Because of their punctuations, neither can see this transactional sequence as a whole, and consequently it becomes more difficult for them to break the pattern. Both get increasingly committed to their individual punctuations.

A classic example of punctuation is in the old joke from experimental psychology about a rat who is trained to run mazes by being reinforced for correct attempts. The rat gets better and better, until the mazes are always negotiated correctly. The rat says, "Ngrt szzrsk mpmrq," rat language for, "I've taught this human to give me pellets."

Punctuation of this type is extremely common. In our culture, at least, we see events in cause-and-effect sequences. Bateson (1972) emphasized how difficult it is to achieve a higher perspective, at least in viewing one's own relations with the world. Similarly, with regard to the transactional model, people typically see themselves as responding to each other, rather than as involved in a reciprocal series in which each cause is also a result and each result is also a cause.

Punctuation and the Linear Cause-and-Effect Model. This tendency to punctuate the stream of events into stimuli and responses, or cause-and-effect sequences, is also seen in the dependence on linear cause-and-effect models in attempting to understand children with learning and language problems. Perhaps the classic example is the concept of minimal brain damage. The child's symptoms are explained as being due to brain damage, but that damage is so subtle or slight that neurologists cannot specify its nature or even state confidently that it is present. The diagnosis of minimal brain damage would be unlikely were it not for the fact that many diagnosticians punctuate causal relationships in a linear cause-and-effect framework.

Extending these notions somewhat, reification again complicates the problem. Minimal brain damage becomes reified; it is a "thing," not a hypothesis. We now have what Watzlawick (1976) refers to as a self-sealing premise. Certain types of behavior in children are explained as being due to minimal brain damage. The concept of minimal brain damage is supported because there are children with those types of behavior! Perhaps the strongest form of this type of thinking is in what Bateson (1972) calls an "explanatory principle." There are some phenomena that scientists refer to and make use of but cannot explain. For example, gravity is an explanatory principle. We explain a great many things with gravity, but no one is explaining gravity. It is surprisingly easy for explanatory principles to sneak into our clinical thinking in comments such as, "That's typical of hyperactive children," or, "Language problems are common in learning-disabled children." Other terms present the same temptations, such as childhood aphasia, perceptual disorder, auditory processing problem, attentional deficit, and emotional problem. The use of such terms as explanatory principles depends on a reciprocal relation be-

tween reification and the linear cause-and-effect model. In my view, however, terms such as these don't explain anything; rather, they themselves need explanation.

Summary of Models of Causation

We began with the relatively simple view of linear cause and effect and ended up with a more complex picture of causation, involving the transactional model and general systems theory. Perhaps two ideas are most important in this presentation. First, human development never stops. Whatever initial factors may be present, the child's experiences over time influence development. Causation, then, is multiply determined. Second, causation in human development is reciprocal and transactional in nature. The child responds to the environment and, concomitantly, the environment responds to the child. Influence and change are mutual in series of transactions that last throughout life. The reciprocity of development and the general systems perspective can be seen in various places in preceding chapters. For example, I have argued that language and concepts are developed interdependently; that language knowledge, language processing, and auditory processing skills are interdependent; and that language use and human relations are similarly interdependent.

It may be tempting at this point to throw up your hands and conclude that everything is related to everything and that it's too complicated to be of practical benefit. Such conclusions miss the point. The transactional model and the assumptions of general systems theory that I have associated with that model point in very useful directions. First, they lead us away from simplistic descriptions of etiology and pat linear cause-and-effect explanations of causation. Second, they offer more than one avenue for intervention with any particular child. Any change in the transactional system that is powerful enough is likely to cause change in the child. Thus, for example, intervention might focus on expression, comprehension, concepts, information processing, human relationships, or the family system. We do not make these choices solely on the basis of the child's needs, although of course those needs are important. Our choice of an intervention is also in response to the following question: Given this child's situation, what type of intervention is most likely to lead to permanent change? It follows from these remarks that another advantage of the transactional and systems views is that they expand our perspectives on what can be involved in intervention. Thus, a theory of causation is also a theory of treatment. Further, it becomes important not only to focus on the child but to look at the system in which the child is functioning and to look at the child as a part of that system. With these ideas in mind let us now consider some specific etiologies for children's language disorders that have been emphasized in the literature.

ETIOLOGICAL CATEGORIES

Historically, a number of etiological categories have received particular attention in the field of children's language disorders. They are: hearing loss, mental retardation, emotional disturbance, childhood aphasia, and auditory processing disorders. In terms of my earlier discussion of constitutional factors, they are second-level causal factors. That is, they are conditions that are associated with language disorders in children, but strictly speaking, they are not causal factors. Rather, they themselves result from

other factors, sometimes with a heavy genetic or disease influence, sometimes from more amorphous origins. Let me now discuss each category separately.

Hearing Loss

The importance of hearing for language development has already been discussed. I must stress here the importance of obtaining competent and thorough hearing assessment. One simply cannot determine whether or not hearing loss is present merely by observing a child or carrying out some informal procedures. Hodgson (1969) illustrates the point nicely. He describes three different types of children with hearing loss. Without careful hearing assessment any one might be misclassified as not having a hearing impairment. The first group includes children with profound hearing loss who are also uncooperative and difficult to test. The conclusion may be made that the child is too retarded or too disturbed to test or that auditory processing problems impair the child's functioning. The second group includes children with a relatively flat hearing loss of moderate severity. Children in this group will respond to sound often enough that observers may conclude that some problem other than hearing is causing the child's difficulty. A third group demonstrates adequate hearing at the low frequencies but a loss at high frequencies. Again, these children respond to many sounds but miss a lot. Children in both the second and third groups are sometimes described as "hearing when they want to." Their responding is inconsistent and may be bizarre at times. It is sometimes easy to misinterpret such a child's behavior as reflecting a learning or perceptual disorder or an emotional disturbance.

Kleffner (1973) has made similar arguments about the significance of hearing loss in children identified as having specific language disability. In particular, he argues that great caution should be employed in concluding that a child's difficulty with language is due to some central disorder over and above the hearing loss itself. In view of the transactional model, one can see why his views make sense.

In sum, hearing loss has a profound impact on language development. Hearing assessment cannot be undertaken superficially, nor can the presence of hearing loss, however mild, be considered unimportant in any child. Further, the hearing-impaired child's language still develops within the framework of the transactional model. In addition to understanding the specifics of a child's loss, then, one should attempt to determine how that hearing loss contributes to the child's transactions with the environment relative to language development and more general communicative behavior.

Mental Retardation

The core attribute of mental retardation is significantly depressed intellectual functioning. Included are the following characteristics (Sloan 1954, quoted in Matthews 1957): maturation at a reduced level, impaired learning ability, and ineffective social functioning. The disorder appears at birth or early in life. There are many types of retardation that have been described as specific medical syndromes. A number of these conditions stem from genetic factors. Many other cases of retardation do not present any particular identifiable causal factors and do not fit any of these specific syndromes. These cases are sometimes referred to as "familial retardation."

The identification of retardation varies with the type of retardation. The specific syndromes are typically identified by medical specialists. One should note, however, that what is identified is the *presence* of retardation rather than its *degree*. Any child with Down's syndrome, for example, is retarded, but the range of retardation varies from very severe to relatively mild. Identification of cases of familial retardation is not as clear-cut by the very nature of the disorder. Typically, assessment involves a team of specialists and a variety of different areas of development in the child.

The labeling of a child as retarded is a sensitive issue, not only because of the personal tragedy involved, but also because of the possible effects of the label itself. Horowitz (1969) has suggested that if outcome is a product of constitution and environment (the interactional model), and the constitution is somehow defective, then unusual variations in the environment might still produce a normal outcome. The Skeels data (Skeels 1966; Skeels and Dye 1939; Skeels, et al. 1938), in which some retarded children were left in an orphanage and others were placed with surrogate mothers, indicates that Horowitz's thesis is at least possible. It is worth noting at this point that all of Skeels's subjects were in the category of familial retardation. On the other hand, the majority of individuals identified as being significantly retarded remain so throughout life, including many who receive superior and innovative interventions.

Many retarded individuals demonstrate impairments in language. These impairments are probably related to two factors. First, language is heavily intertwined with cognition. Second, the communication patterns between the retarded child and the environment may differ from those experienced by normal children (Mahoney 1975). In any case, all but the most severely retarded develop some use of language.

In conclusion, retardation is significantly related to language impairment, but we may gain very little by considering retardation as an etiology for children's language disorders. The causation of retardation is itself problematic in cases of familial retardation. Further, language deficit and retardation interact with each other, particularly in the use of abstraction. Both language and intellectual development depend on the concepts and rules described in Chapter 1 and the human information-processing functions discussed in Chapter 2. In addition, the acquisition of both depends on exchange between the child and the environment. It may be more useful to consider mental retardation and children's language disorders as conditions that may occur in association with each other in the context of the transactional model, rather than attempting to draw definite causal links.

Emotional Disturbance

A major message of Chapter 5 was that emotions, relationships, communication, and language are not separate, independent aspects of the human condition. Because we are in the communication business, it will be profitable for us to interpret emotional disturbance as inseparable from communication, or at least as being manifested through communication. In the field of psychotherapy, Ruesch and Bateson (1951), Szasz (1961), and Watzlawick (1978) have developed similar views.

The causes of emotional disturbance, in children as well as adults, have been notoriously difficult to determine. Research focuses on everything from heredity to family and cultural factors to blood chemistry. Again, the transactional model appears to be the most viable view of causation available at present. Accordingly, like mental retardation, emotional disturbance does not offer much precise explanatory power as an etiology for children's language disorders. Communication, including the use of language, is a central aspect of *both* (although, of course, not necessarily the only aspect of either one). In an individual with emotional problems, it is fair to say that the communication disorder is part of the emotional disturbance; it is equally fair to say that the emotional disturbance is part of the communication disorder.

Emotional disturbance is distributed along a continuum from relatively mild problems, those that impair an individual's functioning but are not totally debilitating, to those that are so severe the individual cannot function in society. The less severe problems in living have received relatively little attention in the literature on children's language disorders. They may occur in association with language disorders, however, because an impairment in the use of language influences the ways one functions in human relationships. A preschool language-delayed child may communicate primarily through tantrums; a sixth-grade language-disordered child may avoid contact with other children. For us it is moot whether or not children such as these are considered as having emotional problems. I'm not sure that they should be. What is important is that their language disorders are not isolated from other aspects of their relationship communication.

Severely disturbed children are referred to as psychotic, schizophrenic, and autistic. For some authors these terms are relatively synonymous. For others they represent different types of disturbances. In any case, the children so identified present profound impairments in the use of language. They may be mute, or they may respond primarily through repeating what is said to them.

They may appear to comprehend at times but not at other times. They frequently avoid interacting with other people.

Autism

The communication disorders associated with autism are particularly dramatic. Consequently, language and communication are central in interventions with these children. The major characteristics of autism have been summarized by Baltaxe and Simmons (1975). Autistic children demonstrate disturbed interpersonal relationships and social behavior. Their intellectual skills are impaired or distorted. They employ many stereotyped behaviors, such as self-stimulation and repetitive movements. Finally, autistic children show disorders of speech and language, including delayed development, echolalia or repetition, mutism, and unusual or bizarre word usage. It takes but a moment's reflection to see that all of these characteristics deeply affect communicative behavior. In fact, they produce communication that is nondiscursive and intuitive to an extreme degree.

It is no surprise, then, that there is considerable disagreement about the nature of autism. Some see it as a psychosis (Baltaxe and Simmons 1975); other authors describe it as a disorder of communication and behavior (National Society for Autistic Children 1973). Some discuss the cognitive impairment associated with the disorder (Byrne and Shervanian 1977), while others stress interpersonal aspects (Richer 1975). As far as I can see, there is some truth in all of these views of autism. An additional factor in understanding the disorder is that the degree of impairment varies from child to child. All things considered, the label becomes less important than a careful assessment of the individual child.

As already suggested, the language clinician plays a major role in intervention with autistic children. However one views the disorder, training focuses on diminishing the child's nondiscursive behavior and developing language skills and other appropriate means of communication.

Returning to our more general perspective, there is a strong connection between emotional disturbance and language impairment in children. As with mental retardation, however, little is gained by invoking this connection as an etiology for disorders of language. Each develops in the context of the other through the transactional model, so that they become inseparable.

Childhood Aphasia and Auditory Processing Disorders

Some children demonstrate impairments in language, and yet there are no indications of hearing loss, retardation, or emotional disturbance. If one thinks with the linear cause-and-effect model, then there still must be a cause. By analogy with aphasia in adults, one possible cause would be some dysfunction in the child's brain. This dysfunction could lead to perceptual or other problems in processing language. Anyone who has had contact with adult aphasic patients cannot help but be impressed with the effects of brain disorders on language functions. These disorders may be dramatic, as when an individual's use of language is virtually wiped out; or they can be subtle, as in the case of an individual who communicates satisfactorily but has some difficulty in retrieving exactly the right vocabulary items during discourse. There is no doubt that language disabilities can be caused by damage to the brain.

Considerable emphasis has been placed on the identification of suspected brain dysfunction in language-disordered children. In some cases such identification is relatively clear-cut. A child may become aphasic just as an adult does, through trauma to the brain or disease. Cooper and Ferry (1978), for example, describe a syndrome of acquired aphasia in children.

Minimal Brain Dysfunction

In many cases, however, a positive identification of the presence of brain dysfunction cannot be made. Linear cause-and-effect reasoning may still be applied in evaluating such children. As I have already noted, the result is sometimes diagnosis of minimal brain dysfunction, which then becomes a reified explanatory principle. While I have been critical of this kind of thinking, we must be careful not to throw out the baby with the bath water. The question is, when is such a determination useful? It may have little benefit when it leads to an empty explanation and a cessation of attempts to look for other causal factors. It may be very useful, though, in other applications, such as research in children's language disorders.

The problem of determining the presence of brain dysfunction in children who are not medically diagnosable as brain impaired presents a great challenge. The solution will have to be inferential, because by definition there are no direct symptoms. At the same time, these inferences must be trustworthy if they are to be of any use. There have been three approaches to this problem. The first involves ruling out other deficits, such as hearing loss, emotional disturbance, and retardation, and then concluding that, in the absence of other causal factors, there must be minimal brain damage. In my view this approach is the least satisfactory. In terms of the transactional model one cannot ever

rule out all other possible causes; one isn't even sure just what all the possibilities might be. The other two approaches depend on a more direct search for brain dysfunction. One involves assessment of one specific aspect of behavior, the other a broad and comprehensive evaluation.

Habituation. Lewis (1975) focused on one particular phenomenon, known as "habituation." The idea is simply this: We are likely to pay attention to a novel stimulus, but with repeated presentations of that stimulus we attend less and less. In other words, we become habituated to that stimulus. Habituation has been measured in a number of ways. Lewis (1975) focused on alterations in heart rate. With the introduction of a novel stimulus, the infant's heart rate changes. As habituation occurs, the heart rate returns to normal. This effect is well documented in the psychological literature. What is to the point here is that Lewis (1975) marshals considerable evidence in support of the view that in babies and young children habituation is a potent indicator of central nervous system dysfunction. Brain dysfunction is associated with a lack of habituation. The baby's heart rate changes with the presentation of a novel stimulus, but it does not show the pattern of return to its previous rate that a normal baby's does. This lack of habituation thus offers a means for identifying brain dysfunction in the very young. Further, the technique has potential for identifying those illusive cases of subclinical or minimal brain damage. So far it has been used primarily in research.

There is a complication in using habituation in the identification of brain dysfunction in young children, however. Recall Sameroff and Chandler's (1975) discussion of prospective studies earlier in the chapter. Generally, the sequelae of high-risk factors present at early ages tend to disappear by the end of elementary school. It is possible that a similar trend will be found in the lack of habituation described by Lewis (1975). In fact Lewis himself subscribes to an interactional view of causation.

Comprehensive Assessment. In contrast to Lewis's focus on one specific aspect of behavior, Reitan (1975; Reitan and Heineman 1968) described an extensive assessment battery, which involves a full day's testing. Included are the *Wechsler Intelligence Scale for Children,* the *Jastak Wide Range Achievement Test,* and the *Reitan-Indiana Neuropsychological Test Battery.* These instruments sample a variety of areas, including comprehension and expression of language, picture and object assembly, mazes, school achievement, strength of grip, and a number of other tests of motor skills; in addition, comparisons are made between left and right sides of the body on various perceptual and motor skills. Other areas of performance may also be sampled. The battery was developed in work with adults with known cerebral lesions. It was later adapted for work with children. In contrast with Lewis, Reitan has concentrated on school-aged children, rather than preschoolers.

Reitan (1975) argues that comparing a child's score with age norms or comparing a child's profile of performances with normative data provides only weak means for inferring the presence of brain damage. Therefore, he gathers a great deal of information about a child and then searches this information for patterns and other clues indicative of brain dysfunction. For example, he looks for signs of deficit on one side of the body, inferring that the opposite hemisphere of the brain may be affected. If impairments in the higher level functions attributed to that hemisphere are also affected, the evidence becomes stronger. If the child also shows specific signs of dysfunction related to that hemisphere, a still more confident conclusion can be made. Thus, Reitan makes his determination through a series of logical inferences based on what is known about the relations between brain and behavior. Interesting case studies will be found in both Reitan (1975) and in Reitan and Heineman (1968). Inferring brain dysfunction from observations of behavior is a tricky business, however. For a critical review of work in this area, see Feuerstein, Ward, and LeBaron (1979).

Clinical Implications. I have described Lewis's and Reitan's work in some detail because it bears on the issue of whether or not there is a condition that can be called minimal brain dysfunction. The evidence so far indicates that such a condition may indeed occur. It is striking, however, that many of Reitan's suggestions for intervention with children he has diagnosed could be developed without ever considering whether or not the child's brain functions normally. They follow directly from the child's behavior. If a child has difficulty with comprehension, for example, use short utterances and avoid a rapid rate of talking. Along these lines, Koupernik, MacKeith and Francis-Williams (1975) suggest that, with learning disabled children, treatment can proceed without identification of the cause. They caution, of course, against this approach in acute disorders, but these cases will be identified through medical diagnosis. With children's language disorders, then, the idea of minimal brain dysfunction may be of more use in research than in day-to-day clinical work and training.

Let us return now to childhood aphasia and auditory processing problems. The two are closely related. Eisenson (1972), in fact, suggests that childhood aphasia consists of disabilities in certain auditory skills. In

Chapter 3, I argued that little is accomplished by reifying auditory processing as existing as an independent set of skills. Similarly, the label childhood aphasic may have some use in putting children into very rough categories, but it does not help in deciding how to intervene with any particular child. As suggested above, neither does the inferred presence of minimal brain dysfunction, which childhood aphasia implies. I know of no research using techniques such as those of Lewis (1975) or Reitan with subjects classified as childhood aphasics. My guess is that when such research is done, some children will show positive signs of brain dysfunction and some won't. In view of the nebulous character of childhood aphasia and of auditory processing deficits, I suggest that the most useful approach to understanding the origins of these disorders will be through the transactional model. The transactions may be subtle and difficult to evaluate during assessment. Nevertheless, investigating the child's transactions with the environment will identify some concrete areas in which to begin intervention.

Summary: Specific Etiological Factors

I have reviewed several etiologies that are often cited in the literature, namely, hearing loss, retardation, emotional disturbance, childhood aphasia, and auditory processing disorders. My general conclusion has been that none of these factors explains fully why a particular child demonstrates difficulties with language. Any child with a possible language deficit should be considered from the perspective of the transactional model. No matter how clearly we can identify a causal factor for a particular child, that child's current communicative functioning is

the result of many transactions with the environment. Thus, two children with similar hearing losses may communicate quite differently. Likewise, two children with equivalent levels of retardation may not be the same in their use of language. Further, our intervention will itself take the form of transactions between the child and individuals in the environment, usually parents, teachers, and clinicians.

It has been argued that the attempt to identify etiologies such as those above is of relatively little merit because no matter what conclusions are made about etiology, we will concentrate on the communicative functioning of the child. In this sense, the etiology becomes irrelevant; we simply "stick to the behaviors." At the same time, such reasoning has led to disastrous blunders in which, for example, hearing-impaired children are misclassified as retarded, disturbed, or aphasic (Hodgson 1969; Kleffner 1973). Further, we have a responsibility to understand any client as fully as possible, particularly because we must make predictions regarding the child's future development. These predictions are important in determining school placements and making referrals, as well as in planning language interventions. In addition, though, it is extremely important that parents develop realistic expectations of what lies ahead for them and their child.

We walk a fine line in this area. It is well documented that labeling children, or making predictions about their future development can literally affect that development (e.g., Rosenthal and Jacobson, 1968). As already mentioned, labels easily become "self-sealing premises." At the same time, parents must plan for the future. In addition, many laws require that children be identified or certified as belonging to a particular etiological category before they can receive special services in the schools. Normally the determination of etiologies for these purposes involves assessment by various specialties, such as pediatrics, audiology, psychology or psychiatry, and education, as well as speech and language pathology. A specific diagnostic label may still be of little use in understanding a child, partly because each child is different and partly because characteristics of different etiological classifications may overlap in the same child. As we will see, what is most important is that adequate follow-up measures be taken to insure that any labels that are offered do not become self-fulfilling prophecies and thus function to the detriment of the child.

CONCLUSIONS

When I was in high school, I wanted to be a lawyer like Clarence Darrow. While arguing a particular case, he would put a larger issue on trial at the same time. Maybe I'm getting there at last. In discussing possible etiologies for children's language disorders, I have also attempted to evaluate our views of causation in human development on a broader scale. While I have no data to support this assertion, it is my guess that most of us apply linear cause-and-effect thinking in many of the situations we encounter. Whorf (1956) might have said that it's in the structure of our language. Korzybski (1948) thought that it is in the structure of our logic. Doubtless, there is much in our culture that supports this view of cause and effect. Generally, it is a punctuation of the stream of events that we are comfortable with.

I have argued, however, that linear cause-and-effect views are likely to be inadequate in understanding the genesis of complex human conditions, such as disorders of language in children. The influences on language development are just not that simple and direct. Consequently, I have espoused the principles of general systems theory, which indeed have the flexibility to encompass the most complex causal relations. At the same time, general systems theory is perhaps a little unwieldy to use as a practical vehicle for approaching etiology in clinical work. Therefore, I have adopted Sameroff's (1975) transactional view of causation as a perspective that can handle the complexity and yet at the same time is not too formidable for practical application.

The transactional model seems to be an appropriate vehicle for understanding the general systems principle of equifinality, that the same beginnings can lead to different ends and vice versa. This way we can resolve the apparent contradictions between the retrospective and prospective studies discussed at the beginning of the chapter. Further, the transactional model provides a way to view the development of disorders associated with language impairment, such as retardation and emotional disturbance, and their relations with language disorders. It also provides a vehicle to approach those cases of "functional language delay" and "ideopathic language disorders," for which we simply can't generate any specific hypotheses about etiology. As Mahoney (1975) says, language development isn't a goal, it's a continually evolving process.

Working through the transactional model forces us to focus on communication of various sorts. Sameroff's (1975) transactions, after all, are a series of exchanges between the child and the environment, a particularly appropriate way to approach disorders of language. Further, it is through these transactions that morphostatic and morphogenic processes, those recurring events that inhibit or encourage change, occur. While we cannot expect to understand all these processes in one hour, by working with a child we can discover ways to intervene in some of the child's transactional patterns that are morphogenic, that accelerate development in the child.

As we will see in the next chapter, our understanding of causation is linked to our approach to assessment, which in turn blends into intervention. The overall intervention strategy, ultimately, is to alter some of the child's transactions with the environment. These transactions, in turn, are discovered and assessed through preliminary work with the child, based on attempting to understand the child through the transactional model. Because of the principles of equifinality and wholeness, we can intervene in different ways, depending on our assessment of the child's situation. Thus, we may focus on conceptual development, relationship functioning, information-processing skills as they relate to language use, environmental factors, or on language structure itself. We choose among these options, and combinations of them, according to our continuing evaluation of which interventions will most efficiently enhance the child's use of language.

7

PRINCIPLES
OF ASSESSMENT

Assessment means appraisal, evaluation, a sizing up of the child and the situation; it means determining what the child does and does not do and then making clinical sense out of that information; it means determining a child's strengths and weaknesses; it is a process in which we take in information about a child and then use that information in making decisions about that child.

There are a great many areas to be considered in assessing a language-impaired child. First, we are interested in the child's communicative functioning. Obviously, we will want to evaluate language use in comprehension as well as expression. Both vocabulary and grammatical options are important. In addition, we are interested in more general relationship communication. How does the child function with the clinician, peers, and family? We are led to nonverbal communication and iconic signs. Overall, we want to evaluate the child's communicative behavior in terms of its degrees of discreteness, discursiveness, and effectiveness. In addition to all these areas of interpersonal communication, we are interested in the child's cognitive functioning. It may be important to know what types of concepts the child uses. Further, we need to be on the lookout for difficulties in the five aspects of human information processing and related areas of perception. In a third vein, we need to search for factors that may have contributed to the development of the language disorder or that are instrumental in maintaining it. Included in this area are both neurophysiological and environmental factors, and related developmental disorders. Finally, we need to interpret all this information from the perspective of the transactional model of causation and derive some options for intervention from that interpretation.

What I have outlined in the preceding paragraph is a tall order indeed. It turns out that the clinician will not need every bit of that information for every child. At the same time, one must be prepared to obtain whatever information is relevant for a particular child. In this chapter I will develop a perspective and discuss assessment procedures. The following chapter will be devoted to language sample analysis.

THE PROCESS OF ASSESSMENT

Assessment continues as long as we have contact with the child. While the goal is always to evaluate the child's functioning, assessment will have somewhat different forms at various times. Generally, an initial assessment is carried out during the first meetings with the child and parents. The goal is to determine if a language disorder is present and, if so what general approaches to intervention might be appropriate. Assessment continues as an intervention strategy develops. The early sessions will concentrate on exploring the child's difficulties with language in more detail and on discovering what specific types of intervention have the most potential for the child. As these interventions develop, their effectiveness is assessed. The child's progress is monitored throughout training so that new goals can be selected and, at an appropriate time, a decision can be reached concerning when the child no longer needs special help.

As long as you know someone, you learn more and more about that person. Assessment is a formalization of that process in the context of the clinical relationship. Let us look in more detail at the points along the way.

Initial Assessment

The first time the clinician sees the child, the major questions are, does the child demonstrate a significant impairment in the use of language, and if so, in what areas? That is, a decision is required concerning whether or not the child is likely to benefit from special treatment of some sort. An initial assessment is usually relatively brief, perhaps an hour or an hour and a half. The evaluation is likely to focus on the levels of functioning demonstrated by the child. The clinician gathers evidence relevant to deciding whether or not the child is operating at age level. The child's performance is often compared with age norms of various sorts.

In an initial assessment, then, we are concerned with the overall communicative effectiveness of the child's language use and with the appropriateness of a variety of language skills for the child's age level. In addition, some first impressions may be made about what areas of the child's functioning may require intervention. Let us assume now that on the basis of an initial assessment, it is determined that a child does indeed demonstrate a language disorder. The child is enrolled for training, and we expand to another level of evaluation.

Continuing Assessment

The purpose of assessment is now different. We want to concentrate on identifying those areas in which the child is having difficulty, describe those difficulties, and determine what strategies for intervention might be most effective. We will assess the child's language skills in more depth. We will investigate environmental factors or relationship factors if the child's communicative functioning leads us in those directions. Similarly, we will explore the conceptual or information-processing components of language use if the child's difficulties point toward those areas. Frequently it will be necessary to gather information in more than one of these domains. In addition, we

will look for signs of related developmental disabilities. From the perspective of the transactional model we seek to find out what changes in the child and/or in the environment are most likely to lead to enhanced language skill.

Continuing assessment differs from initial assessment in several ways. While initial assessments are likely to be similar with different children, at least with those of the same age levels, continuing assessment will be different for each child because the clinician follows the implications in the child's behavior. If comprehension is adequate but expression is poor and, further, expression varies from situation to situation, the clinician would be more likely to explore relationship aspects of the child's language use than information-processing aspects. On the other hand, if a child comprehends very short utterances but gets confused with longer ones and this phenomenon occurs in various situations, the clinician might focus on information processing and language structure.

Another difference is that continuing assessment will explore particular areas in more depth than that required merely to identify the presence of a disorder. In particular, because a person's cognitive and interpersonal strategies both vary across different situations, a particular area of skill such as comprehension will have to be assessed in differing contexts. This observation suggests an additional difference. While structured tests may be used in continuing assessment, there will be more emphasis on informal procedures devised by the clinician. For the most part, structured tests do not assess in sufficient depth.

The assessment needed to develop an intervention strategy may take a few sessions with the child or it may extend over numbers of weeks. This period of assessment often blends into intervention. There is no abrupt shift between the two. As the clinician's assessment gets more and more individualized to the child and increasingly specific to particular areas of functioning, it evolves into training. There is only one caution I would raise about the duration of this intensive assessment. Especially with complicated children, it may be tempting to keep on evaluating for months and months. There is always one more area to check, one more test to give. Some children are surely difficult to understand. Unending assessment, however, frequently becomes a search for a lingui-communicative Holy Grail. Following a period of assessment the clinician may learn more about a puzzling child by moving into intervention and observing the child's reactions, rather than by continuing the evaluation indefinitely. I will discuss this matter in more depth in the section on exploratory teaching.

Finally, in contrast to initial assessment, the context of evaluation is expanded in continuing assessment. In addition to working directly with the child in the clinic, the clinician may observe the parents with the child. We may make home visits or consult with the child's teachers. If signs of related areas of developmental disability are present, we may make referrals and collaborate with other specialists.

Conclusion

In this overview I have tried to illustrate that assessment is not a set of procedures that the clinician selects from, but a problem-solving process that the clinician engages in. The problems to be solved vary with the status of the child. Most commonly they begin with deciding whether or not the child is likely to benefit from special help. If this decision is affirmative, the next questions involve determining as precisely as possible just what difficulties the child is having in using language, how these difficulties fit in the transactional patterns between the child and the environment, and what types of intervention might be most effective. As a clinician learns more about a child, the assessment questions get increasingly precise and specific to that child. Thus evaluation is at least somewhat unique for each child. In addition, as training procedures and goals become established, the assessment problems to be solved become more and more a matter of determining when a particular goal has been sufficiently established or when the focus of intervention can shift from one area to others.

Prediction

If I had to define assessment, evaluation, diagnosis, and similar terms in one word, that word would be *prediction*.[1] During initial assessment the goal is to decide whether or not the child demonstrates a language disorder. The importance of this decision is in the prediction it carries with it. If it is decided that a particular child does not demonstrate significant language impairment, we are really predicting that the child will develop language normally without intervention. Conversely, recommending intervention implies the prediction that the child either will not improve in language skill without special help, or at least that such development will be behind schedule. In the latter case there is the additional prediction that delayed development will lead to further difficulties. Similarly, if we identify specific problem areas, we are predicting that those areas will remain im-

---

[1] I am grateful to Ralph Shelton for first teaching me the importance of prediction in assessment.

paired at least for some time. Further, choosing certain types of intervention on the basis of assessment is a prediction that those approaches are likely to produce change. Even dismissing a child from training is a prediction, this time that the child will not require further special help, or at least that a continuation of the present intervention will not be of benefit.

Ultimately, then, we are interested not only in what individual language-disordered children are like, but equally, in where they are going. The prediction of human events is never easy, as we saw in the discussion of high-risk factors in Chapter 6. Further, it turns out that the younger the child, the more difficult prediction of future development becomes. The irony is that we would like to identify children who will need help in language development as early as possible, the assumption being that early intervention is likely to be more effective in the long run. The transactional model is important here because it helps explain why prediction is so difficult. An individual's future development is never the product solely of past history and the present situation. There are always further transactions down the road. In spite of the difficulties associated with prediction, it is a useful perspective to adopt in evaluating children. While often implicit, prediction is the core of assessment.

AREAS TO BE ASSESSED

Now that we have an idea of the process of assessment, let us identify the areas of information that should be explored. These areas will include not only particular behavioral repertoires but also information about the contexts in which those behaviors occur. Very generally, there are three domains that

we will need to explore: interpersonal relations, neurophysiological status, and the child's knowledge and skills in areas that are directly related to language use. Let us look at each of these three separately.[2]

Interpersonal Aspects of Behavior

The interpersonal aspects of behavior include not only relationship functioning but in addition such things as attitudes, motivation, and emotional factors. In line with Chapter 5, these areas are inseparable from human relationships. Further, relationship rules are "meta" to linguistic rules and to many other areas of behavior as well. In assessing a child, then, it will be necessary to interpret the child's behavior in terms of the relationship. If a client is cooperative, attentive, responsive, and in general appears to be positively motivated, then the relationship is likely to be one in which you can interpret the child's behavior as representing levels of skill and knowledge (assuming you sample in sufficient depth). Your assessment can proceed just as mapped out in the lesson plan. If, however, the client is fearful, hesitant, distractible, hostile, withdrawn, or in other ways not cooperative, attentive, or responsive, then the observable behavior may not represent at all that child's levels of skill and knowledge. It will be necessary to deal with the relationship before you can interpret the child's behavior in other areas related to language.

The relations between language and culture discussed in Chapter 5 are important here. The culturally different child may respond poorly for reasons that have nothing to do with language skill. This child's

---

[2] This section was inspired by the work of Jim Chalfant and Georgia Foster. While I have adapted their ideas considerably, it was Chalfant and Foster who started me thinking in many of these directions.

responses may be inhibited by fear or because of values held by the peer culture concerning behavior in school. In some situations "good" behavior may cause a child to lose status with peers. Again, a child may be operating under different cultural metarules than those of the examiner, for example, in producing only minimal talking in front of an adult or in not allowing eye contact. Thus, interpersonal factors are influenced not only by each child's specific transactional history but also by the larger cultural traditions in which those transactions have occurred.

In this discussion we are focusing on the child's behavior during assessment itself. Obviously, relationship factors will be important at larger levels as well, in accordance with the transactional model. I will discuss this matter in later chapters. Our first and often most direct access to the child's transactions with the environment, however, is in the relationship between the child and the clinician or trainer.

The Physiological Determinants of Behavior

While I have been stressing environmental and relationship factors, there is no doubt that physiological factors play a part in the transactional model. In addition to the neurophysical and genetic contributions to development discussed in Chapter 6, there are other physiological factors that may affect the child's functioning during assessment. Fatigue, medication the child is receiving, poor diet, disease ranging from colds to more serious afflictions, and other physiological factors may influence how the child behaves at any one time.

The treatment and even identification of such physiological factors is often beyond the scope of our professional training and responsibility. Nevertheless, such factors may be very important in trying to understand the behavior of particular children. A teacher friend of mine, for example, once had a sixth-grade boy who might be described as "dull and unresponsive." The child demonstrated little interest in school, although he attended regularly. He participated in classroom activities in minimal fashion, and he sometimes dozed off during class. It turned out that his parents ran a tavern and lived in a small apartment at the back of the building. The child rarely got to sleep before 3:00 A.M., he got himself up in the morning, and ate what he pleased, if anything, for breakfast. Intervention in such a situation may be touchy to say the least, and may be best left to other personnel. At the same time, understanding this boy's pattern of living greatly altered the teacher's assessment of him.

Most of our information about physiological factors comes from three sources. First, we can interview the parents, or the child if old enough. Second, it is sometimes possible to observe a child over time. Suppose a child is particularly distractible or unresponsive. We attempt different relationship tactics, but to no avail. It might be possible at that point to work with the child at different times of the day and notice any differences in behavior. The child may be more amenable to training at certain hours than others. The third source of information is through referrals and consultations with other professionals. This is the avenue through which we find out about hearing loss, for example.

As already mentioned, it is not our function to treat directly the physiological determinants of behavior. Occasionally we can work toward change in some areas, especially in cooperation with other specialists. Physiological factors, however, may have powerful effects on the child's transactions with the environment in general and behavior during assessment and training in particular. Therefore, the more we know about the presence of such factors, the more wisely we can devise an intervention plan.

The Child's Knowledge and Skills

We come now to the bread and butter of language specialists, those areas discussed in Chapters 1 through 4. Conceptual development, information processing and attendant perceptual skills, and knowledge of language are certainly important factors in the child's ability to use language. Let us look at each of these areas briefly.

Conceptual Development

Children use language to represent their knowledge of the world. It is convenient to consider this knowledge as being embodied in concepts. It therefore becomes important to get an idea of how the child operates conceptually. It is not necessary to plumb every aspect of the child's conceptual system. Rather, we are interested in what types of concepts the child appears to employ. It is important to discover if the child seems to know about the world primarily through core concepts, with their attendant functional relations and their emphasis on use. We wonder if the child also has knowledge of perceptual attributes and concrete concepts. Finally, we are interested in the child's use of abstract concepts. To use language fully the child must be conversant with all three types of concepts.

Frequently the clinician can find out if the child uses at least some of each type of concept in a relatively brief period of time. By observing the child in play and using various objects one obtains evidence about core concepts. Similarly, if the child is able to sort or identify various objects and pictures, then at least some concrete concepts are present. Activities such as following directions, defining words, and pretending illustrate aspects of abstract concepts. With many children this type of assessment will be brief or unnecessary. They obviously have a conceptual system sufficiently rich for language learning. With certain children, however, it may be very important to understand how the child knows about the world. Intervention will be different with an immature or retarded child who functions primarily with core concepts than it will be with a child who uses a broader range of concepts.

In addition, with some severely impaired children it may be necessary to ascertain if the child possesses particular areas of conceptual knowledge that are related to grammatical structures. Does the child know some concepts that can be associated with semantic cases such as agent, object, and action? Similarly, does the child have in some form the concepts related to grammatical operators such as future and present, singular and plural? Finally, we may also need to ask if the child demonstrates knowledge that could be described with conceptual rules, relating various concepts with each other. Does the child connect agents with actions? Objects with locations? It is conceptual rules such as these that underlie the relatedness that is the heart of grammar.

By definition, children who are using language, even though it may be impaired in some way, will show at least some affirmative evidence in all of these conceptual areas. On the other hand, children who demonstrate very little or no use of language, or whose language use is somehow bizarre, may also have deficits in these conceptual areas. Usually observation and informal assessment procedures will be of most value in understanding such children.

Information Processing and Perceptual Skills

As discussed in Chapter 2, language development and use depend on sensory systems, attention, intermodal integration, memory, and cognitive strategies. Further, all of these skills are brought to bear in those processes known as auditory perceptual skills. At the same time, these phenomena are influenced by the knowledge and use of language. As we have seen, information processing and perceptual skills have determinants of their own. These various processes, then, can only be assessed relative to particular tasks in particular contexts. The tasks and contexts we are interested in, of course, are those involving the use of language.

The evidence from adult aphasia indicates that brain dysfunction can indeed impair language processing and that these impairments can be fairly specific. Processing impairments in children, however, are extremely nebulous, both in origin and in character. They can only be understood in association with language and other factors in a general systems framework. In this perspective, the processing deficit *per se* may sometimes become an "effect" rather than a "cause," or it may disappear altogether. It is surprising how many deficits in attention, integration, sequencing, and the like turn out to be artifacts of the particular tasks used or due to interpersonal or cultural factors.

In view of this situation, I am inclined to operate as follows. First, look for other possible determinants of behavior before considering information-processing or perceptual disorders. These other possibili-

ties can be investigated through techniques to be discussed later in the chapter. If I do explore information processing or perceptual functioning, it will be through their direct manifestations in language use, rather than in other tasks. Suppose a child does not repeat utterances accurately, evidence of difficulties with "sequencing" or "memory span." Initially I would look at the interpersonal situation. Is the child bored? Threatened? Confused? Then I would ask if the task has meaning for that particular child. If I assessed memory span and sequencing more specifically, it would be through meaningful sentences, not unrelated words, in order to invoke the chunking inherent in language structure. Further, I would make the task as natural as I possibly could, thus approaching the problem-solving and cognitive strategies the child might actually employ in using language in some real situation. Finally, I would use several different tasks in this assessment.

In sum, information-processing and auditory perceptual deficits seem to be inextricable from the use of language and from the tasks in which they are elicited. It is rarely necessary to reify these processes and assess them separately. We cover the same territory and more by focusing directly on the child's problem solving and use of language in the various tasks that we offer within the clinical relationship.

Knowledge of Language

Finally, of course, we are concerned with what the child can do with language itself. We are interested in the child's general effectiveness as a communicator commensurate with age and also in more technical aspects of the child's command of language. At both levels we attempt to discover which options-to-mean a particular child has available and the grammatical and semantic accuracy or precision with which those options are employed. The child's skill in comprehension as well as expression will be evaluated.

It is often helpful to organize the analysis of a child's grammatical knowledge around a language sample. This sample contains a record of grammatical relations and particular structures that the child actually employed. It demonstrates some of the things the child can do with language. Following language sampling, further assessment will concentrate on determining the status of structures not represented in the sample and analysis of errors contained in the sample. In addition, we are interested in pragmatics, or language use. This area can only be assessed during direct interaction with the child, because pragmatics focuses on the use of particular utterances in relation to the larger discourse and communicative situation. In assessing pragmatics the clinician must make inferences about the child's intent in producing various utterances. For this reason, and because of the complexity involved, pragmatic skills are rarely evaluated in detail. Recent discussions of pragmatics in relation to children's language disorders will be found in Miller (1978) and Prutting (1979). I will enlarge on this topic in Chapter 9.

In conclusion, interpreting children's behavior as representing concepts, dimensions of information processing, and knowledge of language is fundamental in language assessment. Our understanding of these areas in any one child may never be complete or totally accurate. We can, however, explore a child's functioning in ways that are helpful in planning intervention. As we discover what a child does and does not do with language, we are better able to devise clinical goals that fit that child's patterns of communication.

Conclusion

I have identified three sets of factors that will require attention during assessment: interpersonal relations, physiological status, and specific knowledge and skills related to language use. Obviously, none of these areas is independent of the others. In the preceding chapter I emphasized a more abstract perspective, focusing on the transactional patterns between child and environment. Assessment of the three areas above, however, contributes to that focus. In looking at interpersonal factors as they occur during assessment, we are considering one set of transactions directly. The other two areas are not transactional patterns of and by themselves, but they contribute to the transactional patterns in which children live and learn. If certain children are continually fatigued or use only one-word utterances, individuals in the environment must respond in terms of those characteristics because that is how those children present themselves in their transactions with the environment. It might be argued, in fact, that transactional patterns are themselves another class of reifications; the idea of such a pattern is certainly an abstract concept. What we can look for during individual assessment of various children, then, are some of the concrete contributions to those patterns. With other techniques we may be able to identify some of the contributors from the larger environment as well.

TECHNIQUES OF ASSESSMENT

It is apparent that there is a wide variety of information that could be included in a language assessment and of procedures that could be used in exploring that information. The focus of any particular assessment will depend on the clinician's purposes, the nature of the child, and, doubtless, the biases of the clinician. In this section I will consider various techniques of assessment with a view toward what types of information they provide and how they can be used.

Sources of Information

To begin with, there are three very general sources of information about children who are possibly impaired in language use. We gather information from parents and caretakers, we obtain information from other professionals who are in contact with the child, and, of course, we look directly at the child's performance. Let us consider each of these sources briefly.

Parents

Parents and caretakers provide an important source of information. Often, talking with parents is the only way we can find out about the child's developmental history and use of language outside of the clinic or school. The family obviously plays an important role in the transactional history of the child's development and in the transactional patterns that are current in the child's life. Because of these roles and the complexity of the family system, I will discuss parents and families in detail later in the book.

For the present it will suffice to note that information can be obtained from parents in several ways. Obviously we may interview the parents directly. Frequently parents are asked to fill out a questionnaire on the child's developmental history and the nature of the language disorder (see, for example, Darley 1978; Byrne 1978b). On some occa-

sions a clinician may observe the parents and child interacting together in a clinic room. Finally, home visits are sometimes arranged, during which the clinician can observe the child's functioning in a "natural habitat" and view interaction between the child and various family members.

Other Professionals

In addition to the child's parents, we frequently obtain information from other specialists. It is important to be aware of the status of the child's hearing, for example. Often the clinician may consult with the child's teachers as well. As the situation warrants, we may also contact pediatricians, neurologists, psychologists, psychiatrists, and other specialists. Alternately, we may be contacted by any of those individuals. In fact, in communities where such arrangements are practical, children with developmental disorders are often seen by interdisciplinary teams of specialists. In the case of children with pervasive disorders such as autism or children with multiple handicaps, the participation of various specialists is essential in developing efficient interventions.

The Child's Performance

The ultimate source of information about children's language is, of course, the children themselves. We observe the child as a communicator and we assess specific aspects of the child's performance. If the child exhibits sufficient expressive language to make it worthwhile, assessment will usually include an analysis of the child's spontaneous talking. Language-sampling techniques will be discussed in the next chapter. The rest of this chapter will focus on procedures for assessing children's skills and knowledge as represented in their behavior. First, we will consider the problem of interpreting the child's behavior in general. We will then look at various techniques for eliciting and interpreting specific aspects of that behavior.

Interpretation of Children's Behavior

Assessment is a process of eliciting behavior from children and then interpreting that behavior. In previous chapters I have built a broad background for interpreting children's behavior. As you well know, it is one thing to elicit a particular behavior and quite another to know just what that behavior means. It is even more difficult to understand a child if various behaviors are not produced at all. In this section we will consider some of the factors involved in interpreting children's behavior.

Multiple Determination of Behavior

The assertion that behavior is multiply determined is by now a standard theme of mine, to be sung in the key of G. I will not dwell on it, but use it as a place to start in interpreting children's behavior. The development of a language disorder is associated with multiple causal factors. The transactional model illustrates this process. Further, one's behavior at any moment is also multiply determined. It follows from both of these observations that the child's behavior during assessment will stem from a variety of factors, in general systems fashion. The question I wish to address is, how can we apply these abstract ideas in interpreting children's behavior?

Selection From a Repertoire

In Chapter 4 we encountered Halliday's (1973) idea of a behavior potential. More specifically, each person has a repertoire of possible behaviors that can be employed in any specific situation. Further, there is a hierarchy of metarules guiding the selection of behaviors from this repertoire on any occasion. As Goodnow (1972) puts it, how one behaves is the result of selection from the individual's repertoire. She goes on to point out that, for the behavior to be appropriate or effective, there must be a match between the demands of the situation and the particular behavior that is selected. The problem-solving aspect of behavior is thus emphasized.

For example, when presented with a set of pictures and the request that each picture be named, the child's repertoire of behavior contains a number of responses that could be selected. The child could name the pictures, say "I don't know," play with the pictures, look away, talk about something else, throw the pictures on the floor, and so on. As just mentioned, a correct response means a match between the behavior the child selects and the demands of the situation, which are defined by the clinician.

There are several possible reasons for a child to respond in a way that does not match the situation (Goodnow 1972). First, the appropriate behavior may not exist in the child's repertoire. The child simply doesn't possess that knowledge or response. Throughout our school years, we have been heavily conditioned to think of errors on tests in this fashion. Similarly, in assessment, if a child does poorly on a test, we may conclude the child doesn't know much in the area covered by that test.

Goodnow describes several other possibilities for a mismatch between the child's behavior and the situation, however. First, there may be too many demands on the child at the same time. For example, an immature child may be unable to sit still long enough to attend to an entire test. In many tests the child has to remember the directions, as well as respond to each item, as well as sit still and inhibit other activity. A second source of mismatches is in ritualized behavior on the part of the child. The same response may be employed in different situations, whether appropriate or not. I recall a child who used to nod and smile no matter what was said to him. A third type of mismatch may occur in situations where the "correct" or "incorrect" behavior is defined in a very restricted way. In some vocabulary tests, for example, the child must choose from a set of pictures the one that matches the word spoken by the examiner. The child who names all the pictures cannot be scored. Further, as pointed out in the discussion of the picture-utterance match task in Chapter 3, a child may possess the appropriate knowledge but be led to a different response by the nature of the task.

Finally, a child's response may not match the demands of the situation because the rules of behavior for the situation are implicit or are assumed by the clinician. Consequently, the child's punctuation of the situation may differ from that of the clinician. Hayes (1972) noted that the examiner is frequently not engaging in normal social interaction with a child. In asking questions the clinician is often not seeking any particular information the child may supply in answering. Rather, the clinician wants to find out if the child knows the answers or is able to verbalize them. For example, a clinician is watching a child who is working on a puzzle. The clinician asks, "What are you doing?" It is patently obvious what the child is doing. A young child may therefore not understand the point of such a question. An older child may recognize the question as an attempt to elicit talking. If this child is already embarrassed about talking, the response may still be silence. Such difficulties may be particularly important with culturally different children.

Many of these difficulties in achieving a match between a child's behavior and the clinician's expectations become particularly acute when the assessment is brief or when a particular area of skill is evaluated with only a few items. The best insurance against errors of interpretation due to problems such as those just described is to sample each area in depth and breadth. We can look at a particular skill, say use of verbs, in both comprehension and expression, in different contexts, using different activities, and on different days. The sections in this chapter on informal procedures and exploratory teaching will expand on this aspect of assessment.

Responses during assessment, then, result from selections from various repertoires the child possesses. We have already identified some influences on that selection, including relationship and physiological factors and the child's knowledge and skills related to language. These areas determine both the repertoires of behaviors the child has available and the metarules that dictate selections among those options. A child might behave inappropriately (that is, not demonstrate desired or "correct" behavior during a language assessment) because the child does not know the desired response, because the procedure does not elicit that response, or because the child elects not to produce it for some other reason. The child's behavioral selections, then, are influenced not only by what options the child has available but also by that child's punctuation and problem-solving decisions in the situation. With these ideas in mind let us now look at some specific procedures for assessment.

Standardized Tests

All assessment begins with observation. We present some sort of situation and then observe the child's behavior in that context. Standardized tests represent one technique for clinical observation, and they have two special characteristics. First, each test provides a specific set of stimuli to elicit behavior from the child and specific standards to evaluate that behavior. Consequently, each child is treated very nearly the same, thus minimizing the chances of children's performances varying because of differences in the testing procedure. Second, standardized tests are designed to provide a means for comparing one child with other children. The standardized test administration makes this goal possible. Toward this end, many tests provide normative data, so that a particular child's performance can be compared with that of a reference group of other children.

A child's performance on a test is usually described with a score or age level, although some tests also provide a profile of subtest scores. Such scores are intended to represent the child's levels of functioning. Because of this focus on a total or overall score, the primary use of most tests is in determining a child's level of functioning in whatever area the test measures. Tests are therefore most useful when the clinician needs to specify these levels for a child, such as in initial assessment. Many special programs for developmentally disabled youngsters require that children have certain characteristics in order to be enrolled. Standardized tests provide a means for certifying or documenting that children meet those criteria.

The interpretation of a child's behavior in terms of a total score leads to another characteristic of standardized tests. They rarely provide the detail necessary for developing an intervention plan. A test may indicate that a child is functioning below age level in a certain area, such as grammar or vocabulary, but tests rarely tell the clinician precisely what the child needs to learn. That is, they do not show what aspects of grammar or vocabulary are deficient, because each aspect is sampled in only minimal fashion. This situation is not necessarily a "fault" of standardized tests. Rather, it is an artifact of the purpose for which most tests are designed, which is to derive an indication of overall functioning.

Validity and Reliability

Validity and reliability are important in any assessment procedure. Good discussions of these ideas will be found in Kelly (1967) and Buros (1972). Students, teachers, and clinicians alike are harangued about these terms, but validity and reliability still remain abstractions to many people. Ultimately they are related to your interpretation of the child's behavior. Can you trust your results?

Validity and reliability are usually considered in academic and intellectual terms. Let me attempt to put more of an emotional cast to them. Think back across your college career to some test that you took that was truly unfair. Almost everyone has encountered at least one such test at some time. Perhaps the instructor asked questions that had nothing to do with the course content (a problem of validity) or asked questions that were so vague they could be answered in many ways but not all of those answers were considered correct (a problem of reliability). How did you feel when that test was returned? Most people feel angry or depressed. You've been robbed, cheated, done in! Your performance in that course was misrepresented. Validity and reliability, then, are not merely academic abstractions; they affect people's lives.

Take this illustration one step further. What can you do when an unfair test is returned to you? In the first place, you are likely to recognize that the test was indeed unfair. Having made this observation, you can take some sort of action. You can complain, lobby for more points, drop the class, see the dean, picket the professor's office, or whatever. Now consider a six-year-old child who is evaluated with procedures that are invalid or unreliable. It is highly unlikely that this child will recognize anything as abstract as a test of language skill as being invalid or unreliable, much less challenge you about it. The result is that a child is evaluated unfairly and *no one knows it,* or at most, only you, the clinician, are aware of it. The solutions to this problem are well known. First, avoid tests for which the validity or reliability is inadequate or which do not report evaluations of these parameters. Second, if you use a procedure of unknown or questionable validity or reliability, be sure to assess the same area in other ways, so that your interpretation is not based only on the one procedure.

In our attempts to develop tests that are reliable, we have developed procedures that control all the stimuli and channel the child toward a very specific response. The picture-utterance match task discussed in Chapter 3 is a good example. Ironically, however, such procedures generate other problems. They can be invalid, for example, because they evoke different problem-solving strategies than those associated with more natural use of language.

Because of the restricted nature of the task they set for the child, language tests are sometimes described as indicating minimum levels of the child's functioning. That is, the number of correct responses a child makes is likely to be a valid indicator of some knowledge the child possesses. The incorrect responses, however, may underestimate the child's command of language.

It was pointed out earlier that many standardized tests provide a basis for comparing a child's performance with other children's through the use of normative data. The problems of trustworthiness arise again, however. Determining the level of a child's functioning by comparing it with norms that are inappropriate or poorly developed may lead to errors in interpreting the behavior of particular children. Weiner and Hoock (1973) have discussed the development of norms in detail. Because of the amount of work and expense involved in developing normative data, many tests are produced in which the quality of the norms does not approach that discussed by Weiner and Hoock.

Finally, structured tests are notorious for eliciting poor responses from culturally different children, particularly when more than one cultural factor is operating. Consider a minority child who either speaks a nonstandard dialect or is bilingual and in addition is living in conditions of poverty. It will be difficult to obtain reliable, valid standardized test results on this child. Not only are there the interpersonal cultural factors mentioned earlier. In addition, test items are typically selected to reflect Standard English. Further, most tests are normed on middle-class children.

Conclusion

Standardized tests may be most useful in providing information on the minimal levels at which children are performing. By their very nature tests cannot pinpoint precisely what a child needs to learn. Some tests, such as the *Illinois Test of Psycholinguistic Abilities,* are designed to give a profile of scores, indicating a child's strengths and weaknesses in a variety of areas. Each of the subscores in such a profile, however, is still a level of performance rather than an analysis of performance. In my judgment, then, a thorough assessment cannot be accomplished on the basis of standardized tests alone. Tests make a useful contribution to initial assessment, in which a major purpose is to determine if the child's level of functioning is such that intervention should be recommended. They may also provide helpful comparisons to some of one's conclusions from informal procedures.

I have not listed and described specific tests because this information is available elsewhere and because individual preferences vary greatly among clinicians. Discussions of relevant tests will be found in Byrne (1978a), Irwin and Marge (1972), and Wiig and Semel (1976). Critical reviews of many tests are included in Buros (1972) and in Darley (1979). Tests, in sum, play a useful but limited role in language assessment. In most evaluations, test results are complemented with informal assessment procedures. It is to this topic that we now turn.

Informal Procedures

Standardized testing developed with the philosophy that each child must be treated exactly the same. The procedures for administering a test must be fully described in the test manual and precisely followed by the clinician. It has been argued that the test procedure must remain the same in order for different children to be evaluated fairly. A consistent administration is certainly needed if children are to be compared with norms. The application of an unvarying procedure, however, might also be unfair to the child. It might not illuminate what the child really knows. The mismatches between the child's behavior and the demands of the situation discussed earlier would be examples of this possibility. Olson (1970a) compares the use of highly specified and consistent procedures with the "clinical method" developed by Piaget. As Olson sees it, the

object of the clinical method is to make sure the child understands what is wanted. The likelihood of a match between the child's behavior and the clinician's expectations is thus enhanced. At the same time, the procedure is no longer standardized. Some children may need more explanation or different kinds of stimulation than others.

Glucksberg, Hay, and Danks (1976) have illustrated very nicely the importance of the clinical method. It has been reported (Donaldson and Wales 1970) that children of certain ages do not differentiate between the words *same* and *different*. They appear to treat the two words alike. Glucksberg, Hay, and Danks studied children's understanding of these words in two different sentence frames. They found that the children confused *same* and *different* in one of these tasks but not in the other. Further, adults showed the same patterns! The task in which the errors occurred was as follows. Five objects were placed on a table, including, say, three pencils and two items from a different class, such as toothbrushes. Two of the pencils were identical and one was different in some detail such as color or length. The experimenter picked up one of the identical pencils and said to the subject, *Show me something different.* Both children and adults frequently chose the nonidentical pencil. Apparently they interpreted the experimenter's remark as a request for another pencil, but one that was different in some detail. Their "error" was in how they interpreted the whole sentence, not in their comprehension of *same* and *different*. Glucksberg, Hay, and Danks (1976) conclude that it is risky to study knowledge of vocabulary items outside of their sentential contexts. I would suggest that similar problems are present in attempting to assess grammatical structures. Glucksberg, Hay, and Danks conclude that, "We are on relatively firm ground when children perform in ways that lead us to infer that they 'know' the meanings of words by responding appropriately to a variety of utterances in widely ranging contexts. Inferences of incompetence, on the other hand, are suspect on the grounds that children may 'fail' one or another test of comprehension for any one of a number of reasons" (1976, p. 740). Again, I would apply this conclusion to grammatical structures as well as words. Whether or not a child "knows" some aspect of language may depend on the specific means employed to test that knowledge. It is precisely because of this problem that the clinical method is of such importance. Standardized procedures, by definition, do not have the flexibility to explore the child's knowledge of particular vocabulary or grammatical items. In my mind, then, making sure the child understands the tasks or what is wanted is a cornerstone of informal procedures in assessment. With older children it may involve explanations, examples of various kinds, and different types of probes. With younger children abstract explanations may be minimized, but various probes and situations can be provided in an attempt to insure that the child's repertoire is fairly sampled.

Informal techniques are subject to the same problems of validity and reliability that structured tests are. It is each clinician's responsibility, therefore, to make the results of informal procedures as trustworthy as possible. Fortunately this goal is inherent in the process. To convince yourself of the validity and reliability of your procedures, you assess the same area with different tasks and in different relationship contexts. Suppose, for example, that a child is inconsistent in demonstrating comprehension. If this inconsistency remains across different tasks, one might shift the focus to the interpersonal context. Perhaps a change in the clini-

cian's relationship behavior will produce a difference in the child's attending and responding. On the other hand, if a child does not demonstrate comprehension of a grammatical structure such as plural in either play or structured activities, whether using pictures or concrete objects, and does not use plurals in expressive language, the clinician begins to feel some confidence that the plural is an area of grammar that this child does not possess.

It is noteworthy that if for any reason structured tests cannot be administered to a particular child, informal procedures are the only source of direct information. If a child does not respond to test items or is too distractible for tests to be administered, we still must make decisions about that child. Toward this end, two areas that can be explored informally are general communicative functioning and overall maturational level.

Assessment of General Communicative Functioning

The idea here is to get a picture of the child as a communicator. Frequently we can get information in this area through parent conferences. We also want to look at the child's communicative behavior directly. The general technique is to engage the child in some sort of social interaction and then observe the child during that exchange. A young child may be offered play materials. I would begin with materials that are social in function, such as a tea set or a group of puppets, so that it is "natural" for the clinician to join in. Some activities are essentially individual in nature but can easily be made social. Building blocks, dollhouses and play workbenches would fit in this category. I would avoid primarily individual activities and those that do not foster social interaction and talking, such as puzzles, painting, and toy cars.

With older children it may not be necessary to use play to establish an avenue for social exchange. In fact, some children may be insulted by play activities you happen to offer. The goal is still the same, though. We want to engage children in discourse that is meaningful to them. I know one clinician who discusses Spider Man comics with some of her junior-high boys. Another asks older children for advice on what movies to see and, of course, why each movie is good. Labov (1972a) asked about the most harrowing or threatening experience each child had encountered.

No matter what techniques are used and what the age of the child, the goal is the same. We want to entice or intrigue the child into talking. The clinician is not the interlocutor, and certainly not the interrogator. Rather, the clinician is someone who is interested in what the child has to say. At the same time, we observe the effectiveness with which the child communicates. Is the use of language discursive? Is it based on a linear logic we can follow? Do the child's utterances represent appropriate pragmatic choices? Do they fit into the flow of discourse? Are sentences employed? Noun phrases? Grammatical morphemes? Does the child appear to comprehend what we say? Are nonverbal iconic gestures used effectively, especially by children who don't talk? Are these gestures discrete and discursive? If engaged in play, does the child's activity demonstrate signs of core concepts? For example, are toys played with appropriately? Conversely, are there signs of abstract symbolic functioning, such as using a block for a car? After a few minutes, one can often engage the child in verbal activities that illustrate abstract use of language. Ask the child to define a few words, or how

to get to the principal's office, or—my favorite—ask the child to tell all the steps in making a peanut butter sandwich. Berry (1969) lists many other areas of behavior that can be observed.

Regardless of their ages and degrees of language deficit, many children will open up in this kind of situation rather quickly, particularly as they perceive that you really are interested in what they have to say. There will be some children, of course, who will not respond, even to our best efforts. Sometimes such a child will participate later in the session or will respond to direct probes such as questions. It is useful to treat unresponsiveness itself as information about the child, rather than as a lack of information, however. We will have to explore the possibility that it is a relationship tactic that is part of the transactional patterns in the child's life. In any case, lack of responsiveness always carries a relationship message along with it. Further, there are degrees of unresponsiveness. Does the child participate in nonverbal activity with the clinician, but without talking, or is the child's participation minimal in any form? If the child participates in any way, does there appear to be much comprehension of language?

In summary, we form a general picture of a child's communicative functioning in the specific situation in which we are evaluating that child. In this sense our observations are valid at the moment, although many children's behavior will change as they become acquainted with the situation.

Developmental Milestones

Another area that can be assessed through informal techniques is the child's overall level of maturation, although the procedure may not be quite as freewheeling as in assessing communicative functioning. There are normative data available on the ages at which a great many skills are achieved. By determining which skills the child is able to perform, we can estimate the child's maturational level. This information is useful in gaining a perspective on a child, particularly during initial assessment. It may be compared with the child's use of language, as evaluated by informal techniques and standardized tests.

Developmental milestones are usually listed in groups according to age level. The items typically attained by three-year-olds are grouped together, those for four-year-olds are grouped together, and so on. In these developmental schedules, individual item validity is generally low (Byrne 1978a). That is, a child cannot be pegged to be a certain age level on the basis of one item, such as "Combines three words." It is the pattern of development as reflected in a variety of developmental items that is important. Similarly, the placement of a particular item at a specific age level does not mean that all children accomplish that milestone at that age. Rather, there is a range of ages associated with each item.

Unfortunately this age range is very large for some of the milestones we are most interested in, such as particular aspects of language. Frankenburg and Dodds (1967) described a series of developmental norms in terms of the percentages of children who demonstrate a particular milestone at different ages. They studied approximately 1,000 children. Consider three examples from their data. "Comprehends three prepositions" was demonstrated by 25 percent of their children at 2.7 years, 50 percent of their children at 3.1 years, 75 percent of their children at 3.4 years, and 90 percent of their children at 4.5 years. The corresponding ages for "Recognizes three colors" were

2.7, 3.0, 3.7, and 4.9 years. For "Follows two of three directions," the ages were 14.8 months, 19.8 months, 22.0 months, and 31 months. These ages cover much of the entire age range during which the most intensive language acquisition occurs in normal children. Further, they encompass virtually half the children's total life spans at the time the testing was done.

It thus becomes difficult to specify precisely at what ages children should achieve specific milestones. Further, there is some evidence that children are attaining at least some developmental milestones earlier than they did twenty or thirty years ago. Garfinkel and Thorndike (1976), for example, compared the 1972 standardization sample of the Stanford-Binet intelligence test with the standardization done in the thirties. They found that many of the items were now passed at earlier ages, particularly those items aimed at younger children. Similarly, Arlt and Goodban (1976) found that children are articulating many sounds correctly at earlier ages than in previously established norms.

One of the most influential sets of developmental norms available was developed by Gesell (1940) and his associates at Yale. These norms have been widely used in fields such as pediatrics and psychology. They contain many items that are relevant to language and communication. More recent editions of the Yale norms have been presented by Knobloch and Pasamanick (1974) in their work on developmental diagnosis, but the original normative data were gathered in the thirties and have thus become quite dated. During the last five years, Knobloch has revised and updated the entire set of norms (Knobloch, Stevens, and Malone 1980), a most welcome addition to the assessment literature.

There are relatively few current norms

relating specifically to language development. Partly, this lack is due to the problems previously mentioned. In addition, this situation reflects the fact that research in language acquisition has turned away from developmental norms to the study of sequences of development, with only general reference to age. An exception is the test by Hedrick, Prather, and Tobin (1975), which contains normative data for many communicative behaviors up to the age of three. The review by Prutting (1979) contains approximate age levels for many areas of semantics, grammar, and pragmatics. Due to the frequently small numbers of children and lack of careful sample selection in the research Prutting drew from, however, these age levels cannot be considered rigorous norms at all. As she suggests, they are better used as tentative guidelines.

Informal Assessment of Language

It has already been pointed out that structured tests do not provide sufficient information about particular aspects of language, such as semantic cases, vocabulary, and grammatical structures. Therefore, the detailed assessment of these areas will be done through informal techniques. We are interested in which options-to-mean the child uses, and how accurately those options are employed.

If the child talks, I would begin with a language-sample analysis. This analysis will vary in how extensive it is, depending on the level of the child's functioning and on the clinician's background and purposes. A language sample seems an efficient place to begin because it supplies concrete information on various aspects of the child's language use. We know what was actually said and the degree of language skill represented by those utterances. Following this first look at the child's talking, we want to explore areas not represented in the language sample and the errors the child produced. The approach to language sampling I will take in the next chapter is based largely on the work of Dever (1978). The sampling technique itself is somewhat informal. While in the early stages the clinician's tasks are to facilitate talking by the child and to listen carefully to that talking, after a while we begin to probe more specific areas. Language sample analysis, then, leads directly to other informal techniques of assessment. Not all aspects of language receive further assessment. Rather, the language sample directs us to those areas we will need to study in more depth.

Perhaps the key concept in these informal techniques is that whatever areas are assessed, they are assessed in multiple ways. Let us consider two examples of multiple assessment of a specific aspect of language from the literature. Washington and Naremore (1978) studied normal preschoolers' acquisition of nine spatial prepositions. Both comprehension and expression were tested for each preposition. In addition, both three-dimensional objects and two-dimensional pictures were used as stimuli. Washington and Naremore found that the number of prepositions the children "knew" (responded correctly to) depended on the testing method. Table 3 illustrates the most dramatic differences, which were with a group of children averaging three years, nine months in age. These data make it very clear that how children exhibit the linguistic information in their repertoires depends on the decision making in the specific communicative task at hand. We simply cannot assess knowledge of language directly.

In another study, Kuczaj II and Maratsos (1975) used other tasks to study the acquisi-

Table 3. Prepositions with at least 70 percent correct responses in four testing situations. N = 20 children, ages 3–6 to 3–11.

Expression		Comprehension	
Objects	Pictures	Objects	Pictures
inside	inside	inside	inside
on	on	on	on
under		under	under
behind		behind	behind
		around	around
		in front of	
		between	
		beside	

Adapted from D. S. Washington and R. C. Naremore, "Children's Use of Spatial Prepositions in Two- and Three-Dimensional Tasks," *J. Speech and Hearing Disorders*, 21, 151–165 (1978).

tion of the prepositions *front, back,* and *side.* Groups of children were asked to demonstrate knowledge of these prepositions relative to their own bodies and to external objects. Further, some of these objects had "intrinsic fronts," such as a toy car or animal, and some did not, such as a drinking glass, a doughnut or a ball. Again, differences were found in the ages at which children responded appropriately to these prepositions, depending on the technique of assessment. As in the Glucksberg, Hay, and Danks (1976) study of *same* and *different* cited earlier, the children's knowledge is not all that is being assessed. In addition, each technique evokes particular problem-solving strategies in the children. These strategies may produce selections from the children's repertoires that do not match the examiner's expectations.

The findings of all three of these studies illustrate the relevance of informal assessment and Piaget's clinical method in general. To understand how well a child

knows a particular grammatical structure, that structure will have to be assessed in multiple ways. Further, these studies underscore the difficulties in attempting to specify age norms for the acquisition of various grammatical structures. Each specific technique produces its own considerable range of ages at which a particular structure occurs, and the range is broadened even further as a variety of techniques are used and the results combined.

Specific Techniques. The next step is to consider some techniques for informal assessment. Leonard, Prutting, Perozzi, and Berkley (1978) discuss several informal tasks that have been employed in research in children's language. Three of these tasks focus on the child's comprehension. First, there is the "identification task." A word or grammatical structure is spoken by the clinician. The child identifies an object or picture that appropriately matches the verbal stimulus. Our famous picture-utterance match task is an example of this category. These authors describe a second receptive task, which they call "acting out." In this case the child demonstrates comprehension by performing whatever event is depicted in the clinician's verbal stimulus. In the third comprehension task the child makes "formal judgments" about the utterances presented by the clinician. The child may be asked if each utterance is correct or acceptable. Alternately, the child may choose which utterance is "better" between pairs of verbal stimuli.

Leonard, Prutting, Perozzi, and Berkley (1978) also describe three tasks for assessing expressive functioning. The first is "imitation." Imitation may be delayed or immediate. The second involves a "completion" task, where a portion of an utterance is presented and the child supplies the missing part. Finally, these authors describe a "paraphrase" task. In one version of this task the clinician tells a brief story to the child, and the child is then asked to tell the story back. The clinician can load the story with a particular grammatical structure, such as past tense markers, and then observe how the child expresses this grammatical category. Dever (1978) has described another paraphrase task, in which he asks a child to tell another child something. In phrasing this directive, the clinician sets up a context in which the child ought to use a particular grammatical structure.

Another dimension in which informal techniques for assessment can be varied involves the structure of the relationship between child and clinician. Obviously, any relationship can vary in many aspects. Perhaps the one of most practical interest is the degree to which the child performs the task because the clinician has directed that it be done. That is, a child may perform a task because it is relevant, useful, or interesting at the moment. On the other hand, the child may perform only as a result of the clinician's directions. In these two situations, the task is punctuated differently by the child. Thus, an identification task might be purely a "test" situation administered by the clinician, or it might be part of a game the child wants very much to play.

While I have described these three dimensions separately, it can be seen that they overlap and, in fact, all three will be represented in some form in any assessment technique. Whatever procedures you use, they will involve both comprehension and some sort of response from the child, they will involve some task or activity that may be more or less abstract, and they will occur in the context of the human relationship between you and the child. The clinician's choices among these alternatives should be based on what will be most efficient with each child. If a child responds well in a heavily directed, testlike situation, you will be able to collect a great deal of information in a short period of time by working in that type of relationship. On the other hand, if the child does not respond in such a situation or you feel that the responses are not representative of a child's skills, you may need to shift to a less structured activity. Some children, for example, may respond minimally if they sense they are being tested. In contrast, the same children may talk freely about favorite topics in a situation where they do not feel stressed.

Similarly, abstract stimuli are an efficient choice, because they are readily available and easily manipulated. If the child does not respond to them, however, one must move to more concrete tasks. I recall attempting to assess general comprehension in a five-year-old boy. I tried giving him commands such as *Stand by the window, Touch the door, Put the book on the table.* No response. He appeared not even to hear me. Notice, though, that there was no point in these commands other than that I wanted him to do various activities. During the next two sessions, I found that he would follow commands quite well if they were functional in the situation from his punctuation. Thus he responded appropriately to commands such as *Take off your coat, Close the door, Turn on the light, Please pick that up* (just after I dropped something), and so on. At first I thought he was responding to the context, rather than to my words. After using different commands and mixing their order during two or three sessions, however, it was apparent that he was responding fairly precisely to what I was saying.

There are still other factors that influence the choice of informal assessment procedures. First, use tasks that are consonant with what you are trying to explore. For example, a paraphrase task may be of little use with a young child who is using primarily two-word utterances. Paraphrase or completion tasks might be very useful in pinpointing the difficulties of older children who use plenty of expressive language but demonstrate specific difficulties in syntax. Imitation is always difficult to interpret because of the special cognitive strategies it evokes, but it may be the only technique that elicits expressive language from some children. The child's preference is another aspect to consider in choosing tasks. If a child prefers a particular type of activity and you're getting useful information with it, obviously you'll want to continue in that vein. Finally, some tasks require more preparation on the part of the clinician than others do. It may not always be easy to devise a concrete, appealing identification task for a twelve-year-old. Again, use the simplest methods that are effective.

Summary

Informal techniques are a rich source of information in assessment. In conjunction with language sampling and exploratory teaching, which is our next topic, they supply the necessary information for moving from an initial assessment to an effective intervention plan. "Informal" simply means not part of a standardized test. A procedure may be devised by the clinician, borrowed from a friend, or taken from the research literature.

While the informal techniques I have described focus on semantics and grammar, similar techniques can be used to explore some of a child's pragmatic decisions. We observe how the child talks in different situations. Similarly, informal techniques are useful in evaluating a child's knowledge

of the different types of concepts described in Chapter 1. Object-sorting tasks such as those described by Sigel and McBane (1967), Goldstein and Scheerer (1941), or Rapaport, Gill, and Schafer (1968) are useful here. By asking children to sort various objects and asking them to explain the sorts they produce, we can explore all levels of concepts and rules.

Through informal techniques we can look at areas that are not included in standardized tests and assess in more depth those areas that are included. It is through informal techniques that the clinician can maximize the chances of obtaining a match between the child's behavior and the demands of the situation. Adapting Piaget's clinical method, the first goal of informal techniques is to make sure the child understands what is wanted, or at least to sample a child's skill and knowledge of an area sufficiently to make a fair assessment. To this end we are likely to use more than one task or technique in evaluating a particular area of skill. The use of various tasks in assessment leads directly to our next topic, exploratory teaching, in which we will take an even more active role in attempting to understand language-disordered children.

EXPLORATORY TEACHING

We have been considering specific techniques of assessment in rather concrete fashion. Let me introduce this next topic with some more abstract notions. On the basis of their work in computer simulation of intelligent behavior, both Simon (1969) and Hunt (1971) have suggested that we should assume that the individual is relatively simple. The processes by which we handle information are very general and not terribly complicated. Rather, the complexity is in the environment, and it is our responses to a complex environment that make us appear complex. Hunt (1971), for example, has shown that a program that will allow a computer to comprehend certain types of sentences is much simpler than the syntax of those sentences. There are limits on behavior, though. An environment can get so complex that human beings simply can't respond effectively. In Simon's (1969) view, these limits somehow result from our neurological makeup. In terms of the chapter on causation, they are constitutional. We know from the transactional model that at least some of these limits can change. Nevertheless, the picture we end up with is one of the human being as an information processor that can respond to increasingly complex environmental stimulation up to a point, that point being determined by limits within the individual.

Let us take a different tack for a moment. Bronfenbrenner (1974, p. 1) quotes one of his early teachers in graduate school, Walter Dearborn, as saying, ". . . if you want to understand something, try to change it." This suggestion is particularly relevant if we view the child's communicative behavior from a general systems perspective and the development of language disorders as occurring through the mechanisms of the transactional model. We cannot "see" transactional patterns. They are abstractions, reifications. We can, however, intervene in situations in which we think transactional patterns are operating. We will be able to observe any changes that our intervention produces. Consider an example from another field. One time I asked a biologist friend how one could study homeostatic mechanisms, such as the maintenance of consistent body temperature, or even prove that homeostatic mechanisms exist. That is, if one merely observes the system, one can't

see the interrelatedness and feedback between components. The system appears to be in a steady state and therefore looks like a set of unrelated parts. His answer was that the biologist has to intervene in the system somehow. Only by instituting change can one become aware of how the system functions. Similarly, if we view language disorders as part of a matrix of cognitive and social factors, subject to both morphostatic and morphogenic processes, we cannot become aware of those processes unless we intrude somehow so that their functions become visible.

These ideas can be combined in considering the assessment of language-disordered children. We can increase the complexity/demands/problem solving in the situation until the child has difficulty. If our sampling of the child's behavior has been sufficient and accurate, we have discovered a limit in the child's functioning. This limit could be constitutional in origin, but it is more likely a reflection of the child's transactional history, including current transactional patterns. This limit in the child's functioning, then, probably has morphostatic functions in the child's transactions and development. Just as with the biologist above, we will have to follow Dearborn's advice: To understand this situation, we will have to try to change it.

Let me recast these theoretical notions now at a more direct clinical level. The central idea was suggested to me by a clinician and teacher by the name of Jim Chalfant: To understand a child's disabilities, teach in the area of deficit.[3] Rather than observing and interpreting the child's behavior in relatively passive fashion, where we reflect on what the child's behavior might mean, we actively try to change the child's com-

---

[3] James Chalfant (1976), personal communication.

municative functioning. I consider this idea a cornerstone of assessment and a very powerful way to understand children with language impairments. The more difficult and complicated the child, the more powerful the technique becomes. Frequently such children have already been assessed very thoroughly, often by different specialists, but with no definitive conclusions. If you attempt to teach such a child, you will find out very quickly how at least some of the impairments function, and in the most meaningful way: interaction with another human being. The same is true of less severely impaired children.

Let us consider the process in more detail. As we make the demands in assessment increasingly complex, the child eventually reaches a "limit." Some children will evidence limits very quickly, while others will perform satisfactorily until the task becomes fairly complicated or subtle. When a child demonstrates such a limit, we try to explore that area in other ways. The child's responses relate to the context. Different situations elicit different punctuations, problem solving, and cognitive strategies. In exploratory teaching the clinician makes changes in the situation or context.

These changes involve alterations in the clinician's relationship behavior and also choices among informal techniques such as those described earlier. Indeed, these interpersonal strategies and informal techniques are not important in assessment only. They are central alternatives for intervention as well. The avenues available for eliciting behavior during assessment are essentially the same as those for eliciting behavior during intervention, although the emphasis may be different.

Consequently, we are exploring both the child's responding and possible ways to intervene in that behavior. Exploratory

teaching, then, takes advantage of the transactional model. The child's behavior can only be understood in terms of the transactional patterns that encompass that behavior. By varying the approach, the clinician generates somewhat different transactional frameworks in which the child can participate. At the same time, certain changes in the child's behavior may also alter the transactional pattern.

Exploratory teaching,[4] then, has two major thrusts. First, it is an important means for assessing the transactional aspects of a child's behavior. These transactions, obviously, are limited to those involving the clinician. Other avenues will be needed to look at the transactional patterns in which the child participates with family and friends. Second, exploratory teaching is a direct bridge between assessment and intervention. As already pointed out, in using different approaches to elicit behavior from a child, we assess not only that behavior but also those approaches. As we find approaches that are effective, we are already involved in intervention.

In discussing exploratory teaching I am not suggesting that the clinician merely improvise, "full muddle ahead." Recall that assessment (and intervention, too) is a problem-solving process. You are attempt-

[4] A few words about terminology might be in order at this point. Readers who are familiar with the literature will quickly realize that the topic of this section is what has been called "diagnostic therapy." We all play word games, though. I didn't want to use the term "diagnostic" because it connotes the medical model. Many speech and language pathologists do not care for the term, "therapy" because it may imply working under prescription. I scratched around for other terms, such as "heuristic habilitation," and finally selected exploratory teaching. This term is not perfect because it requires that teaching be defined more broadly than usual. On the other hand, I like the ambiguity in this expression: Is teaching being used to explore the child's skills, or is teaching itself being explored? As we have seen, the answer is both.

ing to elicit the most competent performance possible from the child. Your problem solving, then, is directed at achieving that goal as efficiently as possible. Thus, the techniques selected will be those the clinician judges most likely to enhance the child's performance.

An Example. A three-and-a-half-year-old girl named Jan will illustrate the process. She was referred because of lack of expressive language. She had been labeled by other specialists as retarded or autistic. It was quickly apparent that standardized tests could not be used. Jan would not attend to the materials for long enough periods of time. The clinician introduced three-dimensional objects that were more playlike in nature, such as blocks and crayons, although still directing Jan's behavior heavily. Jan participated in a number of tasks related to developmental milestones, demonstrating a maturational level roughly equivalent to her chronological age. In the area of language, however, she responded to virtually none of the probes in either comprehension or expression. At the same time, she did demonstrate comprehension on some occasions when the language used was functional in her play. For example, she dropped a puzzle piece on the floor without noticing it. The clinician told her the piece was on the floor, carefully giving no nonverbal cues along with this verbal information. Jan immediately looked on the floor and found the piece. Similarly, she did no vocalization in response to attempts to elicit talking, but suddenly she spoke the numerals one through four as they were printed on a toy.

These observations suggested that a change in the structure of the relationship might be productive. In fact, one could say that Jan was effecting such a change by ignoring most of the clinician's directives.

Two alternatives were considered: move to more control through the use of conditioning techniques, or allow Jan to play relatively freely. The latter course was selected. It seemed probable that heightened control would lead to further resistance and consequently to the use of increasingly powerful reinforcers in order for the clinician to remain one-up. More important, though, channeling and controlling Jan's behavior heavily would limit the areas of functioning that could be observed, and thus what could be learned about her. At this point, it appeared more useful to sample a wide variety of Jan's behavior. Therefore, a number of play activities were made available. It was soon apparent that her short attention span was due to the context. She demonstrated very adequate attention during play, often remaining with favorite activities for long periods of time. She used very little vocalization, however, and (worse yet!) she virtually ignored the clinician.

Therefore, she was offered only activities in which the clinician could easily participate. Together they worked out cooperative play routines with certain activities such as a tool bench. As they mutually defined their relationship in these routines, it was noticed that Jan would frequently follow verbal suggestions regarding such things as use of the tools. As the clinician made use of this fact, it became clear that comprehension was not Jan's major area of difficulty. Expression was still minimal, though, and it was determined that expressive language would be an appropriate goal for intervention. The clinician began to model utterances, sticking to ones that were appropriate in the play activity. After a while Jan began to imitate some of these utterances and use them spontaneously as well. Both from clinical observations and from talking with her mother, it appeared that these utterances were ones Jan had never used before. There was still much the clinician didn't understand about Jan, but intervention appeared to be off on a productive tack. As a point of information, it may be added that the time involved—from when the child was first seen until the work on modeling utterances for expression began—was about five weeks, with the child being seen twice a week.

This example illustrates a number of points. First, it is not clear whether we are talking about assessment or intervention. Exploratory teaching seems a fit title for the activities involved. Second, the changes in clinical approach are a mix of relationship and task factors. Each change is an attempt to optimize the child's responding. Third, each change is devised or selected on the basis of the child's previous responding rather than according to a predetermined plan. Finally, the sequence of events can change as the clinician elects among alternatives along the way. Exploratory teaching is based on clinical judgment and is not infallible. The judgments involved, however, are evaluated in terms of the results they produce.

Assessment of Specific Skills

In the preceding example, the complexity of many of the tasks offered the child was not too great. The same approach would be used with more subtle areas of language functioning, although the exploratory teaching would obviously involve different tasks. Suppose, for example, that a child demonstrates utterance length that is considerably shorter than that of other children of the same age. In addition, the child does poorly on a test of auditory memory span. We might begin by searching for ways to assess these areas that are truly meaningful for the

child. Can a sixth grader remember a best friend's phone number? Can a seventh grader who is a music fan remember many of the tunes that are in the current top ten or many of the lyrics from some of those tunes? Can another child, this time a football fan, remember the starting lineup of a favorite ball team or which teams have won the Super Bowl in the last several years? Does the child's utterance length increase when talking about favorite topics in a relationship context that is conducive to free talk? If you describe a football play to a sports fan, can that child retain it long enough to analyze it for you? If you list statistics about favorite athletes, can the child repeat them back to you?

Similarly, one could explore more technical aspects of the child's performance. Is the child's memory span for unrelated words shorter than that for sentences? If so, exploration of memory span for unrelated words may not tell us much because we can get a more optimal performance through sentences. If they are the same, it might be profitable to look at the child's knowledge of sentence relations, verb phrases, and noun phrases. These areas of grammar are important in the chunking that is involved in memory for sentences. Again, these factors may interact with the degree to which the task is appealing to the child.

In any case, through informal techniques and exploratory teaching the clinician may be able to come a lot closer to the child's optimal performance. In addition, we can identify some of the factors and dynamics involved in the child's performance.

Summary

Exploratory teaching is a matrix in which assessment, training, and the transactional model all come together. By increasing the complexity or demands in the situation, we find out where the child has difficulty. We then try to enhance the child's performance in each area of difficulty. Different approaches are used in attempting to elicit optimal performance from the child. In attempting to go beyond these limits in the child's functioning, we get a richer understanding of those difficulties, and at the same time we discover which approaches to intervention are most effective. The child's responding and the clinician's elicitation techniques are both explored, each in the context of the other.

The approaches employed by the clinician will involve both relationship tactics and informal techniques aimed at more specific aspects of behavior, such as those described in the section on informal procedures. In fact, as already suggested, there is no formal difference between assessment procedures and intervention procedures; both attempt to elicit the maximal levels of functioning the child can attain. Exploratory teaching seeks to develop transactional patterns between clinician and child that will enhance the child's language growth as efficiently as possible.

THE CULTURALLY DIFFERENT CHILD

As mentioned in Chapter 5, the language clinician must be very careful to differentiate between difference and disorder in culturally different children (Williams and Wolfram 1977). Especially in public schools, there may be referrals in which the "problem" turns out to be that the child is bilingual or speaks a nonstandard dialect. With older children and adults, determining the presence of nonstandard dialect or bilingualism is easy; any native speaker can do

it, although perhaps without precision. The difficulty comes in determining that a bilingual or nonstandard speaker demonstrates a disorder. There are two problems here. First, as discussed earlier, interpersonal and cultural factors may lead such children to make insufficient or inappropriate selections from their repertoires. We don't get a valid picture of their language skills. Second, as we will see in the next chapter, options that are acceptable and grammatical in a nonstandard dialect may be errors in Standard English. This situation is particularly true in the nonstandard dialect spoken by inner city blacks.

The difficulties in assessing culturally different children increase with the norm-based approach that underlies the use of standardized tests and developmental milestones. As mentioned earlier, these procedures emphasize Standard English and behavior patterns of the dominant culture. While they may allow the child to exhibit some knowledge of language, they cannot reflect areas of language skill that are different from those of the majority culture. The result is that, through testing, culturally different children may be identified as language deficient when their language skills are actually within the normal range. Tests and norms imply absolute judgments about what is correct; culturally different children force us to make those judgments relative. Language sample analysis carries the same hazard, because it is based on formal Standard English.

As mentioned earlier, the challenge is to distinguish disordered language from culturally different language. Clearly, standardized testing and language sampling will not be enough. We will have to employ informal assessment and exploratory teaching. The thrust will have to be toward assessing the child's effectiveness as a communicator rather than looking for specific errors. Consequently, it will be particularly important to find situations in which the child will talk freely. It should be clear that this goal may take some time.

There are two options for more specific assessment, each with its own problems. First, the clinician can become familiar with the dialect or language the child speaks and with some of the attitudes of the associated culture. While we can get some general ideas from curriculum guides that many school districts have available, it takes years of study to gain full knowledge of another culture or language. Consequently, this goal may not be practical for many clinicians. For example, in the schools in my community there are speakers of Black English vernacular and bilingual speakers representing Spanish, Japanese, Chinese, Filipino, Vietnamese, some American Indian languages, and even a pocket of Russian speakers.

A second option would be to assess the child's language skill in particular situations and tasks. In this way we can have an objective look at communicative effectiveness. Some of the communication tasks in Chapter 10 might be useful here. The problem is that we are likely to end up assessing culturally different children's skill in situations requiring Standard English, precisely the situation we started out to avoid.

No matter how we go about it, the assessment of culturally different children involves difficult problem solving for the clinician. Perhaps the following guidelines will be useful in approaching these children. First, the goal is to identify and explore language disorders; you are looking for those children who manifest language impairment beyond any language difference in dialect or bilingualism. Second, focus on communicative effectiveness, in both comprehension and expression. Employ as many

procedures as appropriate to explore these areas. Third, be patient. Take the time to establish relationship contexts in which these goals can be met. Finally, don't be dismayed if the situation seems complex. Fundamentally these children are no different from others, nor from you and me. Enjoy getting to know them.

CONCLUSIONS

Our goal is to understand each child as best we can and to develop interventions that will help each child achieve maximal language growth. Toward these ends we gather information about the child from parents and other specialists (Note the ambiguity here—are parents specialists?). We also provide various stimuli, tasks, and situations for the child and observe the child's behavior in these contexts. Finally, we interpret that behavior in conjunction with the information we have from other sources. Assessment rests on both observation and interpretation.

This interpretation may be seen as an attempt to answer a series of increasingly specific questions: Is any intervention necessary? If so, in what areas does the child need help? Finally, what types of intervention will be most efficient? All of these questions involve prediction. While we must deal with the child in the present, we are also concerned about future development. We have seen that prediction in human affairs is often a difficult and imperfect process. From the perspective of the transactional model and general systems theory, it could not be otherwise. Therefore, we need to make our predictions tentative and test them out as carefully as we can.

A key concept in understanding human functioning is that behavior is always multiply determined. Along these lines, a central problem in assessment is to sort out the interpersonal and motivational aspects of a child's behavior from those aspects in the cognitive and linguistic domains. All assessment procedures include components of both. This situation may complicate matters, but it is unavoidable. I have emphasized both areas because of our tendency to view other people's behavior from a linear cause-and-effect perspective. I recall one boy who was diagnosed as having a severe perceptual or processing disorder. He could not imitate. This "impairment" was present with verbal stimuli and also with motor activities of various sorts. It finally turned out that this child simply didn't like being told what to do! When the interpersonal context was changed, the processing disorder disappeared. On the other hand, a child who does not possess concepts such as *in, on,* and *under* will not demonstrate knowledge of those concepts no matter how the interpersonal context is manipulated.

We have looked at a number of techniques that can be used in exploring a child's knowledge and skills. Each approach has its purpose, and each purpose can be related to the three questions posed earlier. Standardized tests provide estimates of the child's minimal levels of skill. Because of the emphasis on overall scores in these tests, they may be most useful in relation to questions about whether or not intervention is necessary with a particular child. Informal assessment techniques provide more flexibility than is possible in structured tests. Consequently, they are useful in looking at areas that are not included in standardized tests and, particularly, in evaluating in depth specific aspects of the child's skills. In any kind of assessment one must always deal with the following question: Does lack of performance mean lack of knowledge or skill? Informal techniques approach this problem by assessing the same area in different ways. In line with Piaget's clinical method, they permit a fair sampling of the child's skills.

Employing a variety of techniques leads to another possible problem in assessment. We can only understand the child's behavior in terms of what the clinician is doing. We can turn this reciprocity into an asset rather than a problem, however. In exploring a child's knowledge through different tasks and situations, we are also exploring the efficacy of those particular tasks and situations for that child. Thus, as we learn more about particular children, we also learn more about how to work with them. I have called this process "exploratory teaching." It is through this approach that we can begin to differentiate between the interpersonal and the cognitive contributors to a child's behavior. I take Dearborn's remark as my motto: If you want to understand something, try to change it. This advice is particularly important in attempting to understand the transactional patterns of which the child's behavior is a part. Language use is inseparable from human relationships.

We learn more and more about a child, then, through informal techniques and exploratory teaching. In some form or other, the process continues as long as we know the child. As the child demonstrates new responses, it may sometimes be difficult to tell if the child "already knew" the response or "just learned" it. This question is intriguing, but in a broad sense irrelevant. In both assessment and intervention we attempt to elicit optimal responding from the child. As pointed out in Chapter 4, from the standpoint of transformational grammar we focus on performance, rather than competence.

Much is made of individual differences in

working with children of all ages, but frequently children are plugged into programs which may be only partially appropriate for their needs. Informal assessment and exploratory teaching force us to be responsive to individual differences, at least to some degree. We change according to how the child responds. Our changes are in the direction of seeking optimal performance from the child. In this way assessment not only blends into intervention, it leads to intervention that is individualized for each child. Before looking at intervention in depth, there is one more aspect of assessment to consider in detail. In the next chapter we turn to the matter of language sampling.

8

LANGUAGE SAMPLING AND THE SEQUENCE OF TRAINING

In trying to understand language-disordered children, it is obvious that we should listen to them talk. The section on assessing general communicative functioning in the preceding chapter touched on this matter. We can do much more, however, than merely noting some general features of a child's expressive language during conversation. Obtaining a precise record of a child's spontaneous talking and analyzing that record is known as "language sampling." It provides relevant, concrete data about individual children's use of specific aspects of language. It adds rigor to the assessment of expressive language.

There are some complications in language sampling, however. First, all talking that children do is influenced by many factors. We thus run the risk of sampling error. What children say to us may not be representative of how they talk in other situations. Further, analysis of children's language structures requires some linguistic sophistication and can be very extensive indeed. We need to keep our heads above water, both linguistically and in terms of sheer time involved in evaluating each language sample. Finally, given that we have carried out some sort of analysis, we need to make sense out of it somehow. Once we have an idea of how a child is talking, we have to decide what to do about it.

BASIS OF LANGUAGE-SAMPLE ANALYSIS

Some researchers in children's language acquisition have collected large numbers of utterances from individual children and then written grammars representing how those children organize language. This procedure is not appropriate for most individuals who are working with language-disordered children, however, because of the time and linguistic sophistication required. Therefore, most grammatical analysis in language sampling is based on linguistic work that has already been done. This work is of two kinds. First, there are complete grammars of adult English, which provide a framework for deciding which structures a child is using and which are absent. At the same time, it is obvious that children do not learn all the structures of English at once. Therefore, even though the language-sampling system may be based on a grammar of adult English, there is always a sequence of development implied. Hence, normal language acquisition is the second area of linguistic work that is important in language sampling. Language-impaired children's output can be compared with normal children's talking at various stages of development.

In sum, language sampling is based on two factors: linguistic analyses of adult English and research on developmental sequences. Before looking at language-sampling techniques, we need to consider what is involved in each of these factors.

The Reference Grammar

To begin with, it is necessary to select a particular version of adult grammar as a point of reference. All language-sampling systems available are based on Standard English. In addition, they reflect a relatively formal style, one that might be called "careful English." There are two problems here.

First, it should be clear from the discussions in Chapters 5 and 7 that one cannot evaluate the language skills of bilingual and nonstandard dialect speakers by comparing them with Standard English. All we can do that way is to look at their knowledge of Standard English, which may not reflect at all their larger abilities as language users.

The second problem is more subtle. In using an adult grammar as a reference point, the implication is that people always talk the same, that is, they organize their sentences according to that grammar. The rules are hard and fast. This assumption, however, is false. Many rules are variable in nature. As Dale puts it, "Many aspects of language are fundamentally probabilistic, not absolute. Although we often tend to perceive probabilistic phenomena as 'all or nothing,' the variability is there" (1976, p. 270). Consider some examples from Labov (1969). We can say *He's here* but not *Here's he.* In answer to the question *Who's going?* we could say *He is* but not *He's.* These are examples of absolute rules, ones that always apply. On the other hand, we could say *He's happy* or *He is happy.* Similarly, a speaker might say *It doesn't matter* or *It don't matter* or even *It don't make no never-mind,* depending on the situation. The rules associated with these utterances are variable. They change with the social context and the speaker's purposes. Labov (1969, 1972b) presents numerous examples of variable rules. There are many of them in English. They are the basis for style shifting, and also for shifting between dialects, as some speakers are able to do.

Our adult grammar does not include this variation. Therefore, it provides a reference grammar of formal Standard English. For practical purposes it is a framework for language-sample analysis, not a specification of all acceptable grammatical options. In the terms I will develop in Chapter 13, it is a model of English grammar.

One other point regarding the reference grammar is that in language sampling we pay minimal attention to pragmatics, to the variations in language use just alluded to. Rather, we are concentrating on the repertoire of grammatical options that underlies pragmatics and variations in style. In the larger picture, of course, we are interested in how children use language. That is why I prefer the term "option-to-mean" rather than "linguistic rule." I will return to these matters in Chapter 9.

The Developmental Sequence

Along with adult grammar, the second basis for language-sample analysis is the normal sequence of language development. Both assessment and intervention are tied to this sequence. Language acquisition has to be sequential. Children don't suddenly burst forth with complete knowledge of language. Rather, they learn some things before others, with the later learning building on what was acquired earlier. In assessment we use this sequence in trying to decide the level at which each child is functioning. Similarly, we organize our language training according to the developmental sequence.

In this section I want to urge caution in applying the developmental sequence. The reason is simple. At the present state of the art, the developmental sequence for language development is not well understood. We just don't know specifically what that sequence is. In fact, it appears that normal development may occur through different sequences in different children.

The language acquisition literature does document development, but generally it is broad. Children are described as progressing through a succession of stages or levels (Brown 1973; Dever 1978; Crystal, Fletcher, and Garman 1976). However, the ages at which various stages are reached and the developments within each stage vary among children. Further, it is not the case that a child goes through one stage and then the next. Rather, a stage begins to appear but its development continues over a period of time, during which other stages also begin to appear (Brown 1973; Crystal, Fletcher, and Garman 1976). Similarly, the use of any one structure develops gradually, making it difficult to say just when a child has acquired a particular form and is using it productively. Bloom, Lightbown, and Hood (1975), for example, adopted the arbitrary convention of declaring a structure to be productive in a child's speech if it appeared at least five times in their records of that child's talking.

To further complicate the picture, individual differences in language acquisition abound. In studying only the first fifty different words uttered, Nelson (1973) found that some children concentrated more on an object orientation and others on a person or social orientation. Similarly, in early word combinations, some children appear to rely heavily on the pivot-open construction, and others do not (Bloom 1970). Some children concentrate on pronominal forms before using many category names, but others do just the opposite (Bloom, Lightbown, and Hood 1975). Some children elaborate clause structures before noun phrases; others develop in the opposite order (Crystal, Fletcher, and Garman 1976). There is considerable variation within noun phrase development itself, as documented by Sharf (1972). Just as with the cognitive strategies discussed in Chapter 2, it seems that wherever you look for individual differences in language acquisition, you find them.

There are other difficulties in identifying developmental sequences from the literature. Two kinds of data are relevant: developmental norms and longitudinal studies. Developmental norms have already been discussed in Chapter 7. There are wide and overlapping ranges for the normal attainment of various language structures, making sequences of development difficult to specify. Further, normative data of any

kind do not exist for many aspects of language. The longitudinal studies are not without problems also. First, they have demonstrated many individual differences. In addition, a longitudinal study involves a great deal of time and effort. Consequently, the number of children who have been studied is very small. Most studies have employed three or four children at most. Brown (1973) drew from all the available research in his extensive review, yet the total number of children on which his discussion is based is only about twenty-four. The number of children studied longitudinally continues to grow, but it still seems a risky base on which to plan language interventions affecting thousands of children.

There is one further difficulty with the developmental sequence. Normal developmental errors overlap both with errors made by language-impaired children and with acceptable structures in nonstandard dialects. Suppose a language sample contains many utterances such as *He home, they hungry,* and *Mama gone.* These utterances would be considered normal for children approaching their second birthdays. Alternatively, the same utterances would be considered errors in a language-delayed child of four years. Again, they would be considered appropriate and acceptable by black teen-agers in the inner city.

In conclusion, language sampling is an imperfect process to say the least. Nevertheless, it is worth the attempt because it provides some of the most specific evidence we can get about a child's knowledge of language. In view of the difficulties in applying both the reference grammer and the developmental sequence, my approach will be a compromise. In succeeding sections I will outline a plan for language-sample analysis. Inherent in this outline is both a grammar of Standard English and a developmental sequence. However, it is broad in nature. As mentioned earlier, it is a framework or model for grammatical analysis. Through it we can get general ideas of the options-to-mean a child is using, in terms of the reference grammar, and of the overall level of development at which that child is functioning. We can then use this language-sample analysis as a guide for further informal assessment and exploratory teaching, leading to specific decisions about each child and situation.

LANGUAGE SAMPLING: THE MICROCOSMIC MATRIX

Introduction

We begin with some ideas from Chapter 4. The function of grammar is to indicate relationships within and among parts of the sentence. These relations in turn represent relationships in meaning and reality. The more elaborate the grammar a child is able to employ, the greater the variety, specificity, and subtlety of the relationships that child is able to comprehend and express. From this view, grammatical structures may be thought of as options-to-mean. That is, in choosing a particular grammatical structure, the child is electing to express a certain kind of meaning.

In Chapter 7 the child's behavior was described as selection from a repertoire. This description fits nicely with the idea of options-to-mean. A child has a repertoire of grammatical structures and lexical items. From this repertoire specific items are chosen, depending on both the ideas the child wishes to express and the child's perception of the social situation at the moment. In analyzing a language sample, then, we ask: What options-to-mean does this child employ?

Holland (1975) emphasized that we do not teach the entire language to a child. Rather, we teach a microcosm of the language. As suggested by Holland, this microcosm provides the child with a basic means of communication through language. Through using such a microcosm, the child will frequently develop additional knowledge of language. In view of the importance of this microcosm, it makes sense to focus initially on very general options, those that express fundamental meaning relationships in the sentence. These relations occur at the clause level. Grammatically speaking, they are relations such as those among subject, verb, and object. In the child language acquisition literature of the 1960s, they were referred to as basic grammatical relations. In terms of semantics, as discussed in Chapter 4, they may be thought of as deriving from semantic relations, those basic components of meaning that underlie sentence structure. In any case, these clause relations form a nucleus around which we can view other aspects of grammatical development. Dever (1978) describes the clause as the matrix within which other grammatical learning occurs. It is because of the importance of these notions from Holland and Dever that I call this approach to language sampling the "microcosmic matrix."[1]

My strategy for language sampling is based on the work of Richard Dever (1978). It is a step-by-step process. In looking at a corpus of a child's talking, we first ask if the child is using clauses with all their obligatory relations. (Clauses and other structures will be defined more precisely later; at the moment I am just outlining the general strategy.) Following Dever's procedure, the next step depends on whether or not we find that

---

[1] With enormous exercise of will, I fought off the temptation to title this whole chapter "Mysteries of the Microcosmic Matrix."

the child is using clauses. If the child does not demonstrate use of clauses, we look for preclausal options. These options will take the form of two-term semantic relations similar to those described by Schlesinger (1971) or Brown (1973). If, on the other hand, we find the child is using various types of clauses, we look for increasingly fine levels of detail and sophistication. There are three areas of grammar that we will explore: noun phrase options, verb phrase options, and sentence elaboration.

Before moving into the microcosmic matrix in more detail, let me remind you again that we are not merely identifying grammatical structures; rather, we are examining parts of the child's repertoire-to-mean. Each grammatical structure is an option to express meaning. This distinction is not merely academic. It is a constant reminder that we are interested in pragmatics, in how children communicate with language. Focusing on grammatical structures only as grammatical structures takes the child's knowledge of language out of any context and divorces it from its symbolic and communicative functions.

In the next sections I will discuss each level in more detail. We will look at clause options first. In subsequent sections we will consider preclausal options, noun phrase and verb phrase options, and sentence elaboration.

Clause-Level Options

Crystal, Fletcher, and Garman (1976) make a distinction between major sentences and minor sentences. In their terms, major sentences have subject-predicate structure, whereas minor sentences do not. Minor sentences consist of stereotyped and social utterances such as *See you later, yeah, hello* and *uh-uh.* Generally they are not gram-

matically analyzable but occur as fixed units. (Only a lumberjack could say, *Saw you later.*) Because they are not grammatically productive, they do not contribute much to the microcosm of language we are interested in teaching. Therefore, they are significant in language sampling only when most of the child's talking is in the form of minor sentences.

Major sentences, on the other hand, are grammatically productive. Crystal, Fletcher, and Garman's (1976) description of them as built around the subject-predicate relationships leads us directly to a definition of the term "clause." A clause contains a subject and a predicate, such as, *I want some coffee* or *Eagle Scouts have a dandy time.* It turns out that the subject does not have to be present in an imperative, but we don't need to worry about that for the moment. Sentences and clauses are not the same. A sentence may contain more than one clause, as in, *Eagle Scouts have a dandy time because they do good turns.* Sentences, therefore, are at a higher level than clauses. For the present, we will concentrate on the clause level.

There are two sets of clause-level options, which Dever calls "clause types" and "clause variations." Clause types represent different relations among the basic elements of the clause. These options-to-mean focus on relations within the clause itself, that is, subjects, verbs, objects, complements, and so on. The verb is central in these relations. A transitive clause, with its subject-verb-object construction, is an example of a clause type.

Dever also describes clause variations. Each clause type can occur in different forms. Thus, a transitive clause can occur as a declarative, question, or imperative. These options-to-mean represent different forms of statement that can be directed toward a receiver.

Before describing these various options in detail, there is one more distinction to make. Clauses are composed of both obligatory and optional elements. Obligatory elements must be present. Clause types are defined in terms of their obligatory elements. Optional elements, on the other hand, may or may not be present. For example, in transitive clauses the verb is obligatory, but the use of an adverbial is optional. One can say *Papa cooks dinner* or *Papa cooks dinner frequently,* but one cannot say *Papa dinner.*

Clause Types

Dever (1978) describes three clause types. Ultimately, it turns out that the only component of clauses that is always obligatory is the verb. In addition, the nature of the verb characterizes the clause type.

Intransitive Clauses. An intransitive clause contains a subject and a verb. The verb is intransitive, that is, it does not take an object. Intransitive clauses may also contain adverbials as optional elements. The adverbial may be an adverb or a larger structure such as a prepositional phrase. It will indicate location, manner, time, or the like. Recall now the discussion of function, class, and position in Chapter 4. The three constituents of intransitive clauses can be considered as three grammatical functions. We can then describe intransitive clauses[2] as follows:

$$Cl_{intr} = + \; Subject + Verb$$
$$\pm \; Adverbial$$

This statement identifies the grammatical functions in intransitive clauses and indicates whether each function is obligatory

(+) or optional (±). It also indicates the position of each function in the clause, although adverbials sometimes occur in other positions. We will consider the classes associated with these functions later on. The key to identifying intransitive clauses is that they contain a subject and a verb, but no direct object. Examples include utterances such as the following:

Billy runs.
The old man sits in the sun.
The dog slept soundly.

Note that adverbials may be present, such as *in the sun* and *soundly.* The following would qualify as intransitive clauses, even though they are not in Standard English. The obligatory functions are all present in some form.

Me ranned fast.
Daddy sleep in bed.

On the other hand, the following utterances would not be counted as intransitive clauses in Standard English because some obligatory function is missing:

Me fast.
Daddy in bed.

I have described intransitive clauses first because they are relatively easy to teach. As Dever notes, they have only two obligatory functions.

Transitive Clauses. A transitive clause contains a subject, a verb, and a direct object. Obviously, the verb will be transitive. It will take an object. In addition to these three obligatory functions, transitive clauses may also contain the optional elements of indirect object and adverbial. Thus, the general form of transitive clauses[3] is as follows:

---

[2] Adapted from Richard Dever, *TALK: Teaching the American Language to Kids* (Columbus, Ohio: Charles E. Merrill Publishing Company, 1978), p. 47.

[3] Adapted from Richard Dever, *TALK: Teaching the American Language to Kids* (Columbus, Ohio: Charles E. Merrill Publishing Company, 1978), pp. 42 and 44.

$$Cl_{tr} = \begin{array}{l} + \text{ Subject } + \text{ Verb} \\ \pm \text{ Indirect Object} \\ + \text{ Direct Object } \pm \text{ Adverbial} \end{array}$$

As with the intransitive clause, this statement indicates the grammatical functions in transitive clauses, whether they are obligatory or optional, and their typical position. Following are some examples of transitive clauses:

The boys ate their dinner.
Sam gave Eddie a hard time.
I drove the car all night.
She sent me a letter at last.
We could have been watching television.

Note that while the last example seems complex, it turns out that it contains only the three obligatory components of a transitive clause; the complexity is in the verb phrase. As before, an utterance is counted as a transitive clause as long as it contains all the obligatory functions, whether or not these functions are in formal Standard English.

Dever notes that only transitive clauses can be transformed into passives. This fact can be used as an informal way to determine whether or not a particular clause is transitive or not. Usually, if you can restate it in passive form, it is transitive.

Equative Clauses. An equative clause contains a subject, a linking verb, and a complement. The complement further specifies or completes the subject. The verb performs the function of linking the subject with its complement. The most common linking verb is BE in all its forms. In fact, Dever considers only clauses whose main verb is a form of BE to be equative. However, other verbs may also function as linking verbs, such as *seem, become,* and *appear.* For simplicity we will follow Dever in describing equative clauses as containing

only forms of BE in the verb slot. Equative clauses[4] may be summarized as follows:

$$Cl_{eq} = \begin{array}{l} + \text{ Subject } + \text{ BE } + \text{ Complement} \\ \pm \text{ Adverbial} \end{array}$$

Here are some examples of equative clauses:

My best coat was on the floor.
The cow will be contented.
Eddy am a growing boy.
We were lost for three days.

Note that the complement can be adjectival, adverbial, or nominal. Also, the last example contains an optional adverbial in addition to its obligatory structures. As with the other clause types, an utterance is accepted as an equative clause as long as all obligatory functions are present, however formed. Examples such as the following would not be considered equative clauses in Standard English. They are missing an obligatory constituent. The last two, however, would be acceptable in Black English Vernacular.

I am.
That good.
My bike in the garage.

On the other hand, the following examples are not equative clauses, even though they do contain some form of BE. In these utterances, the BE is an auxiliary to another verb. (I will discuss auxiliaries later in this chapter.)

My mama is working.
I am running away.

Summary of Clause Types. The key factors differentiating among the three clause types are in their obligatory components. Intransitive clauses contain a subject and an

[4] Adapted from Richard Dever, *TALK: Teaching the American Language to Kids* (Columbus, Ohio: Charles E. Merrill Publishing Company, 1978), p. 51.

intransitive verb, whereas transitive clauses contain subject, transitive verb, and, in addition, an object. Equative clauses contain a subject, a form of BE, and a complement to the subject. We begin to see now how these clause types can be described as different options-to-mean. Intransitive clauses codify relations between subjects and verbs where there is no object receiving the force of the verb. In forming an intransitive clause, then, we choose to mean that kind of relationship. In electing to use a transitive clause, on the other hand, we choose to mean a relationship involving an object as well as a subject and a verb. In producing an equative clause, we choose to mean that the subject and its complement are equated in some way. The verb BE merely signals this relationship. The following excerpt will illustrate the clause types and an approach to analysis. Rosie is growing up in an environment of Standard English. Her grammar is immature for a four-and-a-half-year-old.

SAMPLE 1: Rosie CA = 4–5

1. I put my stars on too
2. me do that now
3. baby's on the side
4. now the door opens
5. the stars right here
6. me glue it
7. this go right here
8. the woods way out there outside
9. I'm here
10. it's another bed
11. I want a house now
12. the daddy in the back
13. this is the baby bear
14. baby's walking around
15. I go night-night
16. one outside playing right there
17. me put on circles right now

Let me note at the outset that I do not consider seventeen utterances a sufficient number for language-sample analysis. I have excerpted them from a longer sample to keep the illustration brief. In the analysis that follows I have taken one clause type at a time and listed all its functions across the page. Below this listing I have filled in all of Rosie's clauses that are of that type, so that each component of each clause is in the column representing its function. Beginning with intransitive, I took utterance number 4, put *the door* under *Subject, opens* under *Verb,* and *now* under *Adverbial;* the same procedure was applied with all other clauses.

By arranging the utterances in columnar form, we can tell quickly which components of each clause type are present. We can make use of the relation between function and class here. A grammatical function is represented by a class of items. Conversely, the function may be identified in terms of that class. In our procedure the functions are listed across the top in their typical positions. The columns below are the classes of items Rosie used to represent each function.

We can see that Rosie has all three clause types in her repertoire. In addition, she uses optional adverbials. We do not see any evidence of indirect objects in transitive clauses. We can also note that the subjects of transitive and intransitive clauses are usually represented by pronouns, simple verbs predominate, and that BE in equatives

Intransitive Clauses

	Subject	*Verb*	*Adverbial**
4.	the door	opens	now
7.	this	go	right here
14.	baby	's walking	around
15.	I	go	night-night

* Adverbials do not appear only at the ends of clauses. For clarity, however, we will use only one column for adverbials.

Transitive Clauses

	Subject	Verb	Indirect Object	Direct Object	Adverbial
1.	I	put (on)		my stars	too
2.	me	do		that	now
6.	me	glue		it	
11.	I	want		a house	now
17.	me	put (on)		circles	right now

Equative Clauses

	Subject	BE	Complement	Adverbial
3.	baby	's	on the side	
9.	I	'm	here	
10.	it	's	another bed	
13.	this	is	the baby bear	

is usually in contracted form. At present we do not know if this picture is typical of all of Rosie's talking or if it is an artifact of the situation in which the sample was collected.

From sorting Rosie's utterances into columns, we also see that both objects and complements are sometimes represented by two- and three-word utterances, as well as single words. In fact, a major advantage of this columnar arrangement is that it facilitates later noun phrase and verb phrase analysis.

There are four other utterances in this excerpt, ones which are not complete clauses of any type:

5. the stars right here
8. the woods way out there outside
12. the daddy in the back
16. one outside playing right there

While producing these utterances, Rosie was arranging various play objects around the room. Each utterance contains a "subject" and a locative expression. In view of the fact that Rosie is learning Standard English, it is tempting to call them incomplete equatives, but notice that they could also be incomplete intransitive clauses. All we know for sure is that the errors are in the area of the verb.

These incomplete utterances raise a larger issue. In many language samples there will be some utterances that are unclassifiable, no matter what analysis system you use. Other utterances may seem to be classifiable into more than one category. For my purposes we do not need to worry about every single utterance. We want to understand what types of options the child does employ and what patterns of errors are present, so that we can determine goals for intervention. A few individual utterances shouldn't sway these decisions one way or the other. We are interested in more general trends.

Clause Variations

One set of options-to-mean involves relations within the clause. These are the clause types just discussed. In addition, there is a set of options related to the form of statement and how the utterance is used in discourse. Thus, each clause type can occur in different variations, depending on the speaker's purposes. Of course, there is no one-to-one correspondence between the grammatical variations of statement, question and imperative on the one hand, and the pragmatic functions of dealing with people on the other. For example, Ervin-Tripp

(1977) describes six different types of directives, each employing a statement, question or imperative. Pragmatics is the art of using the variant that will best accomplish your purpose in the situation. Nevertheless, following the discussion of Halliday's (1973) ideas in Chapter 4, each of these three clause variations carries a somewhat different relationship message. It is precisely for this reason that so many pragmatic variants become necessary. As Bolinger says, "The important thing is that a social criterion establishes a grammatical class. Once grammaticalized . . . the social functions in turn become more elaborate, for one can use a question to express a command, mitigating the force of it just as by using a more wheedling intonation. The protocols of using one (clause variation) or another become quite elaborate" (1975, p. 329). I continue to draw from Dever (1978) in describing the clause variations.

Declaratives. A declarative makes a statement; it declares. All the clause types discussed above have been described in their declarative form. Semanticists often describe the declarative as making a proposition.

Imperatives. An imperative expresses a command. Imperatives are similar in construction to declaratives except for two things. First, the subject is usually not expressed in an imperative. Second, the verb is tenseless. That is, it cannot be marked as future, past, or present. We cannot tell someone, *Sits down!* or, *Sat down!* It is rarely necessary to teach a child imperatives. As any parent will tell you, children seem to be born using this option.

Questions. Questions seek information. In addition, they constrain the type of response that the listener should make (Leach 1972). The formation of questions requires changes both at the clause level and within the verb phrase. There are three types of questions.

First, there are yes/no questions. In general, these questions seek agreement or disagreement and consequently limit the receiver to responses that confirm or deny the question. As with all the clause variations, though, one general descriptive statement such as this will not always apply. If you ask someone, *Can you pass the salt?* a response consisting solely of the word *Yes* would not be satisfactory. Your burger still needs salt. In this case the yes/no question clause variation is being used as a directive rather than to solicit information.

Second, there are wh- questions, so called because they contain a word beginning with *wh-*. These questions seek information about some specific aspect of the situation, rather than simply agreement or disagreement. That aspect may be related to any of the clause level functions, such as subject, object, verb, or adverbial. Whatever function we wish to inquire about is represented by a wh- word, such as *what, where, when* or *how*. To an extent, the form of the wh-question dictates the form of the response, but again pragmatic considerations introduce considerable flexibility. *Why don't we have our snack now?* may function as a gently put directive rather than as a question.

Finally, there are tag questions, which are added onto declarative clauses: *You do love ice cream, don't you?* These questions seem to seek agreement, rather than seeking new information, as the other questions do. Again, their functions are broader than this statement implies. Parents of young children sometimes use numerous tag questions in an apparent effort to elicit responding from the child. More generally, tags often have a politeness function. Tag questions appear fairly early in normal children's language development in simple forms such as *Right?* and *OK?* At the same time, they are a relatively subtle option and consequently are rarely taught to language-impaired children. I will make the half-arbitrary decision that tag questions are outside of the microcosm of language it will be necessary to teach.

Passives. Transitive clauses can also occur as passives. What would be the grammatical object in a transitive clause functions as the subject in the passive, and the subject of the transitive clause acts as an adverbial representing agent or instrument. A transitive clause such as *Bill purchased a Porsche* becomes *A Porsche was purchased by Bill* in the passive. The passive construction is a very subtle option-to-mean. It is primarily used for emphasis and to meet the discourse requirements of various interpersonal situations. Loban (1963) found its use relatively rare in elementary-school children. For these reasons the passive is rarely taught to language-disordered children. In my judgment it is beyond the microcosm that we typically need to be concerned with.

Summary of Clause Variations. We have seen that there are three clause variations and a few subvariations. Rather than representing different relations within the clause, each variation represents a different choice of form of statement that can be addressed to a receiver. Consequently, these options-to-mean are of particular importance in pragmatics, where language structure is put to work in dealing with people. One clause variation is the declarative, which makes a statement. A second clause variation is the imperative, which represents a command. Finally, there are questions, which are subdivided into three additional options. In asking a yes/no question, you solicit affirmation or denial. With a wh-question, you go after more specific information. Tag questions, on the other hand, generally seek agreement.

Summary of Clause-Level Options

Following Dever (1978), I have described three clause types and three clause variations. These structures are basic options-to-mean in the language. They provide a grammatical framework through which semantic relations are realized and through which utterances are used to transmit and seek information and direct other people's activity. We can relate agents and objects with actions, states, and qualities through clauses. Not only do we make statements about these relations, we ask questions about them and give commands related to them. I am in agreement with Dever that these options truly form a matrix in which other language learning occurs.

Children develop elements of both variations and types simultaneously and interdependently, and both sets of options begin to develop very early. Whatever else, one should not interpret the above discussion of clause types and clause variations as implying that once the clause types develop, clause variations then develop through transforming those clause types in various ways. There is no way to determine that the types are somehow more basic than the variations or vice versa.

Returning to more practical matters, the structure of a clause may take nine different general forms: Each of the three types may occur in any of three variations. Typically, a language sample will not contain all of these forms in equivalent number. Usually some are much more frequent than others, and often some are not present at all or are minimally represented.

Recall now the overall strategy of the

microcosmic matrix method as adapted from Dever (1978). The first focus is on the clause level. If a child demonstrates productive use of clauses, we then move to levels of more detail and sophistication, namely noun phrases, verb phrases, and sentence elaboration. If, conversely, the child is not using clauses, we begin looking for preclausal options. Let us consider this second possibility in the next section.

Preclausal Options

We are looking now for the precursors of the clause types and variations. By precursors I do not mean structures that a child *must* have before clauses can develop. It is difficult to identify specific structures of this type for individual children. Rather, I want to focus on options that will serve the child's communicative efforts at the moment, but that will also be functional in complete clauses. These preclausal options will form a matrix for learning clauses. We will look at single words first, then at two-word combinations, and finally at longer nonclausal utterances.

Single-Word Utterances

A number of semantic roles were defined in Chapter 4. These roles represent basic components of meaning that are assumed to underlie sentence structure, such as agent, location, patient, state, and action. In that chapter it was pointed out that these semantic roles have proven very useful in characterizing young children's early word combinations. Similarly, Bloom and Lahey (1978) have argued that early intervention should be organized around basic semantic categories that normal children exhibit in their utterances. The aspects of reality represented by semantic roles are present in the lives of virtually every child. Bloom and Lahey (1978) list semantic functions such as the following as occurring at the one-word level: existence, nonexistence, recurrence, rejection, denial, attribution, possession, action, and locative. These categories were developed from intensive study of a small number of children. While they are not precisely the same as the semantic cases of Fillmore (1968) or Chafe (1970) discussed in Chapter 4, the idea is similar.

Identification of categories such as those of Bloom and Lahey requires a great deal of interpretation by the observer. As noted in Chapter 4, the type and amount of interpretation in language analysis has been a central issue in linguistics. Further, as we saw in Chapter 7, interpreting children's behavior is not always straightforward. Along these lines, Starr (1975) found that she could not reliably identify many semantic functions in children's one-word utterances. Similarly, Howe (1976) argued that adult interpretation of young children's semantic intentions is likely to be in error because we make the assumption that children see the world the same way we do. That is, our interpretations are in answer to the question, what would *we* mean in the same situation. In fact, Crystal, Fletcher, and Garman (1976) argue that the interpretation of specific semantic intent from one- and two-word utterances is too nebulous to be of value in language-sample analysis.

Let us take a middle road. We will take semantic functions into account, but we will use only categories on which there is fairly general agreement in the literature and which Starr (1975) found could be reliably applied in analyzing children's one-word utterances. The following categories fit these requirements.

Agent—words that symbolize animate beings.

Action—words that symbolize actions; typically verbs.

Object—words that symbolize inanimate entities.

Modifier—words that describe, symbolize an attribute, or that could be modifiers in other ways.

Interjection—minor sentences, such as *yes, no, wow, thank you, OK,* and *ouch.* Many interjections are socially oriented.

These five categories form a framework for classifying children's one-word utterances. In developing a perspective on vocabulary work, though, there are two other distinctions to keep in mind. The first has been nicely described by Bloom and Lahey (1978). It is the difference between substantives and relational words. Substantives are names of entities, both animate and inanimate, such as *house, dog, daddy,* etc. Relational words are not associated with particular entities, but with relations among entities. This idea will be familiar from the discussion of relational concepts in Chapter 1. Bloom and Lahey mention several classes of relational words. First, there are general relations, such as negation, possession, and recurrence. We have already met these relations in the discussion of semantic functions above. Second, there are general actions, such as *put, go, make, get, do, give.* Finally, there are general descriptive terms, such as *good, big, high, dirty.* As should be clear from earlier chapters, the distinction in training is that substantives have referents, but relationals don't. You can show children what a *block* is, but you can't show them a *put.*

A second distinction has been described by Nelson (1973). Her research indicated that the early vocabulary of some children emphasizes names and things. Other children focus more on socially oriented terms, ones used in relation to the self and others. Not only do children use both substantive and relational words of various kinds, but their use of words reflects their interests in both the "thing" world and the "interpersonal" world. This distinction could have significance from the point of view of the transactional model. Both Nelson (1973) and Zlatin and Phelps (1975) noted a match between the emphasis in the child's vocabulary and aspects of the parent's talking.

It is probably not possible to characterize reliably each child's talking in terms of all of these variables. Therefore, it might be best to stick with the five categories listed earlier in analyzing children's one-word utterances. At the same time, the distinctions described by Bloom and Lahey and by Nelson become very important in selecting words for training and in how we organize that training. Words do function differently, and so do children. The more we can adjust our intervention techniques to match these functions, the more effective that training can be.

Holland (1975) suggested a possible list of words for early vocabulary training. Her goal was to provide the child with a repertoire for expression in a number of basic areas. Lahey and Bloom (1977), on the other hand, argued that selection of particular words will have to depend on the child and the situation. In any case, we are looking for words that meet two criteria. First, they must be immediately functional for the child. One should not teach colors and shapes to a child who cannot use language for such basic purposes as to ask for a drink of water or to go to the bathroom. Ecological validity is an appropriate watchword here: Words selected for training should be meaningful and useful in the child's daily living. The second criterion is that most words we decide to train should lend themselves to later use in word combinations. In order to understand this goal better, let us consider two-word combinations now.

Two-Word Combinations

Researchers in language acquisition have described a number of two-term semantic relations in young children's talking. I will combine and redefine these relations into six categories. These categories represent a compromise between semantic relations and clause-level grammatical structures. Again, they are a microcosm in which the child can develop more elaborate language structures.

Agent + Action. In analyzing a language sample, I would interpret both agent and action rather broadly. Agent + Action is directly parallel with the intransitive clause type described earlier, although young children may also use transitive verbs in this construction. Agent + Action is also a component of transitive clauses. Examples include the following.

> *me eat*
> *mama go*
> *baby cry*

Action + Object. Object is also a broad category. From the perspective of semantic roles, it will frequently be a patient. Crystal, Fletcher, and Garman (1976) lump both objects and complements together at this stage. Action + Object is a component of transitive clauses generally and is directly parallel with transitive imperatives. Here are a few examples of Action + Object:

> *see ball*
> *want cookie*
> *fix that*

In my view, two-word options such as Agent + Action and Action + Object provide a direct link between semantic roles and the grammatical structure of clauses. They are taken from the semantic relations described by Brown (1973) and Schlesinger (1971), but they foreshadow specifically the obligatory grammatical relations of transitive and intransitive clauses. I am not proposing this link at a theoretical level in normal language acquisition; rather, I want to take advantage of it in intervention with language-impaired youngsters.

Modifier + X. The X stands for anything that can be modified, but most commonly it will be a noun. This combination includes similar semantic relations that have been described in the normal acquisition literature, such as Entity + Attribute, Demonstrative + Entity, Possessor + Possession, and Nomination, that Brown (1973) has described, and Modifier + Head and Introducer + X, both described by Schlesinger (1971). Thus, in language sampling we will consider all kinds of modification together at the two-word level. Individual children may show differences in which types they emphasize. Probably these differences are unimportant in moving a child toward clause-level constructions. Finally, it is important to notice that this combination can occur in either order, that is, Modifier + X, or X + Modifier. Some examples of Modifier + X follow.

> *the ball*
> *my spoon*
> *face dirty*
> *big car*

Modifier + X is obviously a precursor to noun phrases, as in *Good boy*. It relates an attribute to an entity. But equative clauses can also relate attributes to entities, although with the opposite word order: *The boy is good*. Thus, there is some ambiguity in relating Modifier + X to higher levels in the microcosmic matrix. Fortunately this ambiguity need not paralyze us. Both word orders will be important in later training.

Locative + X. Locative refers to location, both in the sense of position or location and in that of direction of movement. Bloom and Lahey (1978) differentiate between locatives relating to action and those relating to state, but again their conclusions are based on data from a very small number of children. As with Modifier + X, Locative + X can occur in either word order. It is a precursor to the optional adverbial functions in clauses. In the order X + Locative it may foreshadow certain equative clauses, as in *Billy here* and intransitive clauses such as *Walk here*. Additional examples of Locative + X follow.

me chair
here ball
mama there

Negative + X. All authors stress that the expression of negation is an important and early-appearing function. Many follow Bloom's (1970) description of three types of negation in early utterances: nonexistence, rejection, and denial. Negation, however, is not a direct precursor of clause-level constructions. Rather, as we will see, it is ultimately part of the verb phrase. Detailed analysis of negation, therefore, can wait until the child's grammatical system is advanced enough that careful investigation of verb phrases is warranted. At the preclausal level we simply want to know if the child's repertoire includes negation. Here are some examples of Negative + X.

not go
don't want
not broken

Question + X. Question includes all wh- words, mostly *what* and *where* in young children, and questioning inflections in the child's prosody. Strictly speaking, this combination is not a semantic relation. It is more akin to the clause variations than to the semantic relations that underlie the clause types. There is evidence that all three variations occur very early. Hedrick, Prather, and Tobin (1975) report that prosodic inflections for statements, commands, and questions are being used by sixteen months. Because Question + X is not a semantic relation, you may wish to omit it from your preclausal analyses. I find it useful for the following reasons. First, some language samples I have encountered contain numerous wh- words. While they can often be categorized as semantic relations (*where* = Locative, *who* = Agent, and so on), somehow I think that misses the point. *Where* may be Locative, but in addition, the child is seeking information relating to semantic roles. Further, because of my emphasis on the transactional model, I am interested in what the child is doing to elicit talking from people in the environment. Doubtless, children employ many techniques toward this end. Asking questions, however, is particularly important because the answers that are evoked often provide specific information about language. As Synder-McLean and McLean (1978) point out, questioning is an important information-gathering strategy for the child. The following are examples of Question + X. I will follow the convention of using a question mark to indicate the presence of prosodic features indicating questions, such as terminal rising inflection.

what that?
daddy allgone?
where cookie?

Longer Preclausal Utterances

As Miller and Yoder (1974) point out, longer utterances are produced primarily by combining the various relations present in two-word combinations. Many of these longer utterances will be clauses, resulting from combinations of Agent + Action and Action + Object:

me want dolly
daddy eat cake

In addition, some utterances will involve other two-term relations:

see mama there
not my soup
what mama doing?

Some of these utterances will be clauses and some will not. There are no data indicating which of these multiple combinations will lead most efficiently to further language growth. Doubtless, it will vary from child to child. I would encourage any such combinations, but emphasize transitive and intransitive clause types.

Example of Preclausal Analysis

Before beginning the analysis, let me make a few general comments. Earlier in this chapter I noted that there can be considerable overlap between "disordered" grammar, nonstandard dialects, and developmental errors, that is, errors that are normal at certain stages of development. Elise is a case in point. We cannot distinguish among these possibilities solely on the basis of a written language sample. If Elise is learning a nonstandard dialect, there will probably be indicators other than grammar that this is the case. She will show phonological characteristics of that dialect, unless her articulation is too poor. She is likely to demonstrate pro-

sodic characteristics of the dialect as well. Further, we can talk with people in her home environment and note the dialect they speak. (She is too young to be influenced by peer culture, so there is no point in checking there.)

We can also compare Elise's performance with normative data: What should a child three years and ten months old be doing? We will have to select norms that will not penalize nonstandard speakers. These norms will have to be broad in nature, rather than focusing on specific items that vary among dialects. Until we know that

---

SAMPLE 2: Elise   CA = 3–10

1. some missing right here
2. not fit my baby
3. bath
4. where soap?
5. not now
6. don't know
7. it broke
8. you dummy
9. can't off it
10. here put it
11. yipe not that
12. there
13. whoa
14. what this?
15. cook egg
16. nope
17. paper on there
18. yeah
19. oh not see
20. baby seat
21. big boy
22. oh-oh
23. dunno
24. on that side
25. hear me on here right now

Elise is not a nonstandard dialect speaker, we would not use items such as plurals and pronouns. Comparison with broader norms, however, does suggest that Elise is behind. According to Prutting (1979), children between two and three years of age develop all three clause types. Even allowing for nonstandard dialects, Elise is just beginning to use these options, and she is almost four. Further, a child her age should be using complex verb phrases and clause combinations, areas that will be discussed later in the chapter. One could also look at mean length of utterance, another topic to be considered later in the chapter. This normative measure also places Elise significantly behind age level. Finally, standardized tests may be of value, as long as we recognize their limitations with culturally different children. In Elise's case, scores on comprehension were not far below her age level.

With the exception of the standardized testing, all of the variables discussed in the preceding paragraph would be applicable with a child speaking any dialect of English. Thus, we have a basis for concluding that Elise is delayed in expressive language, except for one thing. It could have been that this language sample was obtained in an interpersonal context that inhibited Elise's talking. As already stressed, the potential for this kind of sampling error is particularly great with culturally different children. With any child, however, it may take several sessions and some exploration of different relationship strategies before the clinician judges that a valid language sample has been obtained. In the present case, you will have to trust me that this sample is representative of Elise's talking. Having used this child as a springboard to discuss the overlaps among nonstandard dialects, developmental errors, and "disordered" language, let me now

point out that Elise was growing up in an environment of Standard English and that she was significantly impaired in expressive language.

Let us return to the microcosmic matrix. The analysis into columns illustrated earlier for clause types is not necessary with preclausal combinations. We need simply list all the utterances that represent each of the six combinations.

Agent + Action. Elise did not produce any utterances that clearly represent this category. There are two constructions that come close:

1. some missing right here
7. it broke

The first fits if you're willing to count *missing* as a verb rather than a modifier. Note that this utterance also has a locative. The second belongs in this category only if you consider *it* an agent.

Action + Object. The evidence for Elise's use of this option is more convincing.

10. here put it
15. cook egg
25. hear me on here right now

All of these contain Action + Object and all but *cook egg* contain other relations as well. Note particularly that the last utterance, said as the tape recorder was turned off, also contains a locational and a temporal. It is the longest utterance in the excerpt, but it is still not a complete clause.

Modifier + X. The following utterances seem to represent this category:

8. you dummy
20. baby seat
21. big boy
24. on that side

The first one may be a percursor to an equative clause, while the others seem more like noun phrases. The last one is clearly referring to location, but I classified it as Modifier + X because it does not identify what is to be *on that side.*

Locative + X.

1. some missing right here
10. here put it
17. paper on there
25. hear me on here right now

Again, all but number 17 contain more than one semantic relation. All of these locatives involve *here* and *there.* Some children (and Elise as well, on another occasion) might indicate location with a wider variety of terms, such as *table, floor, pocket,* and *outside.*

Negative + X.

2. not fit my baby
5. not now
6. don't know
9. can't off it
11. yipe not that
19. oh not see

You may be tempted to classify number 9 under Action + Object as well as under negation. Note, however, that there is no real action here. The utterance has more the flavor of *state* than of *action,* as those terms were defined in the discussion of semantically based grammars in Chapter 4. Knowledge of the situation would help in deciding if *off* is functioning as a verb. Also notice that the last two utterances contain interjections.

Question + X. There are two utterances that would be classified here.

4. where soap?
14. what this?

Finally, there are a few single-word utterances in the sample. One of them, number 3, *bath,* I'd call an object. Number 12, *there,* is best considered a modifier. The others I would place in the interjection category.

13. whoa
16. nope
18. yeah
22. oh-oh
23. dunno

Interjections are particularly important when they are the dominant type of utterance in a child's talking. Because of their minor sentence quality, they do not provide much opportunity for language growth.

As with the previous excerpt, we don't have a large enough sample to make definitive judgments about Elise. If further sampling parallels what we have, I think she is probably ready to begin work on clauses. Before moving in that direction, however, I would want to explore Agent + Action further and make sure that three-word utterances are frequent in her talking.

Conclusion

I have tried to described preclausal utterances with the minimum number of categories possible. More important, I have attempted to develop a sequence that builds directly from single words to word combinations to clauses. While lacking detail, this sequence is generally consonant with the language development literature. When you attempt to analyze samples with this framework, however, you may conclude that the categories I have described look fine until you try to use them! Some utterances will fall between the cracks and cannot be classified, and some will be ambiguous and can be classified in more than one way. In my experience the same is true of all systems for categorizing children's utterances. Similar difficulties are not uncommon among linguists working with much more sophisticated samples of talking. Perhaps what we are up against here is what the linguist Jim Hoard calls "the natural perversity of language."

Fortunately, however, we are only seeking evidence about the presence of those basic relations that are the foundation for language development at higher levels in the matrix. We don't need to be terribly concerned if some utterances cannot be classified with confidence, as long as we can get the larger picture that we need. Further, we should avoid taking ourselves too seriously in interpreting young children's semantic intentions, which, after all, involves reading the children's minds. Howe (1976) suggests that we are more than likely projecting our own interpretations on the child's utterances, rather than truly divining what the child is thinking.

Whatever the difficulties in identifying instances of the various semantic roles and relations in children's preclausal speech, these ideas do provide a basis for organizing language intervention, as Miller and Yoder (1974) have pointed out. MacDonald and his associates (MacDonald and Blott 1974; MacDonald, Blott, Gordon, Spiegel, and Hartmann 1974; MacDonald and Horstmeier 1978) have developed an intensive assessment and training programing based on two-term semantic relations.

Return now to the grand plan accompanying the microcosmic matrix. In looking at a language sample, we begin by looking for clauses. If we find the child is not using clauses, we analyze preclausal structures as detailed above. If, on the other hand, we find the child is using primarily complete clauses, there is little point in considering preclausal options. Rather, we look for

more sophisticated and subtle options that occur within the clause functions. Let us begin with noun phrases.

Noun Phrases

English noun phrases can be very complicated. In fact, Dever (1978) describes nine different components of noun phrases. Following Crystal, Fletcher, and Garman (1976), however, we will analyze the noun phrase into five different constituents. As with the clauses, these five components can be described in terms of function, class, and position. I will describe each component separately, listing them according to their position in the noun phrase.

1. Initiators, such as *just, at least, only, all, both, one-fifth, one-third.* An initiator may have several functions. It may limit a noun, as in *only the best.* It may express certain kinds of quantity, such as *one-fifth* or *all.* Finally, it may function as an intensifier, as in *quite a surprise.* In view of these different functions, there is some appeal in using an imprecise word such as *initiators* to label the whole group. Words that can function as initiators can often function in other ways as well. For example, *just* and *only* can be adverbials; *all* and *both* can be adjectivals. Perhaps the easiest way to identify initiators is by virtue of the fact that they are the only component of the noun phrase that can occur in front of a determiner.
2. Determiners, such as *the, this, that, a, each, some, my, your, no.* Determiners are grammatical morphemes that specify or identify nouns in some way. Employing both initiators and determiners, we can have noun phrases such as *just a cat,* or *only my car.*
3. Adjectivals. Crystal, Fletcher, and Garman (1976) list five types of adjectivals:
   adjectives, such as *good, high, sweet, perfidious.*
   quantifiers, such as *three, seventy-two.*
   ordinals, such as *third, fifth.*
   nouns, such as *horse* in *horse cart, barn* in *barn door.*

nouns marked for possession, such as *Eddy's* in *Eddy's book* and *citizens'* in *citizens' band*.

Adding adjectivals to our previous noun phrases, we could have, *just a frumpy cat* or *only my green car*. More than one adjectival can occur in the same noun phrase, so we could also have *just a frumpy old cat* or *only my grandfather's third green touring car*.

4. Head. Finally we get to the noun itself. It is called the *head* because it is the core or central component of the noun phrase. It may be a noun or a more complex nominal expression.

5. Postmodifiers. These options follow the head noun. They are of three types:

Prepositional phrases, such as in *the picture on the wall;*

clauses, such as in *the picture that grandma sent us;*

adjectives or *adverbs,* such as in *that picture there.*

Adding postmodifiers to the noun phrase examples above would produce statements such as *just a frumpy old cat trying to maintain her dignity* or *only my grandfather's third green touring car with three flat tires*. It can be seen that the noun phrase functions offer an extremely rich set of options-to-mean, one that children will be developing well beyond elementary school.

Summarizing, the noun phrase has the following organization.[5]

$$NP = \pm \text{ Initiator } \pm \text{ Determiner}$$
$$\pm \text{ Adjectival } + \text{ Head}$$
$$\pm \text{ Postmodifier}$$

Note that only the head is obligatory. All other options may or may not be present in any particular noun phrase. Following is a brief example of noun phrase analysis.

These utterances were excerpted from a longer sample. Not all of Judy's talking was

[5] Adapted from David Crystal, Paul Fletcher, and Michael Garman, *The Grammatical Analysis of Language Disability* (New York: Elsevier, 1976), p. 53.

SAMPLE 3: Judy   CA = 12–0

1. one played a horn and all sorts of things
2. then they had to sneak in the refrigerator again for a piece of cheese
3. the cat was a teacher to this dog
4. this girl named Susie came in and saw her dog named Moose
5. then this fish thinks this is a fishing line but it isn't
6. the baby bear takes a heavy stick used for a bat
7. once there was this fly that had an umbrella
8. it was just a little stream

---

this rich in noun phrases. In the normal situation, you would first analyze the clause into columns as before. Identifying noun phrases is then much easier. You need merely run through each column in the clausal analysis that is likely to contain noun phrases, particularly subjects, objects, and adverbials.

I have made no mention of prepositional phrases so far. Sometimes a prepositional phrase contains a noun phrase, as in *in the old, rusty barrel*. In fact, Crystal, Fletcher, and Garman (1976) include prepositions in their noun phrases. For further discussion and a list of English prepositions, see Dever (1978), pp. 95–97. In any case, I am including a column for prepositions in the following analysis because they occurred in Judy's talking. The numbers for each item in the analysis correspond to the sentence numbers above.

Several things are apparent from this layout of Judy's noun phrases. First, she uses all the functions of the noun phrase. That is, all the columns have entries in them. She sometimes uses more than one noun phrase in the same clause. Further, Judy uses noun phrases within noun phrases in the postmodifier slot. The postmodifier in number

	(Preposition)	Initiator	Determiner	Adjectival	Head	Postmodifier
1a			a		horn	
1b		all			sorts	of things
2a	in		the		refrigerator	
2b	for		a		piece	of cheese
3a			the		cat	
3b			a		teacher	to this dog
4a			this		girl	named Susie
4b			her		dog	named Moose
5a			this		fish	
5b			a	fishing	line	
6a			the	baby	bear	
6b			a	heavy	stick	used for a bat
7			this	fly		that had an umbrella
8		just	a	little	stream	

6b, for example, contains the prepositional phrase, *for a bat,* which in turn contains the noun phrase, *a bat.* I have not listed these smaller prepositional phrases and noun phrases separately because it is clear Judy's talking contains constructions considerably beyond these simple options.

There are no dramatic errors in these noun phrases. Some readers may object to the use of *this* in numbers 3b, 4a, and 5a. However, we would need to know the context to be sure. Further, this kind of *this* may well be a dialectical variation, in which case it would demonstrate some sensitivity to grammar, rather than suggesting language disorder. In addition to possible errors, we can look for aspects of noun phrases that Judy did not employ. There are no examples of multiple use of a particular function within the same phrase, such as *a little plastic fishing line,* which contains multiple adjectivals. Other options within the noun phrase could also be more complex, such as the head and postmodifier functions. Finally, there are only two examples of *Initiators.* We might want to explore that area further.

Before moving on, I should make two qualifications. First, as before, this excerpt is much too short to form a basis for decisions about Judy's use of noun phrases. It does outline an approach to noun phrases that I have found useful. Second, the noun phrases in some language samples will be more complicated than can readily be analyzed with five functions. Dever (1978), especially Chapter 4, contains background for more detailed analysis.

The order of acquisition of the elements of the noun phrase is not well understood. Individual differences abound, as has been illustrated by Sharf (1972). We still need a sequence for teaching, however. Both Dever and Crystal, Fletcher, and Garman have proposed tentative developmental sequences. Based on their work, we can say the following. First, make sure the child is using nouns before worrying about other aspects of the noun phrase. Not only do nouns function as *head* in the noun phrase, but in addition they can function the same way more elaborate noun phrases can in the clause matrix. The next development includes both adjectivals and determiners.

Some members of these classes are used considerably earlier than others, however, such as in the two-word combination Modifier + X. The last functions to appear are postmodifiers and initiators. As already noted, the complexity of postmodifiers varies greatly and depends partly on skill in other areas of grammar, such as clause structure.

In summary, noun phrases grow in three ways. First, they grow in length. This increase reflects two other changes. The child begins to use more of the components of the noun phrase and begins to elaborate the use of different components. It is well to remember again that these changes are not merely in grammatical skill. Rather, the child develops an increasingly rich set of options-to-mean involving noun phrase structures. Generally speaking, good command of noun phrases reflects specificity, flexibility, and sophistication in the expression of ideas.

Verb Phrases

The English verb phrase is both simpler and more complicated than the noun phrase. It is simpler because the classes that represent each function are smaller and there is less possibility of overlap. It is more complicated because the position of various elements in verb phrases does not follow as simple a linear order as that of noun phrases. This situation will make it more difficult to analyze verb phrases in neat columns as I have recommended for clause types and noun phrases. It will be helpful to approach the verb phrase in two steps. In the first step we will look at five constituents of verb phrases. These components do occur in a linear order and we will consider them in that order. My discussion follows Dever (1978) closely.

1. Modals are words such as *may, can, should, will, would, might,* and *must.* Modals indicate mood or attitude, such as obligation *(must, should)* or expectation *(will).*
2. Perfective. The perfective is used to specify certain types of action in the past. It is usually represented as *HAVE + en.* This symbolization is used to indicate that the perfective has two components, but they are discontinuous. After a form of *HAVE* another verb appears as a past participle. This participle is symbolized by *en.* Thus we have *has been, had thrown,* and *have looked.*
3. Continuum. The continuum indicates continuing action. It is the famous "is verbing" that many language trainers have focused on. In parallel with the perfective, it is symbolized by *BE + ing.* Examples include *is thinking, are running,* and *was doing.*
4. Passive. As mentioned in the discussion of clauses, the passive is a subtle option and frequently is not taught. We need to be aware of it, however, so that it can be recognized when it occurs in language samples. In the verb phrase, the passive is symbolized by *BE + en,* as in *was fixed, is carried,* and *are seen.* An agent or instrument is always either present or implied in a passive clause: *was fixed by my brother, is carried by the railroad,* and so on.
5. Head. Just as in the noun phrase, the head is the core or central component of the verb phrase. It is often called the main verb. It may be any verb, such as *run, see, think, do, want,* etc.

With these five options, the verb phrase is described as follows.[6]

$$VP = \pm \text{ Modal} \pm \text{Perfective} \\ \pm \text{ Continuum} \\ \pm \text{ Passive} + \text{Head}$$

As with noun phrases, only the head is obligatory. All the preceding components are optional. Frequently these optional elements are referred to collectively as aux-

[6] Adapted from Richard Dever, *TALK: Teaching the American Language to Kids* (Columbus, Ohio: Charles E. Merrill Publishing Company, 1978), p. 66.

iliaries. With this set of options we could say any of the following.

> *Becky plays the banjo,* which includes only the head of the verb phrase.
> *Becky will play the banjo,* which includes a modal also.
> *Becky has played the banjo,* which includes the perfective.
> *Becky is playing the banjo,* which includes the continuum.
> *The banjo was played by Becky,* which includes the passive.
> *Becky will have been playing the banjo,* which includes all but the passive.

Any other combination could also occur, as long as the same order is maintained.

Thus, the first step in analyzing verb phrases is to look for these five components. These structures can be sorted into columns as were the clauses types and noun phrases, although this procedure is a little cumbersome with discontinuous elements such as *BE + ing.*

The second step in looking at verb phrases focuses on two options that do not fit into the column analysis at all. These options are *tense* and *negation.* Tense is used here in a technical grammatical sense, rather than with the common ideas of past, present, and future. Tense refers only to the use of the past-tense marker, *-ED, (work-worked; go-went)* and the third-person-singular marker *(work-works; go-goes).* Other aspects of tense in the common meaning of the term are expressed through auxiliaries, such as future: *I will see you tomorrow.* Regarding position, the tense marker is always attached to the first element in a verb phrase, whatever that element might be.

Negation, often represented by "NEG," includes *not* and its contractions. NEG always immediately follows tense, that is, whatever tense is attached to, NEG will be the next thing. In some cases, a "Dummy DO" is inserted at the beginning of the verb phrase. This Dummy DO then takes tense and then NEG. It is called Dummy DO because it has no semantic meaning. For example, we say *she works,* but in the negative we say *she does not work.* The *does* contributes no meaning of its own, but functions only as a grammatical operator. It is not an option-to-mean in the sense that modal, perfective, and tense are. It is merely a "dummy" form that is required in certain negatives and certain forms of questions as well.

Summarizing our language-sample procedure for verb phrases, first, I would look to see which of the five "step one" components the child is using. This analysis will tell you not only which options the child is using but also which co-occur in the same verb phrases, and how many elements the child puts into one verb phrase. The second step involves scanning the child's verb phrases, looking for the following: *past-tense marker, third-person marker, not, n't,* and *Dummy DO.*

Infinitives have not been included in the above analysis. Lee (1974) places infinitives in a category she calls *secondary verbs.* Dever (1978), on the other hand, analyzes infinitives as one type of clause that can be combined with other clauses. Following his lead, I will include infinitives in the next section on sentence constructions. Let us now consider an example of verb phrase analysis.

Again, a clause analysis into columns is helpful because it identifies all the verb phrases and lists them in the same column. Let us assume that clause analysis has been done, and proceed with the first step of verb phrase analysis.

As before, these utterances were ex-

SAMPLE 4: Karen   CA = 10-2

1. those animals could swim in water
2. the water was deep
3. they would drown
4. the dog didn't know anything
5. he should say stuff
6. I don't have any animals
7. I'm talking on the cassette
8. it won't get worse
9. he's sleeping on a little seaweed
10. the movie was showing today
11. someone's been rocking in my rocking chair
12. someone's been sleeping in my bed

cerpted from a longer sample. With this limited evidence, Karen appears to be using modals, continuum, and head appropriately. There are two examples of the perfective, the last two items. These two utterances, though, occurred as Karen was telling the story of the Three Bears. The language sample contained no other perfectives, so it may be that these two resulted from a stereotyped telling of the story, rather than from productive use of the perfective. It can also be noted that Karen did not use any passives. A final observation is that Karen does not employ all the verb

phrase options she has available to her in the same verb phrase. With the exception of those from the Three Bears, her verb phrases consist of one or two elements, while she has at least three in her repertoire.

In the second step of verb phrase analysis, we look for tense and negation. There is evidence of past tense, such as number 2, but there are no instances of the regular past-tense marker. Similarly, there are no regular third-person markers, but Karen shows sensitivity to third person in items 2, 9, and 10. Regarding negatives, we notice three contracted forms of *not* in items 4, 6, and 8. The first two of these items also employ Dummy DO.

The developmental sequence for verb phrases has been more thoroughly studied than that of noun phrases. It has been discussed by Lee (1974), Crystal, Fletcher, and Garman (1976), and Dever (1978). The sequence seems to be as follows.

1. Head (uninflected verb)
2. Continuum; past and third-person markers; *not* and *n't*.
3. Modals; negatives and questions with Dummy DO
4. Passives and perfectives.

	Modal	Perfective	Continuum	Passive	Head
1.	could				swim
2.					was
3.	would				drown
4.					know
5.	should				say
6.					have
7.			'm + ing		talk
8.	won't				get
9.			's + ing		sleep
10.			was + ing		show
11.		's + en	be + ing		rock
12.		's + en	be + ing		sleep

Note that more than one component of the verb phrase is developing at the same time. Further, just as with the noun phrases, these developments occur gradually, and there is a lot of overlap among them. For example, passives with certain verbs may develop years before passives with all verbs (Lempert 1978). Thus, with both noun phrases and verb phrases we do not have a specific order delineating what to teach first, second, third, and so on. Rather, we find a generalized sequence within which the clinician will have to make decisions regarding which training goals seem most appropriate for individual children.

Sentence Constructions

In the preceding two sections we have been looking at the major components of the clause, namely noun phrases and verb phrases. In turn, though, clauses can be combined into larger structures. We will call these clause combinations *sentences.* Clause combinations provide another rich source of options-to-mean. They facilitate the expression of detail and logical relations, and they enhance the flexibility and subtlety with which ideas can be communicated. There are two major aspects of clause combinations: the relative grammatical status of the clauses that are combined and the completeness of those clauses. I will consider each separately.

Regarding grammatical status, the key ideas are subordination and coordination. Each refers to a different relation between clauses in a sentence. In subordination one clause is said to be dependent or subordinate to another. What "dependent" means is that the subordinate clause plays one grammatical role within the matrix clause. In *My friend waited until the bus drove out of sight,* the clause *until the bus drove out of*

sight plays an adverbial role in the matrix clause, *My friend waited.* In *Whoever ate the last peanut should get some more,* the clause *Whoever ate the last peanut* serves as the subject of the matrix clause. In these examples, the subordinate clause has filled a grammatical role in the matrix clause. Subordinate clauses may also fill a role in noun phrases, namely postmodifier. In the sentence *The boy who ran the fastest got first prize,* the clause *who ran the fastest* is a postmodifier attached to *boy.* Such postmodifiers are often called relative clauses.

As suggested in the section on verb phrases, infinitives also form subordinate clauses. In *I want you to be happy,* the infinitive clause, *you to be happy,* is the complement of the verb in the matrix clause. Similarly, in *To love you is my only desire, To love you* is the subject of the matrix clause. We can, therefore, analyze infinitives as one sort of subordinate clause.

However, Lee (1974) identified five early-occurring infinitival constructions, namely, *wanna, gonna, gotta, lemme,* and *let's.* To me, these early infinitives have an almost modal quality. In Lee's data, general use of infinitives occurs some time after the appearance of these five. In language sample analysis, then, it may be useful to note whether the child uses a range of infinitives or employs only these five early-appearing options. In the latter case, it may be that those infinitives are used as single words, and the child's use of infinitives is not really grammatically productive.

We turn now to coordination. Coordinate clauses do not show the "dependency" relationship inherent in subordinate clause relationships. In a coordinated sentence, each clause has equal grammatical status with the other clauses. In the sentence *I ate peanut butter and I ate bananas,* neither clause performs a grammatical function within the other clause. Each has equal grammatical status and is therefore "independent" of the other. Coordination occurs at other levels as well, as when we coordinate nouns, as in *I bought bread, lettuce, milk, and cheese.*

The discussion so far has concentrated on grammatical relationships. These relationships parallel conceptual relationships. Typically, the "main" idea of a sentence is expressed in the matrix clause, and ideas of "lesser" importance are relegated to subordinate clauses. Similarly, the ideas in a sequence of coordinated clauses have equal weight. I have emphasized the grammatical aspects because I sometimes encounter difficulty in deciding which of two ideas in a sentence is the "main" idea.

I have not found the analysis by columns employed previously to be of much use in analyzing subordinate and coordinate clause combinations. I simply collect the exemplars of each from a language sample and list them together. In differentiating between subordinate and coordinate constructions, it is helpful to note the conjunctions that join them. Different conjunctions are used to introduce each.

The following words precede independent or coordinated clauses:

Coordinating conjunctions: *and, but, for, nor, or, yet, while*
Conjunctive adverbs: *therefore, however,* etc.

Generally speaking, other conjunctions introduce subordinate clauses. Of course, there is no guarantee that every child will know which conjunctions are to be used with which clauses!

In introducing this section, I pointed out that clause combinations are very important in the expression of meaning. In this regard, Brown (1973) emphasized the parallels between logical relations and conjunctions. He

cites the following examples of logical relations and their corresponding conjunctions:

Conjunctive: *and*
Disjunctive: *or*
Contrastive: *but, although,* etc.
Causal: *because,* etc.
Conditional: *if . . . then,* etc.

Thus, as children learn to combine clauses with conjunctions, they begin to express the associated logical relations. Again, it is obvious that grammar alone won't suffice. Learning a conjunction isn't the point. The goal is to express these relational concepts with the aid of appropriate conjunctions.

The second major characteristic of sentences composed of more than one clause is that both clauses do not always appear in complete form. For an example with coordinated clauses, one could say either, *Bill went home and then he went fishing* or *Bill went home and then went fishing.* Similarly with subordination, *When he was done, he left the river* or *When done, he left the river.* The material that is missing from one clause is still present in the other clause. Only redundant information can be deleted. Crystal, Fletcher, and Garman (1976) describe other types of incomplete clauses.

There is relatively little in the literature about the language structures of older language-impaired children. Sentence elaboration seems to be a major concern, however. Sentence elaboration continues to develop in normal children well beyond elementary school. Studies by Hass and Wepman (1974), Loban (1968), and O'Donnell, Griffin, and Norris (1967) all support this conclusion. Loban (1968, quoted in Byrne 1978a) has done extensive longitudinal research on language development in children from the early years through high school. His conclusion is that the difference between effective and noneffective language users is in their expression of ideas, rather than in grammatical skill. It's not simply that children learn grammar. Rather, they increase in their ability to *use* grammar in the service of communication. Ervin-Tripp (1977) makes the same point from the perspective of pragmatics. Finally, Naremore and Dever's (1975) study of retarded children suggests that many language-impaired children at older ages know most of the grammar of English. One might say that their knowledge of the microcosmic matrix is fairly complete. Their errors tend to be on points of detail. Where they have major difficulty is in areas such as sentence elaboration, that is, the fluent expression of ideas in discourse. One might interpret this situation from the perspective of Chapter 1. Many older language-impaired children possess sufficient grammatical structures; the trouble is in the meta-rules and problem solving associated with using those structures efficiently for communication. We will return to sentence elaboration in Chapter 10.

I will close this section with two very brief excerpts of children's clause combinations. Both Amy and Denise are using subordination and coordination, and both children employ incomplete as well as complete clauses. Also, both children show appropriate use of the logical relations underlying clause combinations. At the same time, note

---

SAMPLE 5: Amy   CA = 3–4

1. then I went home and then I opened the ice box and got out a cup and something to eat
2. and then I taked a nap and when I woke up my mommy maked some cookies
3. when I knock on the door he barks
4. he ate one of those but he didn't get sick

SAMPLE 6: Denise   CA = 5–6

1. well you're tape-recording me because you want to take it to your teacher but I don't know what he's going to do with it
2. we should move up a little bit so we won't get soaking wet like I did before
3. I think he's hiding under a rock so no one can see him and catch him

---

that the two girls represent quite different levels of language skill.

A Framework for Developing Sequences of Training

This approach to language-sample analysis emphasizes decision making by the teacher or clinician. Eventually you must decide about whether or not specific grammatical structures ought to be a focus of intervention and, if so, which structures. An overall view of the microcosmic matrix and the developmental sequences it entails will be useful in making these decisions. Table 4 presents this information in outline form. It borrows heavily from Dever (1978) and also from Crystal, Fletcher, and Garman (1976).

Recall that there is simultaneous development among clauses, phrases, and morphology, as well as at the higher levels of sentence and discourse. To reflect this fact, the chart is divided into columns for clause, verb phrase, and noun phrase. I did not include a separate column for morphology because I want to focus on the microcosmic matrix of language development, rather than on grammatical detail. Where appropriate, I have included certain morphological items in the verb phrase column.

The chart is also divided into rows. Preclausal structures are not included on the

Table 4 The Microcosmic Matrix Model.

Clause	Verb Phrase	Noun Phrase
Row A: Intransitive Transitive Equative Declarative Imperative Interrogative (simple or poorly formed)	Uninflected verb *is*	Two-element NP's including adjectivals and determiners

Row B:
Adverbials
Indirect Objects
	Continuum
	Development of BE (Requires
	    pronouns *he, she, it, I, we,*
	    you, they)
	Past marker
	Third-person marker
	Negative: *not, n't*
		Three-element NP's including
		adjectivals and determiners

Row C:
Questions (fully formed):
    Interrogative reversal
    Wh- words
    Dummy DO
Coordinate clauses
	Modals: *can, will, may*
	Dummy DO:
	    In negatives
	    In questions
		Four-element NP's including
		adjectivals and determiners

Row D:
Subordinate clauses:
    Infinitival
    Noninfinitival
	Modals: *must, could, should,*
	might, would, shall
		Postmodifiers
		Initiators

Row E: Passive	Perfective: *have, has, had*	Initiators Postmodifiers

Adapted from Dever, Richard, *TALK: Teaching the American Language to Kids* (Columbus, Ohio: Charles E. Merrill, 1978) pp. 174–175, and David Crystal, Paul Fletcher, and Michael Garman, *The Grammatical Analysis of Language Disability* (New York: Elsevier, 1976), p. 85.

chart, but as children begin using clauses, they enter *Row A*. The rows down the page indicate a developmental sequence. The grid of rows and columns, then, shows concurrent developments in clauses, noun phrases, and verb phrases.

I think, however, that it would be too strong to call these rows developmental stages. First, some areas of the developmental sequences are not yet clear in the literature. For example, in the noun phrase column I have listed postmodifiers and initiators in both *Row D* and *Row E*. All we know for sure is that their development is gradual and that it begins fairly late in the sequence. Further, while each row represents developments that are occurring roughly simultaneously, we can expect individual variations among children. One child may have transitive and intransitive clauses and adverbials and be beginning to use three-element noun phrases, all from *Row B.* At the same time, this child may not be using any form of *BE,* and thus not have any equative clauses from *Row A.* Another may be using all three clause types, but virtually no noun phrases, while still another is doing just the opposite, and so on.

The structures in each row seem appropriate training goals for a child who is using most of the options in the preceding row. However, specific choices of structures for training will be based on many things beyond this generalized developmental sequence. Recall that the microcosmic matrix is intended as a framework in which continued language learning can occur. The same is true of each row. In previous chapters I have urged that we consider children as active learners, operating within the transactional model of development. Therefore we must ask: Which options in the matrix will facilitate the child's language use and development the most? One child may have great difficulty learning morphological detail. For this child it might be better to sidestep the verb phrase structures in *Row B,* with their low salience and high dependence on relational concepts, and emphasize clause and noun phrase options with more immediate communicative potential. Another child may be doing well with structures dependent on lexical morphemes and respond to a focus on those very grammatical operators we avoided with the first child. Always we must ask, what structures will have the most impact on this child's development as a communicator? These are difficult questions, to be sure. Perhaps they are unanswerable. It is better to ask questions such as these, though, than to assume that training a predetermined sequence of grammatical structures will significantly enhance each child's life as a communicator.

Conclusion

The microcosmic matrix is a framework for language-sample analysis and for developing sequences of training. While it is based on the work of Dever (1978) and Crystal, Fletcher, and Garman (1976), it incorporates many themes from the present book. The child is seen as an active decision maker, selecting grammatical options to represent intended meanings. The idea of a microcosm suggests that we focus, not on every detail of language, but on the basic framework of language that children can use to communicate. At whatever level a child is functioning, this framework forms a matrix in which continued language learning can occur.

The microcosmic matrix has been described as a series of vaguely defined levels. The child uses single words, then word combinations, and finally clauses. While there is much individual variation along the way, the clinical focus is on words that lead to word combinations, and word combinations that lead to clauses. Once the child is using clauses, they become the matrix for developing verb phrases, noun phrases, and sentence constructions. As shown in Table 4, development is simultaneous among these areas, but again follows a rough developmental sequence. Each level forms not only a grammatical matrix for later learning but a communicative repertoire in which more subtle grammatical options can become relevant.

Our technique of language-sample analysis is organized around the ideas from Chapter 4 of function, class, and position. We begin with a generalized function or option-to-mean, such as the transitive clause type. We then note the functions within that general option. In most cases, these functions can be listed across a page according to position, e.g., *subject, verb, indirect object, direct object,* and *adverbial* for transitive clauses. We can then form columns below each of these positions or functions and list the class of items that the child used to represent each function. The focus is thus on the different repertoires the child has: words and word combinations to represent grammatical functions, and both words and grammatical functions to express meaning.

In conclusion, I encourage you to try different procedures for language-sample analysis. Don't be afraid to make a few mistakes as you gain experience. See what each approach has to offer and how much work is involved. The ultimate language-sampling system may never exist. In fact, it may turn out that language-sampling techniques should be quite different for various groups of children. A system for clausal children, those knowing some basic structures of language and learning a more elaborate grammar, may not be appropriate for preclausal children showing minimal knowledge of the adult grammatical system. Again, children who know most of the grammatical system but who have difficulty expressing ideas or in academic learning related to language may be best understood through still another approach. As the marathon runner said, we've come a long way but we've hardly begun to move.

THE CULTURALLY DIFFERENT CHILD

As discussed in Chapters 5 and 7, there are additional difficulties in sampling the grammatical skills of culturally different children. First, these children may not demonstrate much of their language repertoires because of cultural and relationship factors. If language disorder is suspected in such a child, there is no substitute for patience and ingenuity in obtaining as representative a sample as possible. As we will see in the next section, the primary variable that the clinician will have to concentrate on in eliciting language samples is the human relationship context.

A second difficulty lies in the fact that language-sample analysis is based on Standard English and formal style. The best we can do with the microcosmic matrix, then, is to get an idea of a child's skill in that dialect. As already pointed out, knowledge of Standard English may or may not be equivalent with language skill in general. The more a child's knowledge of language is based on other languages or dialects, the less likely it becomes that the microcosmic matrix will be able to reflect the child's overall language skill.

This problem is particularly pressing in evaluating children who are growing up in the dialect of inner city blacks, which Labov (1972a) refers to as Black English Vernacular. Particularly in the verb phrase, this dialect uses constructions that would be considered errors in Standard English. For example, wherever *is* or *are* can be contracted in Standard English, they may be omitted in Black English Vernacular: *He gone* for *He is gone.* In other instances, *be* is used rather than *is: He be gone* for *He is gone* (regularly). Similarly, past-tense markers and third-person-singular markers are used differently. Double and triple negatives occur. There are numerous other differences between Black English Vernacular and Standard English. They are conveniently summarized in the excellent booklet by Williams and Wolfram (1977). Other discussions appear in K. Johnson (1970), Baratz and Shuy (1969), Bolinger (1975), and elsewhere.

Two points about Black English Vernacular are particularly important in relation to children's language disorders. First, as noted above, Black English Vernacular employs the same forms as Standard English but uses some of them differently. The result is that it is easy to confuse errors in Standard English with appropriate utterances in Black English Vernacular. This unfortunate situation has been the source of much misunderstanding, particularly in the schools. The second point is that the majority of the differences between the two dialects are in the area of grammatical detail; many are morphological. Consequently, we can still look at the larger elements of the microcosmic matrix in Black English Vernacular speakers. The more fundamental options-to-mean are similar in both dialects.

In sum, keep the larger picture in mind. With all children, but particularly children growing up in Black English Vernacular, concentrate on overall communicative effectiveness and command of language. A significant language disorder will show up in many ways other than whether or not *is* always appears in equative clauses and continuum constructions. Look beyond the details of grammar. Recall that our fundamental question is, how rich a set of options-to-mean does each child employ? Dialectal differences are irrelevant to this question. If a child uses dialectal nonstandard *BE,* so be it.

UTTERANCE LENGTH

We have been concentrating on grammatical analysis in language sampling. A more global measure may also be extracted from a language sample, namely, mean length of utterance. Both average number of words per utterance (e.g. Templin 1957; Mac-Donald and Horstmeier 1978) and average number of morphemes per utterance (e.g., Brown 1973; Morehead and Ingram 1973) have been used to calculate mean length of utterance. Much of the interest in mean length of utterance in words was focused on the development of age norms. Templin (1957) published norms for ages three through eight. No norms have been developed for mean length of utterance in morphemes. In fact, following Brown (1973), the tendency has been to use this measure as an indicator of language level irrespective of age, the argument being that age norms are relatively uninformative.

The data are fairly convincing, however, that degree of grammatical skill is reflected by mean length of utterance in words or morphemes at the early stages of language development (Brown 1973; MacDonald and Horstmeier 1978; Morehead and Ingram 1973; Shipley, Smith, and Gleitman 1969; Sharf 1972). Bloom and Lahey (1978) suggest that the maximum length at which utterances reflect grammatical development is probably five morphemes, which might be equivalent to between two and a half and three years of age. Using quite a different method of calculation, however, O'Donnell, Griffin, and Norris (1967) demonstrated that length continues to increase at least as far as the seventh grade. Instead of focusing on all utterances, these authors adopted the method proposed by Hunt (1965) and calculated average length of complete sentences, including any subordinate clauses.

In sum, mean length of utterance does parallel language growth. This parallel, however, is very general. It does not reflect any of the individual differences in grammatical development discussed at the beginning of this chapter (e.g., Sharf 1972). The very fact that it is a global measure may be of value, however. Brown (1973) characterized five stages in early language development, based on utterance length. These stages have been adopted by many other authors as reference points (e.g., Morehead and Ingram 1973). Similarly, Tyack and Gottsleben (1974) combine the means for words and morphemes into one index.

The measures just discussed consider utterance length without reference to age but as indicating levels of language skill. Age norms for length of utterance may also be of value. Recall Language Sample numbers 1 and 2. As noted already, the errors in both of these children's talking are developmental. Whether or not these children should be considered language impaired, then, depends on their ages (as well as other types of assessment beyond language sampling). Mean length of utterance would be useful here. According to Templin's norms (1957), the first child is below, but within one standard deviation of, her age norm. The second child is significantly below age level (over two standard deviations).

Another area where length measures might be useful is in evaluating nonstandard dialect and bilingual speakers. Differences in grammatical detail could not penalize the child because, by their very nature, length measures are insensitive to such detail. Similarly, the procedure employed by O'Donnell, Griffin, and Norris (1967) could be used with school-aged children, whether Standard English speakers or not.

In sum, mean length of utterance measures cannot provide the specifics required for assessing grammatical structures. Still, they do provide one global measure of language development, particularly at the early stages. Used judiciously in conjunction with other assessment procedures, length measures can provide useful information. One additional problem remains, however. Length measures are easily influenced by the immediate situation. That is, they are influenced not only by grammatical skill, but also by the child's response to the environment (Muma 1978). This observation leads directly to our next topic.

OBTAINING LANGUAGE SAMPLES

Now that we have an idea of what we're looking for in language samples, we can consider questions about how to gather those samples. In this section I will discuss two factors involved in collecting samples of children's talking. The first is techniques for eliciting talking. The second is concerned with the number of utterances that should be included in a language sample.

Eliciting a Language Sample

As has been emphasized, especially in Chapters 4 and 5, the way a person talks is always affected by the situation. As much as possible, then, we need to be aware of the effects of the particular techniques we use in gathering language samples. There are many possible variations. The sample can be elicited by the clinician or by a parent. It can be obtained in the home or in the school or clinic. The stimuli can emphasize pictures, objects, or focus directly on conversation without external materials. The session can be in the form of an interview or unstructured play, or the child can be asked to tell a narrative of some sort.

It is most important that a language sample be as representative and valid as possible. Our goal is a true picture of the child's language ability. However, "representative" can be taken in two ways. First, it may mean that the language sample is a fair reflection of the child's knowledge of language. Second, it can mean that the sample is typical of how the child talks in situations similar to the one in which the language sample was collected.

Several studies suggest that both of these interpretations may apply at once. Children may use approximately the same language structures in different language-sampling contexts, but the frequencies of different structures may vary with the situation. Thus, Olswang and Carpenter (1978) reported that language samples elicited by mothers and by speech clinicians were equivalent in terms of language structures but that mothers elicited a larger number of utterances. Similarly, Scott and Taylor (1978) found that language samples elicited in the clinic and in the home contained about the same structures, but the frequencies of various structures varied between the two situations. Children used more complex utterances, questions, and modals at home. In the clinic their talking focused more on here-and-now activities. Again, Mein (1961) compared two techniques for eliciting talking from retarded individuals. Describing pictures produced more nouns, while a conversational setting produced more word types, particularly verbs.

Other work, however, shows the situation to be more complex. Leach (1972) has shown that questioning limits the variety of responses the child may produce. At the same time, Turnure, Buium, and Thurlow (1976) found that questioning enhances verbal elaboration in children's responses. It may be that questions restrict the listener to certain types of responses but encourage elaboration in those areas. We often use concrete stimuli with young children, but Blank (1975) found that eliciting talking with the stimuli in view decreased the richness of preschoolers' talking. Perhaps this situation involves one aspect of what Cook-Gumperz (1977) has called situated mean-

ing. When an object is in view, certain things are apparent and simply don't need to be said, or at least don't need elaboration. Further, it has been shown that the social status of the listener affects the grammatical structures employed by retarded individuals (Bedrosian and Prutting 1978), and children (Ervin-Tripp 1977; Labov 1972a).

We can conclude from the above studies that a definitive procedure for eliciting language samples has not been identified and is not likely to appear. Do not despair, however. We can use the fact that different language-sampling procedures produce different results to our advantage. Return to the idea that the sample should be representative of the child's language use. We can choose techniques with this idea in mind. I would try to choose situations that are representative of recurring aspects of the child's life outside of the clinic. For a young child it might be play or household routines such as mealtime; for an older child it might involve discussion of favorite activities such as sports, hobbies, or special interests in school. By focusing on real events and themes we increase the ecological validity of the situation for the child. Cazden (1970) has shown that children's talking is enhanced when the topic of discussion is of immediate interest to the child. Similarly, Labov (1972a) demonstrated that talking is enriched when the child has an intense personal involvement in the topic.

Finally, I would try to obtain the language sample in a situation that is parallel with that in which language training is likely to be done. In supervising language intervention I have sometimes noticed that the language sample is gathered in one context and the training occurs in quite another. Both situations are rather artificial and far different from anything typical of the child's life. The result is that the talking the child does in each situation is almost irrelevant to that in the others.

The interpersonal context is tremendously important in language sampling. How we behave influences how the child will behave. If we communicate primarily through questions, we restrict the child to certain types of utterances. In addition, because frequently the answers to questions are incomplete sentences, we may artificially shorten the child's average length of utterance. On a broader scale, by placing many demands to talk on a child we may effectively drive that child into silence or other resistance. This possibility is particularly important with culturally different children. Overall, the type of relationship we offer a child profoundly influences the nature of the language sample we obtain. In Chapter 11 I will discuss structuring relationships to enhance talking. Some of that information will be very relevant to language sampling.

Language-Sample Length

There are conflicting views on the number of utterances that should be included in a language sample. Again, the goal is that the sample be representative. Too short a sample may not allow children to demonstrate what they can do, while too long a sample puts a heavy burden of work on the teacher or clinician.

From the perspective outlined in this chapter, we want to "place" the child in the microcosmic matrix. That is, we have a series of questions about which grammatical options the child is using. There is no set number of utterances to analyze, then. Following Dever (1978), we analyze until our questions are answered. I do not mean that one should go on sampling until every detail of the child's grammar has been specified. Remember that usually language-sample analysis will be followed by informal assessment. If some information is still in doubt after a reasonable amount of sampling, it can be pursued at that time. Occasionally it will be found during informal assessment that further language sampling would be useful, for example, with a child who was very reticent during earlier sampling. Again, we do not need a rigid procedure. We need the flexibility to understand each child as best we can.

CONCLUSIONS

This chapter has presented a framework for evaluating the grammatical structures in children's talking and for developing sequences for training grammatical structures. It is only a framework. Within it, the clinician can make a rough determination of the levels at which a child is functioning and narrow down the choices of grammatical structures that might be appropriate for training. Language sampling is rarely, if ever, the only factor in determining goals for intervention.

I have called this framework the microcosmic matrix to call attention to the fact that we typically do not teach children the entire language. Rather, we teach each child a microcosm, a set of options that form a matrix for further language learning. Some of this further learning may occur through our guidance, but much of it often occurs outside any special help we may provide. This learning is part of children's attempts to communicate in various situations in their lives. The child's communicative problem solving and the forces inherent in the transactional model enhance this learning beyond what we have taught.

In view of these ideas, it is important that grammatical structures for training be selected with care. The concept of "option-to-mean" is relevant here. Given that a child is already using certain structures, what grammatical options could we teach that would enhance that child's effectiveness as a communicator the most? An imponderable question, and yet one that we must face. Some choices are certainly better than others.

Table 4, summarizing the microcosmic matrix, is organized into both columns and rows. The columns represent different areas of grammar that are developing simultaneously. The rows suggest that development is sequential, although it will vary from child to child. I have argued that the developmental sequence is not well enough specified to be applied precisely in designing training sequences. Nevertheless, it makes sense to follow a developmental sequence in language teaching, however general that sequence may be.

The microcosmic matrix is based on Standard English and formal talking. It does not include variations in style or dialect. However, decisions about which structures are appropriate for a given child are left up to the person doing the assessment. Depending on the situation, the clinician may have to differentiate errors that represent language impairment from normal developmental errors and variations in dialect. The analysis is primarily descriptive: What kinds of grammatical options is the child using? Ultimately we are less interested in the fine points of grammar than in discovering the child's repertoire for using language as a communicator.

I have emphasized the importance of decision making by the teacher or clinician, both in language-sample analysis and in determining the goals of intervention. After wading through this chapter, your decision may be to leave language sampling to someone else. I think that would be a mistake. Language sampling provides some of the best information we can get about how children are using language. If you are having difficulty with language-sample analysis, work on one thing at a time. Focus only on clause variations first. Then work on the clause types. Ignore all other detail. When you have clauses in hand, look at verb phrases or noun phrases. Consult other sources, such as Dever (1978), Crystal, Fletcher, and Garman (1976), Tyack and Gottsleben (1974), and Lee (1974). Keep practicing. Eventually you can master the microcosmic matrix method and go beyond it (Dare I say into the communicative cosmos?).

In assessment we attempt to decide whether or not a child needs special help with language and, if so, what that help might be. We saw in the preceding chapter that these decisions become increasingly precise as we understand a child more thoroughly. After initial assessment, language sampling gives us a great deal of information. We still have questions, though, about errors and gaps in the language sample, about the most efficient approach for each child, and about other factors related to intervention. We see now how language sampling fits into the larger assessment plan from the preceding chapter. Language-sample analysis provides one set of questions that can be pursued through informal assessment and exploratory teaching. Sometimes further sampling will be helpful. Ultimately, assessment evolves into treatment. In the next chapter I will describe some general principles that underlie intervention with language-impaired children.

9

PRINCIPLES OF INTERVENTION

What I wish to do in this chapter is to integrate more fully some of the information from previous chapters and develop some more specific perspectives on intervention. I will begin by expanding the notion of language use as a problem-solving task. This subject will be tied in with a comparison of comprehension and expression, which are fundamental in the child's transactions with the environment. Problem solving also leads to cognitive strategies. In this chapter I will explore cognitive strategies in terms of their implications for training language-disordered children. Finally, in the third portion of the chapter, I will develop a point of view concerning the process of language training. How can we structure transactions with the child that will contribute maximally to language learning?

PROBLEM SOLVING AND LANGUAGE USE

We begin with problem solving. In working with language-disordered children the goal is not merely to teach language, that is, to deposit knowledge about language in the child's head. Rather, the aim is to foster the *use* of language by the child, in both comprehension and expression. The use of language involves active problem solving. Children have to decide what the utterances they hear mean; in addition, they have to decide what to say themselves, and how to say it.

The relation between problem solving and language use has been developed at various points along the way. In Chapter 3 it was emphasized that perception involves choice. More specifically, language comprehension is a process in which the listener develops or chooses an interpretation for an utterance. In Chapter 4 I developed the idea that the nature of language itself lends itself nicely to this idea of choice. Following Olson (1970b), the meaning of an utterance is in how it differentiates among the alternatives that are available. These alternatives are represented by the concepts and rules of Chapter 1. In parallel fashion, Halliday (1973) describes grammatical structures as options-to-mean. Alternatives, options . . . these terms only make sense if we think of the language user as making choices. Further, in Chapter 5, it was suggested that these choices also involve the relationship aspects of human communication. Finally, in Chapter 2 we looked at cognitive strategies. In short, all of these chapters converge in the same direction, that of viewing the language-learning child as an active problem solver or decision maker.

Interesting evidence of problem solving in language acquisition comes from Braine's (1976) description of groping patterns. In studying children's early word combinations, he found that individual children would use varying word orders to express a grammatical relation for some period of time. He termed these usages groping patterns, and hypothesized that the child had not yet learned the rule governing the specific relation involved. Consequently, the child tries various word orders. At a later time the variation ceases as the rule becomes established.

If we define problem solving as making decisions, it is hard to deny that children engage in problem solving during language learning and use. The next step is to investigate just what the problems to solve might be. I will approach this matter by comparing the processes of comprehension and expression.

COMPREHENSION
AND EXPRESSION

It has been proposed that comprehension precedes or at least parallels expression (Ingram 1974; Winitz and Reeds 1975). There have been some arguments, however, that expression may precede comprehension in certain instances (Chapman and Miller 1975). This debate has important implications for working with language-disordered children. The majority of clinicians and teachers focus their training directly on expression (for example, Dever 1978; Crystal, Fletcher, and Garman 1976; Lee, Koenigsknecht, and Mulhern 1975). The argument has been made, however, that training should concentrate on comprehension (Winitz 1973; Winitz and Reeds 1975).

Bloom (1974) presented another viewpoint, that comprehension and expression are different but related processes. Further, she suggests that both are subject to many factors. I would like to explore what some of those factors might be. It seems to me that there are two fundamental differences between comprehension and expression. They differ in their information-processing requirements and in the human relationship decisions that are involved. I will discuss these two areas separately.

Information Processing

Comprehension and expression differ in both the amount and nature of the information that is processed. In comprehension one needs to process only that information necessary to make an interpretation of an utterance. Through analysis by synthesis the listener makes use of top-down constraints and the context to predict which information will need to be attended to carefully and which information can be passed by. The effect is that the listener does not have to process every aspect of a sentence thoroughly. We listen for gist.

In expression, on the other hand, one cannot "talk for gist." A speaker must decide exactly what the form of an utterance will be and structure the component parts accordingly. The speaker puts all the detail into the sentence. Let me elaborate on this contrast.

Comprehension and Information Processing

The major decision making in comprehension is in selecting an interpretation for each utterance. I have already discussed this process in Chapter 3. Olson (1970a) has argued that recognition is a basic component of comprehension. That is, we match the utterance with other information we have available, both in memory and in the context. Olson argues that recognition is an incomplete process. In studies of visual perception in which the movements of the subjects' eyes were tracked, Olson and others he cites found that children do not process the entire stimulus configuration. They only look for relevant or salient cues within the stimulus. These cues are based at least partially on the contrast set that is either present or implied. Suppose you take three different colored blocks and hide a nickel under one. Then you tell a child, "It's under the red one." The child does not have to process *under* very thoroughly, and *it's, the* and *one* even less, if at all. On the other hand, you might use a small box and tell the child the nickel is in the box. This time, assuming there are no other containers present, the child need attend carefully only to *in.*

We see here very directly the problem solving described in Chapter 3, involving the utterance and the situation, each forming the context for the other. In interpreting utterances, the listener relies on grammatical structure, meaning, the nonverbal situation, previous utterances, and general knowledge from past experience. The relative importance of these variables will change from moment to moment, topic to topic, and person to person. The idea of equifinality from general systems theory comes to mind. There are a lot of roads to comprehension. The interplay among these factors is related to the cognitive strategies employed by an individual during any comprehension task, as well as the character of the message and the situation.

One factor affecting the difficulty with decision making in comprehension is the number of alternatives that are available. In contrast to the utterances to the child a paragraph ago, suppose I look deeply into your eyes and say, "All life is a metaphor." It would be hard to know what I meant, because there are so many possible alternatives. What is *all life*? What did I mean by *metaphor*? The context is no help. All that it tells you is that I must think the statement profound, because of my compelling gaze. In clinical work we frequently control the number of alternatives available to a child. For example, in vocabulary training a clinician will vary the number of objects in front of the child according to the difficulty of the task for that child. With some children only one object may be presented: "Jerry, show me the ball," when the nonverbal stimulus consists of only a single ball. If Jerry responds appropriately at all, the clinician has insured that the correct alternative will be selected. A child working at a more advanced level might be asked to choose among several stimuli, and perhaps those stimuli will be very similar to each other.

Another factor affecting the difficulty of comprehension is the listener's awareness of the alternatives in the situation. If a child does not know what the alternatives are, adequate comprehension is not possible. If I ask a child to go outside and pick me a loquat and the child is not knowledgeable about such things, I may get a strawberry or a rose in return, or the child may come back empty-handed. A more common example would be in trying to explain to a young child that daddy will be back at 2:15. The child simply does not know our numerical system for measuring time. Consequently, that set of alternatives is not available for use. After several attempts at explanation, usually including elaborate pointing at a watch, we give up and say, "Daddy will be back after a while." The child is probably crying by now, anyway, or has lost interest in the whole matter.

The idea of recognition as a cornerstone of comprehension can carry us a long way, but it seems to me that in certain cases comprehension entails something more. In these situations the listener must grasp a relationship that is new or unfamiliar. Thus, you may have several pieces of information floating around, and a particular sentence you read or hear shows you how those pieces fit together. A gap in your knowledge is filled (Gagné 1970). In such instances comprehension goes beyond recognition to the acquisition of new knowledge. In Olson's terms, the utterance directs your perceptions in new ways. New alternatives become available. This type of learning is common in most people's lives. It is at the heart of formal education, from elementary school on up through the use of texts such as this one.

In summary, the problem solving in comprehension centers around selecting an interpretation of an utterance from a set of alternatives. Typically this decision does not require processing all the detail in the utterance. Rather, the listener attends to those aspects of the utterance that seem relevant or salient. The problem solving used in this task will vary with a number of factors, including the situation and the listener's purposes.

Expression and Information Processing

Utterances are patterned stimuli. The patterns are those described by linguistic rules. Following Olson, I have stressed that in perceiving a pattern the child extracts only some of the information in that pattern. Add to this now the conclusion from Chapter 3 that in comprehension, linguistic structure is frequently less important than semantics and the context. We can now see a major contrast between comprehension and expression. In expression all linguistic detail must be accounted for by the speaker. Expression requires continuous decision making at all levels of language throughout the utterance. While some aspects of grammar may be considered automatic (see, for example, Kirk and Kirk 1971), nevertheless the speaker puts all the detail into the utterance. The listener may select only those cues that seem relevant, whereas the speaker must control all the cues present, including not only grammar and semantics but also matters of melodic contour, stress, rate of talking, and degree of precision of articulation.

The speaker chooses grammatical categories and structures to communicate ideas and relations. Included will be choices about functions to be represented, choices of items from the classes that are associated with those functions, and decisions about position. As Bloom (1974) points out, the child needs some knowledge of grammar to produce an utterance in this fashion, whereas the same utterance might be comprehended with less awareness of grammatical structure. From this point of view, the development of language involves the acquisition of increasing numbers of options-to-mean, parallel with the development of information-processing skills and conceptual relations. In the early stages of expression, both language-disordered and normally developing children will omit much of the grammatical detail. The child communicates without the redundancy in language and without many of the details of structure and nuances of meaning. These communicative efforts are relatively successful because listeners typically do not need all the grammatical detail to decide on an interpretation for an utterance. Further, when they can't comprehend, they can elicit additional utterances from the child.

As the options get finer and finer, their importance in meaning diminishes; their relevance becomes increasingly grammatical. For example, two-word combinations, clause types, and variations from the microcosmic matrix carry heavy meaning potential. Classifying stimuli as agents, actions, and objects and specifying the relations among them are basic in using language to communicate knowledge. Telegrams —a highly successful means of communication—are based on expression at this level. At a later stage grammatical morphemes such as plurals and tense markers are acquired. They represent different options-to-mean, but those meanings are frequently redundant. Finally, there are grammatical morphemes such as the *to* in *I want to read,* where their importance is entirely in the area of grammatical detail. They have no semantic function. It is precisely these levels of redundancy and grammatical detail that can be easily passed over in comprehension. At the same time, these areas are often impaired in language-disordered children. I will return to this matter shortly.

Clinical Implications

In summary, we see that comprehension and expression are indeed quite different information-processing tasks. They differ in both the quantity and quality of information to be processed. It appears that comprehension is more flexible in both areas. The amount of detail attended to in comprehension varies with the situation and the listener's purposes, but frequently some of the detail present in the utterance is not actively processed. In this sense, perception of the grammatical pattern of an utterance is often incomplete. Expression is complete, however; all detail must be actively processed.

Winitz and Reeds (1975) observed that expression requires retrieval of linguistic information, whereas comprehension employs only recognition. Huttenlocher (1974) discussed this matter in some detail. To begin with, ". . . [receptive language] involves *recognition* of words and *recall* of the objects, acts and relations for which they stand, whereas [expressive language] involves *recognition* of the objects, acts and relations and *recall* of the words that stand for them" (p. 335, italics in original). An individual's experiences are important in their own right, but language is only important to the extent that it is related to those experiences. Further, Huttenlocher notes, "Given a familiar word, retrieval of meaning may well be obligatory or automatic ex-

cept when interfering events occur during the retrieval process. The link from a particular perceptual experience to a particular word is almost certainly less direct" (p. 335). Following Olson (1970b), as discussed in Chapter 4, there are many ways we can refer to a single event or object. Not only must speakers retrieve vocabulary and grammatical options from their repertoires, they must retrieve precisely the right options, and in rapid succession. Expression requires search from memory, a process that is not always easy, as you know from taking exams, studying foreign languages, and general "It's on the tip of my tongue" phenomena.

The implications of these conclusions for language intervention are several and, I believe, far-reaching. It could be argued that learning a grammatical structure through comprehension might be easier for a child than learning that same structure through expression, because of the lighter information-processing load. At the same time, remember that grammatical operators, an area often requiring remediation, are just the type of linguistic details that are likely to be glossed over in comprehension. A possible approach to this dilemma would be to arrange comprehension training so that the grammatical structure of interest is a highly relevant feature of the utterance. Thus, the structure to be trained would differentiate among the alternatives in the situation. The plural morpheme could be taught in situations where only that morpheme differentiates between alternatives involving one item or several items (*penny, pennies; shoe, shoes*).

Training expression, on the other hand, may be problematical in that, at some level, the child must always be attending to all the detail in the utterance, not just the particular aspect being trained. Also, the child must actively retrieve both the target structure and familiar parts of the utterance. The information-processing differences between expression and comprehension also help in understanding why, as noted in Chapter 5, a culturally different child may comprehend Standard English fairly well and yet demonstrate little skill with expression in that formal style.

I will be further developing the implications of this section in following chapters. At present, it is time to turn our attention to the second major difference between comprehension and expression.

Interpersonal Behavior

The second fundamental difference between comprehension and expression arises from looking at language use as an aspect of human relationships. Talking is always an overt interpersonal act (given that a receiver is present). From Chapter 5 we know that an utterance is always a comment on the relationship in which it is produced. Relationships are established and maintained through communication. Communicative behavior, in turn, is regulated by the rules governing any particular relationship. Thus, expressive language is always subject to the metarules of whatever relationships are involved in a particular exchange. These metarules relate closely to the transactional patterns previously discussed. In contrast, comprehension is covert; it does not involve any observable behavior and is thus in and of itself not a relationship message. Of course, comprehension is not devoid of relationship implications, as in situations in which you must take directions from someone. However, the point is that, by definition, expression is inseparable from relationship functioning. As with the information-processing section, we will explore the differences between comprehension and expression as interpersonal processes by looking at each separately. We will begin with comprehension.

Interpersonal Behavior and Comprehension

The major interpersonal factor in comprehension is the fact that the listener must direct attention to the speaker. In so doing the listener accepts a relationship with the speaker in which the listener will indeed listen. The relationship may be defined as a complementary one in which each participant has equal status. Relationships are defined in this way, for example, when two friends or two fellow language trainers, talk together. On the other hand, the relationship may be one in which the listener has one-down status and takes orders or instruction from the speaker. The child in clinic is typically in this position.

These relationship aspects of comprehension are of direct importance in training. If a child chooses not to attend to your verbal stimuli, then the question of whether that child comprehends or not becomes irrelevant, because there is no opportunity for comprehension. It can be seen, then, that the definition of the relationship establishes a set of metarules that influences the use of linguistic and conceptual rules. Children must be willing to attempt comprehension before their knowledge of language can come into play.

Again, it is worth remembering that comprehension is an internal, rather than an observable, process. Attending is also primarily covert, although it is often associated with certain iconic behaviors, such as direction of gaze and orientation of the body. Obviously, these behaviors in a listener do not necessarily mean that the listener is attending, much less comprehending, what is being said.

Finally, once an interpretation of an utterance has been chosen, the listener must decide whether to accept it or not. Such decisions are made partly on a relationship basis and partly on the basis of one's knowledge about the topic. It may be argued that these decisions are not really part of comprehension, but part of whatever evaluation or thought processes follow comprehension. I can certainly think of times that I have decided what an utterance means and then gone on to make a decision about its truth value (usually too late). As a practical matter, this level of decision adds another difficulty to the assessment of children's language comprehension. Unless the child emits the appropriate information, one cannot tell whether the child does not comprehend something or comprehends it but chooses not to accept its content, either for relationship or conceptual reasons. A clinician says to a child, ''Betty, it's time to put the toys away.'' Betty goes right on playing . . .

I have been almost unable to discuss comprehension as a relationship process without referring to overt signs of attention and of acceptance or rejection of messages. These signs illustrate the simultaneous nature of comprehension and expression.

Interpersonal Behavior and Expression

There appears to be a hierarchy of rules governing language expression. I will describe four levels that are components of this hierarchy. Most of these rules are in the area of pragmatics, the relations between language and language users.

Relationship Rules. At the highest level in the hierarchy, there are relationship rules.

How you communicate depends on the relationship you are participating in at that moment. This point was abundantly made previously, but consider it now in this light: Relationship rules include a set of metarules that govern the use of linguistic rules. That is, the types of utterances one generates, including their grammatical structure, are influenced by the human relationship in which one is communicating. For example, an adult is likely to use a more formal style of grammar when talking with an important dignitary than when talking with friends around a campfire. As discussed in earlier chapters, relationship rules are also influenced by cultural patterns. Of particular importance to us are those patterns relating to peer culture and to children from different subcultures within our society.

The interplay between relationship rules and talking has direct relevance in working with language-disordered children. I recall one child who talked in multiword utterances outside the clinic but was silent while in the clinic. I have known two children who were particularly striking in a similar way. During individual sessions they would talk during play activities, but when asked to produce specific utterances, they resisted vigorously, shouting, ''No,'' or ''No more pictures!'' One of them even punched the clinician in the nose! Another little boy, who was observed both in the clinic and at home, was found to talk at the lowest rate in his home, more in the clinic, and the most in his own backyard, where no one was there but him and the observer.

Choice of Medium of Expression. A second level in the rule hierarchy governing expression is related to the channel or medium of expression. In many situations, one can decide whether to communicate through talking or through nonverbal means. Consequently, these decisions involve another set of metarules governing the use of linguistic rules. If one decides to communicate nonverbally, one literally rules out the use of linguistic rules. This level is also important with language-disordered children. At the relationship level, a child may decide to communicate willingly with the clinician. At the channel level, though, that child may choose to communicate nonverbally. Recall the child in Chapter 5 whose nonverbal communication was rich, with many conventional gestures and iconic signs. Although his expressive skills were poor, this child could talk, but he rarely elected to do so. In a parallel vein, some stutterers prefer to write notes in certain situations rather than talk. We cannot avoid communicating, as pointed out in Chapter 5, but we do have some leeway in deciding how to go about it.

Social Codes. A third level in the hierarchy consists of rules related to the social code (Krauss and Glucksberg 1977). At the end of Chapter 4 it was pointed out that we structure our utterances with a listener in mind. As illustrated in Chapter 6, there is abundant evidence that parents structure their utterances differently when talking to young children than when talking to adults. While some of this variation is a consequence of relationship rules, much of it is due to social code rules. Parents learn to structure utterances to their children in ways that those children are likely to comprehend. Similarly, it has been found that four-year-olds alter the structure of their utterances while talking to younger children as opposed to other four-year-olds (Shatz and Gelman 1973). It is easy to see this level of rules operating in observing clinicians and teachers talk with language-disordered children. We select certain kinds of vocabulary items, keep utterance length short, and so on. In fact, a special set of social code rules exists in the training session itself. A verbal exchange is going on, but it may not be a conversation in the typical sense. The clinician may not be particularly interested in what the child says, but in how it is said. In some cases the child is asked to imitate rather than communicate. Young children may not appreciate these special rules in the social code.

This code is an interesting example of the social nature of talking. The speaker selects vocabulary and grammatical options that will identify the intended alternative in the situation. All these decisions are influenced by knowledge of what the listener is like. From the perspective being developed here, the major point is that social coding involves another set of metarules governing linguistic choices. Grammatical structure (the linguistic rule system) is subservient to, or governed by, the social determinants in structuring a message.

Discourse Rules. Discourse rules form a fourth set of metarules that govern the use of grammatical rules. Each utterance is affected by the content and structure of utterances preceding it. As noted in the previous chapter, we often respond to questions with elliptical, or incomplete, utterances. A question seeking affirmation or denial often requires only a *yes* or *no* for an answer. A *wh-* question often requires only that whatever is represented by the *wh-* word be identified. Pronominal reference similarly depends on discourse rules. An individual who has already been identified may be referred to as *he* or *she*. Further, in an ongoing conversation there will be frequent changes in the referents for words such as *I, me,* and *you,* according to who is speaking. In the same vein, there is the more general process referred to by Chafe (1972) as "foregrounding." In a verbal exchange certain topics become identified as central to the exchange. These topics are foregrounded and, as such, do not need to be continually identified. For example, if we are talking about a baseball game, many utterances may be exchanged that do not mention or name that game directly. At the same time, we know we're talking about the game. Chafe notes that a speaker may assume that foregrounded topics are on the listener's mind at the moment. This statement is noteworthy because it emphasizes the interconnections between discourse and social coding.

Relationships among the Four Levels. We can get further perspective on social code and discourse rules by returning to the work of Marslen-Wilson and Welsh (1978), discussed in Chapter 3. They described both top-down and bottom-up processes in language perception. Top-down processes involve constraints in what an utterance might be. These constraints stem from the individual's knowledge of language and the world. Bottom-up processes involve extracting information from the message itself. These authors have hypothesized that related processing might occur during expression. On the basis of previous utterances and knowledge of the listener, the speaker can generate a message that contains only the minimal bottom-up information necessary for the listener to comprehend the message in the context. Thus, the speaker predicts, through top-down processing, that a simple *no* will be enough to answer a particular question. On the other hand, if the question is *Didn't you say you don't like lemon in your tea?*, a more elaborate answer may be required to clarify the individual's taste in tea. Clearly, we are looking at a problem-solving process. A speaker decides how best to differentiate the focus of the utterance from its contrast set for the par-

ticular listener who is being addressed. The speaker then selects grammatical options to represent that meaning, again taking that listener into consideration. While social coding and discourse rules are not the same, they interact heavily in this decision making.

It can also be seen that the relationship and the medium-of-expression levels are not independent of each other. The choice of nonverbal rather than verbal means to send messages is itself an iconic sign about the relationship involved. When I was a boy, I had a friend who told me he was never afraid of his father's wrath, no matter how angry the father became, until the father stopped talking! Further, the decision to use verbal or nonverbal means of expression may be made on either social code or relationship grounds. If a child asks me where something is, I may point silently as the most efficient way to transmit that information to the child, or I may point silently because I am too angry to grace that child with my words.

Finally, social code decisions are heavily influenced by relationship considerations. A father may talk to a young child in a certain way in order to increase the chances of the child's understanding, but in addition he may talk that way because he loves his child. Similarly, the nuances of how we talk to other people result from both social code and relationship decisions. More generally, we can select and combine among verbal and nonverbal behaviors to vary the discreteness, discursiveness, and linearity of our messages to a virtually infinite degree.

Permit me one more example of the importance of metarules in governing grammatical structure. This one involves my son when he was in kindergarten. Halfway through dinner he announced, "I ain't got no meat." We gently corrected him: "That's, I don't have any meat." He responded, "I ain't got, I doesn't got, and I never did got any meat!" Knowing a structure and using it in a particular interpersonal context are not the same thing.

Summary

In the chapter on assessment I characterized behavior as selection from a repertoire. Knowledge of language is one such repertoire. In the language sampling chapter I described that repertoire as a set of grammatical options. Now I have outlined some of the forces that influence selections from that repertoire. My central goal has been to emphasize the interpersonal nature of expression. The four levels of rules form a very loose hierarchy at best. In principle, each is a separate level and can be studied as such. In practice, all four blend and interact together.

In summary, expression is determined by a host of factors. Ultimately, it is an interpersonal process that takes place in specific situations over a background of transactional patterns between child and environment. The major thrust of the decision making in expression is in developing an utterance that will accomplish the speaker's intentions. Included in these intentions are relationship as well as content factors.

More generally, I concur with Bloom (1974) that comprehension and expression are quite different processes. Debates about which comes first now seem less relevant than questions about what is involved in each. The metaphor of problem solving as a way to look at both comprehension and expression appears useful, as long as one doesn't take it too literally. Problem solving implies the utilization of cognitive strategies. It is to the relationship between these two that we now turn.

THE CHILD AS A LANGUAGE LEARNER

I have been arguing that language use is an active problem-solving process. It follows that children are active learners. The child is not a *tabula rasa* upon which the structures of language are writ by the environment. Children participate in their own learning. They try things out, observe the consequences of their actions, and monitor the activities of models closely.

It seems probable that the child has to be an active learner if language intervention is going to be successful in a broad sense. There are too many rules to teach, too many situations to cover, particularly if the child is seen for only a few sessions each week. It was with these ideas in mind that I proposed the microcosmic matrix in the preceding chapter. We do not teach the whole language (Imagine teaching children enough vocabulary to get through junior high or enough skill in pragmatics to get through their first dates!). Rather, we teach a carefully selected sample, a microcosm, a basic repertoire. In light of these considerations, my guess is that many of our successes in language intervention may be due partly to the trainer's work but also partly due to the child's own active problem solving, in and out of the training session. I do not make these remarks to be critical of current training procedures in any way. Rather, I hope to take advantage of the child's propensities toward active learning to enhance the efficiency of language intervention.

Cognitive Strategies

The work on children's information processing reviewed in Chapter 2 suggests that children's capacities don't change as their skills develop as much as their techniques for processing information change. A straightforward conclusion from this observation is that we should encourage and enhance our clients' active processing and attendant cognitive strategies during language intervention.

A preliminary question to ask is, can cognitive strategies be taught? The tentative answer seems to be yes, at least to some degree. We saw some evidence bearing on this question in Chapter 2. Flavell (1970) was able to get young children to name objects in a memory task, a strategy that resulted in improved recall in the task. In the work by Belmont and Butterfield (1969, 1971; Butterfield and Belmont 1975; Butterfield, Wambold, and Belmont 1973) retardates were trained in the use of very specific cognitive strategies, again in a memory task. As before, the training resulted in enhanced performance on the task. Other work in training cognitive strategies has been summarized in a review by Denney (1973). In general, it appears that the way a child approaches a problem-solving task can be changed, although there are some contradictory findings in this relatively new field of research. One interesting finding relevant to our interests is that children's accuracy in problem-solving tasks can be enhanced by teaching more efficient perceptual strategies (Meichenbaum and Goodman 1971; Ridberg, Parke, and Hetherington 1971). These studies are of interest because of the importance of perceptual strategies in comprehension and, as we shall see, in problem solving in general. Unfortunately all three studies employed visual tasks, so that the results are merely suggestive for auditory language processing.

There are a number of problems to be dealt with, however, before we begin training cognitive strategies for language learning. First, also demonstrated in Chapter 2,

there is the problem of metarules governing the use of particular cognitive strategies. In both the work by Flavell and that by Belmont and Butterfield, the subjects did not apply on their own the cognitive strategies they had been taught. During experimental sessions following the training sessions, they reverted to their previous strategies. A second problem is that we simply don't know what the appropriate strategies to teach would be. Chunking and analysis-by-synthesis might be likely candidates, but most children are probably employing these strategies in some form already. We might want to take advantage of them in training, rather than teach them. Beyond such very general strategies it is hard to conceive just which strategies should be taught. This matter is further complicated by a third problem: All the evidence available suggests that cognitive strategies vary between individuals and between tasks and that individuals are likely to switch strategies during the same task. Finally, strategies for comprehension will not be the same as those for expression, given the differences between those two processes. Hence, I must conclude that teaching cognitive strategies for language learning, however attractive in principle, does not appear to be a practical option at present.[1]

Problem Solving

We face a dilemma: Cognitive strategies are important in language learning and use, but we cannot teach those strategies directly. One approach to this problem would be

[1] This picture may change eventually with the development of the new field of cognitive behavior modification. Ironically, however, efforts so far in this field have depended on the child's language skill. Children are taught to modify other areas of decision making through self-talk (Meichenbaum 1977a, 1977b).

to involve the child in problem-solving activities. These activities, by definition, would invoke the application of cognitive strategies by the child, although we couldn't precisely characterize those strategies. Winitz and Reeds describe a language-training program that works in this way, although they do not discuss cognitive strategies directly. They define problem solving as the "... induction of grammatical rules" (1975, p. 24). In their program an utterance is presented to the subject and then an array of pictures. The subject selects the picture that matches the utterance. The verbal stimuli are varied systematically as the program progresses, so that the subject is confronted with a series of grammatical options. The problem solving, then, involves selecting alternatives to match various grammatical options. Thus, grammatical rules are induced by the learner, rather than being explained by the teacher.

Winitz and Reeds's program employs a picture-utterance match task, although they do not suggest that their approach must employ that task. As discussed in Chapter 3, this task evokes what may be some fairly specialized cognitive strategies. What is needed at this point is a more general perspective in which to view problem solving. We turn now to another notion from David Olson.

Performatory Acts

In discussing cognitive development and its relations to perception and behavior, Olson (1970a) describes a very general mechanism called the "performatory act." While Olson's focus is not on problem solving *per se,* it will provide an excellent framework for considering problem solving of various types. The idea is that the child acts on the environment in ways that reveal the alter-

natives that are available in the situation. Thus, perception and action are interdependent in the child's learning. The ways the child acts may be relatively unorganized, as in the exploration behavior of a one-year-old playing with blocks, or they may be highly planful, as in the search behavior of a fourteen-year-old figuring out how to use a new set of fishing tackle. The point is that through performatory acts, the child becomes aware of the alternatives in the situation and, ultimately, which alternatives to choose on which occasions.

I recall offering a little boy in clinic some glue one time. The glue was in an open tub, and there was a paint brush to apply it with. There was also an assortment of blocks of wood and pieces of cardboard for the child to glue together. First, he dipped the brush in the glue and stirred it around for a while. Then he noticed that when he took the brush out of the tub, it dripped. He began to dip the brush and then lift it higher and higher, watching the drips fall back into the tub. Soon he was making lines of drops across the wood and cardboard. Then he began to paint pieces of wood vigorously. Then he tried a drop on the back of his hand, then on his shirt sleeve, then on my hand. Through this activity he was exploring the alternatives available with glue and a brush. I had to stop him shortly because he was beginning to demonstrate a little too much enthusiasm. Further, he began to explore the interpersonal alternatives, not merely what glue does, but what would I allow him to do with glue. We spent a few minutes of each session with the glue. It was several days before he discovered the "major" alternative, gluing things together. Then, after sticking with this activity for several sessions, he began to explore different shapes that he could construct by gluing pieces of wood together. This example illustrates the idea of performatory acts. Through acting on the glue he learned the alternatives available in using glue. The learning is neither motor nor perceptual; it is both, each in complement with the other.

Olson points out that language learning requires learning new cues. These cues include both various alternatives of meaning and various grammatical and lexical options for representing those alternatives. Talking, then, could be described as performatory activity in which children produce utterances and observe their consequences. The groping patterns described by Braine (1976) come to mind as examples of performatory acts in the area of grammar. Comprehension could also be viewed in terms of performatory acts. Upon hearing an utterance, a child may respond in some way. Through the responses of others to many such actions, the child becomes aware of alternatives of meaning and grammar.

As Olson notes, when first carrying out some performance the child may not know what the alternatives are regarding each component of that act. If a child is not aware of the appropriate alternatives, it will be difficult for that child to obtain that information simply by looking at a model. Olson (1970a) has shown, for example, that children may recognize diagonals on a checkerboard and yet be unable to construct a diagonal. As a child becomes aware of what the alternatives in a situation are, that child becomes able to obtain usable information from a model concerning what the important cues are and which alternatives to choose. This is precisely the situation we should strive for in language training. As illustrated with the various levels of the microcosmic matrix, children should learn enough about language so that they can extract further information on their own from models in the natural environment. This ex-

traction process, in turn, will involve many additional performatory acts.

One final point concerning performatory acts. The process is not merely one in which the child acquires increasing amounts of information or becomes aware of increasing numbers of alternatives. Rather, this information is acquired in the service of performatory acts. That is, it develops in the context of the child's own purposeful activity and transactions with the environment. Consequently, such information is likely to possess ecological validity for the child and is likely to be retained through automatic memory.

Summary

We have considered the possibility of training children to use particular cognitive strategies for language learning. It seems that any such ideas are premature. We simply don't know enough about cognitive strategies to operate wisely in this area. It does seem reasonable, however, to devise interventions that will evoke active problem solving from the child. Such problem solving may be viewed from the general perspective of performatory acts. The child's activities vis-à-vis the environment reveal the alternatives in the situation. Further performatory acts illuminate appropriate choices among the alternatives available. The process depends on the interaction between action and perception.

The challenge in clinical work, then, is to devise situations that will elicit appropriate performatory acts from each child. These situations would involve the active participation of the child in a special set of transactions with the environment. They would center on language in communicative contexts, in order to evoke appropriate problem solving and cognitive strategies. So far we have been considering the child's activity during language learning. Let us enlarge the scope now, and look at the training environment.

THE STRUCTURE OF INTERVENTION

Feedback

The whole idea of performatory acts implies the presence of feedback from the environment. In some instances this feedback is passive in the sense that children merely note the effects of their actions with inanimate objects, as did the child with the glue. In other cases the feedback is active in that individuals in the environment initiate actions of their own in relation to the child's activity. In language training we are concerned primarily with the second possibility.

In discussing general systems theory I have already emphasized the centrality of feedback in the child's transactions with the environment. For the present let us focus on the feedback that occurs in language training. From a practical standpoint, it seems to me that feedback varies in two ways. It varies in its ecological validity to the child and in the amount of information it contains that is relevant to the child's task. Concerning ecological validity, the most obvious example is reinforcement. The selection of a reinforcer is based on identifying some event that is important in the child's life. For example, a clinician may provide nickels or bits of food, assuming, of course, the child's behavior indicates these objects are valued. In other cases the ecological validity of feedback may be more directly related to the task. In this case the information in the feedback must be important to the child, as in providing corrective feedback to a child who wants very much to become skilled at pitching baseball.

Knowledge of Results

The second dimension of feedback concerns the amount of information it contains that is useful to the child in the task (Annett 1969). This aspect of feedback, often referred to as knowledge of results, is best illustrated with an example. Suppose you are showing pictures to a child, and the child is to tell you what's in each picture. You show a picture of a barn and the child says, "House." You say, "Nope." The next picture is of a truck, which the child labels as a car. Again you respond with, "Nope." Your feedback is minimally helpful to the child in identifying other possible alternatives in the situation. Contrast such feedback for "House" as, "Well, it's a building, yes, but not a house," for "Car," "What else goes down the road?" In general, the effectiveness of this feedback varies with the number of alternatives that it clarifies for the child. One can see that this aspect of feedback dovetails nicely with the idea of performatory acts.

There has been considerable discussion about the relationship between knowledge of results and reinforcement (Annett 1969). Is knowledge of results reinforcing of and by itself? We do not need to enter this debate. In the ideal situation the language trainer will provide feedback to the child that possesses both ecological validity and information about the alternatives in the task. If a child asks for a banana, we can ask, "Peeled or unpeeled?" and supply whichever the child prefers.

Autotelic Responsive Environments

For a more comprehensive view of the training environment, we turn to the work of Moore and Anderson (Moore 1966; Moore and Anderson 1968, 1969). These individuals have developed a special learning situation that they call an "autotelic responsive environment." The terms autotelic and responsive will be discussed separately.

Responsive Environments

A responsive environment is one that clarifies the alternatives and relationships in the situation, but it goes beyond the processes of feedback discussed above. Moore (1966) lists the following characteristics of a responsive environment:

1. It permits the learner to explore freely.
2. It informs the learner immediately about the consequences of his actions.
3. It is self-pacing, i.e., events happen within the environment at a rate determined by the learner.
4. It permits the learner to make full use of his capacity for discovering relations of various kinds.
5. Its structure is such that the learner is likely to make a series of interconnected discoveries about the physical, cultural or social world.[2]

These conditions represent an extremely efficient environment in which to carry out performatory acts. The first and third allow the child to engage in such acts and problem solving in individualized fashion. As Moore puts it, the children are not robbed of the opportunities to make their own discoveries. The second provides the feedback necessary for these activities. The last two are particularly important in language learning. Recall again that grammatical rules are relations and that language use involves relations among conceptual, linguistic, and interpersonal factors. It may not be possible

[2] Omar Khayyam Moore, "Autotelic Responsive Environments and Exceptional Children," in *Experience, Structure and Adaptability*, ed., O. J. Harvey (New York: Springer Publishing Company, 1966), p. 170.

to meet all five of these conditions in all training situations. At the same time, I would propose that all five are present in partial degrees in the natural environments in which most children learn language.

Autotelic Activities

Returning to the first term, Moore and Anderson coined the word "autotelic" to refer to activities in which the goals and rewards of the activity are intrinsic to that activity. Anything that you do for its own sake is autotelic. Playing bridge or tennis is autotelic unless you are playing for something beyond the game itself, such as money. You may read one book because you enjoy it, an autotelic activity, and another book only because you have to pass an exam on its contents. The latter reading is not likely to be autotelic.

I find the term autotelic appealing for two reasons. First, it incorporates the idea of ecological validity, so important in automatic memory and in motivation. In fact, one could say that what Moore and Anderson have done in devising their autotelic environment is to develop a set of activities that are so appealing that they have ecological validity for virtually every child. Second, much of language use, by both children and adults, is autotelic in nature. To be sure, we use language to accomplish many purposes that are extrinsic to language. We ask for the mayonnaise, we tell the boss we need a raise, we have a meeting to discuss plans for a new business venture; children produce utterances to obtain reinforcers and a host of other things. But beyond these variegated purposes, we talk to be talking. There is no doubt in my mind that children do the same. If you are not convinced, eavesdrop on a group of children at play. Opie and Opie (1959) have charmingly documented the use of language for its own sake by British schoolchildren, including many rhymes, ditties, and language games. From a very different point of view, Lovaas, Varni, Koegel, and Lorsch (1977) have discussed the autotelic nature of child language in an article entitled "Some observations on the nonextinguishability of children's speech." It seems obvious, although perhaps a little idealistic, that if we can design interventions in which language use becomes autotelic for the child, our difficulties with generalization of training (Harris 1975) should diminish.

By now you're probably wondering just what kind of a learning situation Moore and Anderson devised that is both responsive and autotelic. First, their approach is aimed primarily at preschool and primary-grade children, such as those in Head Start programs. Second, they focused on the printed word—reading and writing—rather than on auditory-vocal language. The heart of their learning environment is a teaching machine. The machine consists of a typewriter keyboard that has been programmed in various ways. When a child types in a word, a picture of that word may appear on a screen, or the word may be heard auditorily. The machine is flexible so that words a particular child is heard using in spontaneous talking can be programmed into the machine for that child. The keyboard can be programmed so that only certain keys or functions can be depressed. Altogether a wonderful machine.

The child is given absolutely no instruction on how to operate the machine or what to do. Rather, each child is given permission to explore the machine for as long as desired, up to a maximum set by the adult. Each child gets an individual session with the machine every school day. Some children pound on it, some pick at it systematically, some just look at it at first, but no child has stopped returning for further sessions with the "talking typewriter." Thus, the machine is truly autotelic. In addition, it is responsive. It allows free exploration, provides feedback, and allows discoveries of relations such as spelling out words and relating words to each other in statements. For additional description of the machine, and descriptions of children using it, the reader is referred to Moore (1966) and Moore and Anderson (1969). Young children have been very successful in learning to read and to type out stories with versions of this machine.

Allen (1965) describes another autotelic responsive device, this time designed for learning mathematical logic. It consists of a series of games called *WFF'N PROOF*. The games will not be described, other than to point out that they consist of a set of printed instructions and a set of specially marked cubes similar to dice. Thus, autotelic responsive learning does not have to depend on sophisticated programmable equipment. Allen emphasizes that an autotelic activity should be fun. Similarly, Moore and Anderson (1969) stress the importance of play and of games in a more formal sense in the learning and acculturation of the child.

Allen (1965) notes that the problem in designing autotelic responsive learning situations is in developing an activity in which some aspect of intellectual development is the focus but participants engage in that activity primarily for enjoyment. We face the same challenge in working with language-disordered children. It may be argued that because of the complexity of language and the fleeting nature of auditory-vocal language, we cannot devise language interventions that conform to Moore and Anderson's model. I would answer that, in the main, we haven't tried. We have the components. In play-oriented interventions children explore on their own. In a program such as Winitz and Reeds's, children discover relations on their own. In many programs children progress at their own rate, and virtually all programs provide feedback of varying sorts. Thus, we are familiar with all the conditions for responsive environments.

We are also familiar with the autotelic component, although perhaps under different names. Permit me to illustrate with an example. I once knew a language-delayed four-year-old boy who resisted clinical training mightily. He would knock things on the floor, shout, strike the clinician, refuse to cooperate, and above all, cry, cry, cry. The clinician was working on comprehension of prepositions such as *in, on,* and *under,* using a structured approach. Several consequences had been attempted, such as tokens and food, but the child continued to resist and cry. Abruptly, one day the clinician switched to a play format. The theme was still spatial relations, but the child was no longer heavily directed. He stopped crying within a few minutes and played cooperatively and enthusiastically from then on. He did not demonstrate crying in subsequent sessions except occasionally when it was time to go!

In summary, this section has focused on training environments that are responsive to the child's performatory acts and at the same time provide the child both appropriate stimulation and useful feedback, all within activities that are meaningful or useful in the child's life. In the case of language intervention, it follows that the activities are more likely to be functional and communicative than strictly drill. In slanting our training in this direction, we increase the probabilities of engaging the child actively in learning and of lessening the gap between the child's language responses in training

and language use in the world. As stated earlier, the aim is to foster transactions between the child and the environment that will lead to enhanced language skill in the child.

PRAGMATICS

Perhaps I can summarize most of this chapter with a model of pragmatics. The term refers to language in use, language in context, rather than language as an abstract system. In its largest sense it is concerned with the relations between communication and behavior. Miller (1978) has summarized some of the technical literature and discussed implications of pragmatics for working with language-impaired children. I will present a broader view of pragmatics.

Many clinicians operate with a view of language use similar to that in Model 1. Each person has a repertoire of options, including words and grammatical structures, as well as nonverbal behaviors. This repertoire is the basis for that person's communicative behavior, through both language and nonverbal means. There is a linear relationship between repertoire and behavior. Whatever behavior is produced must be in the repertoire; whatever options are in the repertoire can be realized as behavior. This model underlies the common procedure of teaching grammatical structures through drill on expression. The assumption is that if a child says some structure enough times, it will become part of that child's repertoire. Well and good, but not enough. In the chapter on assessment, behavior was characterized as selection from a repertoire. Model 1 ignores this decision-making aspect of language use. Look at Model 2.

Here decision making is inserted between

Model 1   Language and Behavior

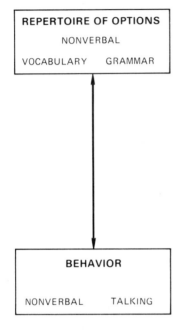

Model 2   Language Use

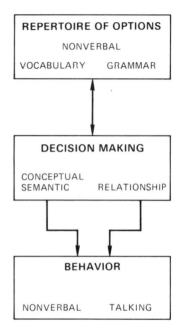

the repertoire and the behavior. In this way, Model 2 is a visual metaphor of language use. Selection lies *between* repertoire and behavior. Note that there are both conceptual-semantic decisions and also relationship decisions. Both types of decision influence behavior, indicated by the fact that each has its own arrow connecting it with behavior. Merely training grammatical structures puts the focus on Model 1. In Model 2 we emphasize language use and thus evoke the decision making that is inherent in human communication. The more those decisions are ecologically valid for the child, the more powerful the learning and generalization should be. However, Model 2 is still inadequate. I have argued that we cannot understand the decision making underlying communication without considering the environment.

In Model 3, I have added the environment or context in which communicative decisions are made. *Environment* here is an all-inclusive term for whatever is present in the communication situation, including listeners and all other stimuli. Notice the reciprocal nature of the model now. Decisions affect behavior, which affects the environment. At the same time, the environment affects both conceptual-semantic and relationship decisions. Both expression and comprehension are represented, depending on whether you read the model down the page or up the page. Performatory acts are represented by the links between decision making and feedback from the environment. The environment can vary in how responsive it is, thus influencing the degree and efficiency with which decisions involve new learning. It is of great clinical

Model 3 Pragmatics Model

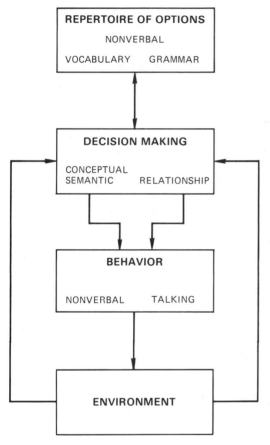

REPERTOIRE OF OPTIONS

NONVERBAL

VOCABULARY   GRAMMAR

DECISION MAKING

CONCEPTUAL
SEMANTIC   RELATIONSHIP

BEHAVIOR

NONVERBAL   TALKING

ENVIRONMENT

importance that listeners themselves can be responsive environments.

The pragmatics model emphasizes the probabilistic or variable linguistic rules discussed at the beginning of Chapter 8. The repertoire will have to include much more than the formal style and Standard English of the microcosmic matrix. Similarly with semantics, the repertoire must be rich enough to allow selections of words to differentiate many referents from an enormous number of contrast sets. With both grammar and vocabulary we see the interaction

among repertoire, decision making, and context that is the heart of pragmatics.

We can also view culturally different children with the pragmatics model. Their repertoire may be different, especially if another language is dominant in their culture. They may view us (the environment) differently, so that their interpretations of our behavior may not be the same as those of middle-class children. In addition, the hierarchy of rules governing expression will differ somewhat from mainstream culture, thus influencing the communicative decisions these children make. Taking all three factors in combination, culturally different children may behave in ways that we do not expect and that may be difficult for us to interpret. Of course, middle-class children may do the same.

You may note some parallel between this model of pragmatics and the transactional model of causation. The two complement each other, but they are not the same. The transactional model encompasses many more variables than those in the pragmatics model. More important, the transactional model can only be understood in relation to the passage of time. There are moment-to-moment adjustments between child and environment, but transactional patterns develop and change over time, and the child's state at any one time is always influenced by the history of those transactions. The pragmatics model focuses on those moment-to-moment interactions. Still, time is important in this model. There is a set of metarules that guide "on line" decisions in interaction. I described these metarules earlier as a hierarchy governing expression. These metarules develop through each person's history of communicative problem solving or decision making. Perhaps the pragmatics model is best seen in the context of the transactional model.

This model of pragmatics highlights four areas that are at the heart of intervention: the child's repertoire, conceptual-semantic decisions, relationship decisions, and the environment. Communicative behavior is where we can see the dynamic ties among these four. In order to change that behavior, we have to change the repertoire, decision making, or environment, or some combination of these three. As trainers and clinicians, we are a special part of the environment in which that behavior occurs.

CONCLUSIONS

This chapter began with a recapitulation of the view that language use is problem-solving activity. We then compared the decision making in comprehension and in expression. It is my view that the two are quite different, both in terms of cognitive strategies and interpersonal strategies. The cognitive decisions in comprehension focus on making an interpretation of the utterance. One needs to process only enough detail in an utterance to choose an interpretation. Consequently, a fair amount of detail is not actively processed. At the same time, the interpersonal decision making in comprehension centers on whether to attend to the listener or not. Other than that associated with attention, there is little relationship communication associated with comprehension *per se;* it is a covert process. In contrast, expression involves more decisions at both levels. It requires linguistic decisions concerning all components of the utterance. A speaker controls all the detail in an utterance, whether or not the listener uses it. In addition, the speaker is very active in making interpersonal decisions during talking, ranging from weighing relationship factors, to structuring the utterance to com-

municate to a particular listener, to assuring discourse agreement.

While comprehension and expression are thus different processes, it does not follow that each will have to be trained separately. What is important is that training strategies should reflect the differences between them. With its emphasis on selecting an interpretation for each utterance, comprehension training fits well in the problem-solving mode. Because of its tendency to minimize detail, the grammatical structure being trained will have to be made salient by making the choice of an interpretation hinge on that structure. Attention can be maintained through employing either an autotelic activity or structured reinforcement. In focusing on expression, major importance will have to be placed on the human relationship factors. Ideally, talking to the clinician will be autotelic for the child. We will consider this matter in Chapter 11. Additionally, relationship factors as well as specific training goals may involve the child's family. At a grammatical level, the child's productions would appear to be excellent examples of performatory acts, and the child should receive feedback in the communicative context. Particular grammatical structures can still be made salient. Because the child must control all the detail in the utterance, it makes sense to focus on a sequence of grammatical structures, such as that in the microcosmic matrix. Finally, it may be more efficient to introduce and train a new grammatical structure through comprehension, precisely because the child's attention can be focused on that particular aspect of the utterance.

I do not believe there is any one Best Approach to intervention with language-disordered children. I do believe that intervention should derive from an optimal theoretical base, and I have been searching for principles that can contribute to that base. The transactional model and related aspects of general systems theory provide one set of principles. It seems to me that problem solving is another such principle. It is consonant with the view presented in Chapter 4, where language use was described in terms of decision making. Involved are both alternatives of meaning and options in the language for representing those alternatives. In addition, problem solving is related to cognitive strategies and performatory acts, as well as to relationship strategies. All these factors are brought together in the pragmatics model, Model 3, in this chapter. All carry the assumption that each child is not merely a bag to fill up with language or a lump of clay to be molded into a language user; rather, children participate in their own learning and development. A further set of principles is to be found in environments that are responsive and autotelic, with their clarifying feedback, stimulation, and ecological validity.

What is most important is that these principles complement each other to a high degree. Each functions best in the presence of the others. Problem solving and responsive environments are almost mirror images of each other. Together they comprise a transactional pattern that enhances learning and development in the child. To the extent that these processes are autotelic, they occur on their own, rather than only when engineered by the trainer.

As concluded in Chapter 6, a theory of causation should also be a theory of assessment and intervention. In my view transactions between the child and the environment are the common denominator for all three. In Chapter 7, I attempted to show how we might look at what the child brings into those transactions and how we might investigate transactions between child and clinician directly through exploratory teaching. The pragmatics model allows us to focus directly on the transactions of the moment and their attendant problem solving. In the next two chapters I will consider intervention as it relates to the child's conceptual-semantic decisions and interpersonal decisions. We will then be ready to expand our transactional view to a very special communicative environment, the family.

10

INTERVENTION: LANGUAGE AS A LINGUISTIC PHENOMENON

GUIDING PRINCIPLES

All through this book, I have been trying to develop principles to guide our work with language-disordered children. The preceding chapter reviewed some of these principles and proposed an idealized view of intervention. It is time to put these abstractions to work. Let me begin by reviewing six Guiding Principles for language intervention.

1. Ecological validity. Whatever we teach should be immediately functional in the child's life. This requirement necessitates that we focus on meaning and communication, that we teach options-to-mean, not merely options-to-say. There is an even greater challenge in this principle. In order to have any idea of what is functional for a child, we will have to know something about that child's life and the ecosystems it is a part of. This assertion brings us to the second principle.

2. Transactional model. It is through their transactions with the environment that children have opportunities to mean and to grow as communicators. Change does not occur in the child alone, though. In reciprocal fashion, it is related to change in the environment. Transactional patterns may be thought of as metarules guiding each individual's decision making in dealing with other people. This view suggests the third principle.

3. Problem solving. We approach the child as an active learner and decision maker. The pragmatics model in Chapter 9 illustrates this principle. Problem solving occurs both in conceptual-semantic decision making and in relationship decisions. We engage the child in cognitive and interpersonal strategies that are relevant to using language for communication. The idea of

performatory acts is a useful metaphor here. It is through children's problem solving in communication situations that they can go beyond whatever levels of the microcosmic matrix we have taught them. Performatory acts have no utility except in contexts, however, which leads us to the fourth principle.

4. Responsive environments. Clinicians and teachers are also involved in problem solving in seeking the most effective ways to help each child grow. Generally, our intervention strategies should allow the child room to make decisions and provide feedback to maximize the learning from that problem solving. Responsive environments are the perfect match for active learners. They allow children to discover relationships and grow at their own rate. In order for children to participate fully in their own learning, though, we need still another principle.

5. Autotelic activities. Ideally, we arrange situations where children engage in ecologically valid communicative problem solving for its own sake—because it is appealing, interesting, and fun. Using extrinsic motivators or reinforcers means that you, the clinician, will have to engineer generalization. If the use of new language skills is autotelic in the child's transactions with the environment, including the clinician, generalization occurs "spontaneously." These last two principles have emphasized clinician decision making, which brings us to our last principle.

6. Exploratory teaching. We develop an intervention strategy for each child through our own problem solving in exploratory teaching. In this process we change our own behavior in order to discover how best to help the child change. In so doing, we focus

on the transactional nature of language learning. Further, exploratory teaching forces us to be responsive to individual differences among children. We can't simply plug them all into the same program.

I have suggested repeatedly that language, cognition, human relationships, and the environment are all inseparable in language learning. Nevertheless, I would like to limit our field of view somewhat so that we can concentrate on specific issues. In the present chapter we will explore ways to move toward the above ideals in teaching the repertoire: grammatical structures. I will emphasize the conceptual-semantic decisions associated with language use. We will begin with a particular communication arrange-

ment that embodies many of the principles stated above.

THE REFERENTIAL COMMUNICATION TASK

Language teaching is always an interaction between clinician and child. We can define it as a specific set of transactional patterns in which both child and clinician influence each other. In line with our guiding principles, it must emphasize communication between the participants. Let us consider one such situation, which was developed for research in interpersonal communication. Look at Figure 7. Two children are seated

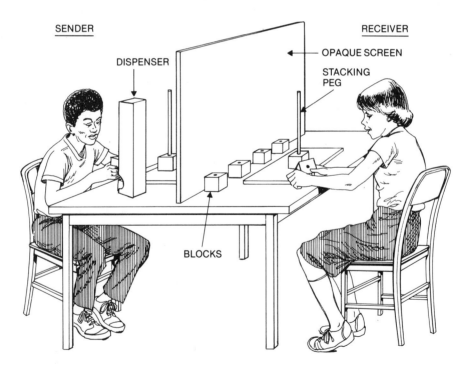

Figure 7. The referential communication task. (Adapted from Sam Glucksberg and Robert Krauss, What do people say after they have learned to talk? Studies of the development of referential communication. *Merrill-Palmer Quarterly,* 13 [1967], 309–316. Figure 2, p. 311.)

opposite each other at a table. There is an opaque screen across the middle of the table, so that the children cannot see each other. Each child has a set of blocks with different designs on them. Identical sets of blocks are given to both children, so that each child has the same set of designs.

In the classic version of the task, one child is designated the *sender* and the other the *receiver*. The sender's blocks are in a dispenser so that they can only be removed in a certain order, while the receiver's blocks are spread out in view. The sender takes the first block and puts it on the stacking peg. (Each block has a hole so that it will stack on the peg.) The task is for the two children to talk back and forth until the receiver can select the same design as the sender's. After it is stacked, the sender takes the second block, and the process continues until all six blocks have been discussed. The goal is to finish with the blocks stacked in the same order on both pegs.

This task emphasizes referential communication. Recall from Chapter 4 that referential meaning involves specifying particular objects. Reference is always specific to the situation. In the communication task described above, the children's purpose is to agree on which designs they are referring to. This task may seem easy, and indeed it is, if the designs are familiar, such as those in Figure 8.

What makes the task interesting (and fun) is that the designs usually employed are novel, nonrepresentational ones such as those in Figure 9. These designs were specifically chosen because they are difficult to name.

Both sender and receiver are very much involved in problem solving. The sender must select words that will best identify the target design. The receiver must similarly match those words with a design. Both must also decide when to ask questions or provide other feedback. A number of the ideas I have discussed earlier appear in concrete form in this task. The sender literally makes selections from a repertoire of options-to-mean. That is, each child chooses words

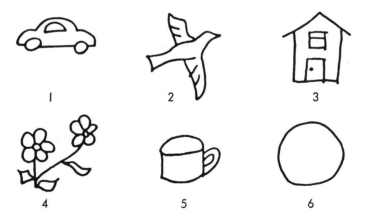

Figure 8. Training pictures for the referential communication task. (From Robert Hubbell, A study of verbal feedback in families with young children. Paper presented at the annual convention of the American Speech and Hearing Association, Detroit, 1973.)

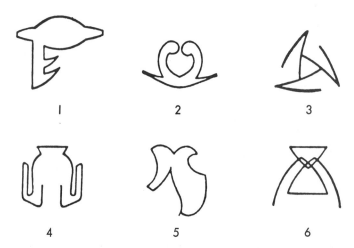

Figure 9. Graphic designs employed in Glucksberg and Krauss's referential communication research. (From Sam Glucksberg and Robert Krauss, What do people say after they have learned to talk? Studies of the development of referential communication. *Merrill-Palmer Quarterly,* 13, [1967], 309–316. Figure 1, p. 311.)

from his vocabulary pool that will best indicate the intended design. Now recall Olson's (1970b) view of referential meaning from Chapter 4. The (referential) meaning of an utterance rests in how it differentiates among the alternatives in a contrast set. Again, that is literally the case in this communication task. The receiver's job is to select one design from the array of designs on the table.

In sum, this task fits nicely with the pragmatics model presented in the preceding chapter. All four components of the model are represented: repertoire, decision making, behavior, and environment. Conceptual-semantic decisions are emphasized, although relationship decisions are also involved. The children must agree to participate in the task and to work together. Sometimes the sender will appear to be in charge, because only the sender knows which design is the target. Other times the task turns into a game of Twenty Questions, and the receiver appears to lead. In general systems fashion, however, both must participate or the task cannot be completed.

Usually the sender's first message isn't precise enough for the receiver to select a design, and so the receiver must ask questions. Hence, the task generates feedback processes. In fact, each participant may be seen as a (more or less) responsive environment for the other's attempts at communication. Young children neither provide nor use feedback efficiently (Glucksberg and Krauss 1967), but the point here is that both sender and receiver roles have the potential of serving as responsive environments for each other. A clinician, in taking one role, can enhance the child's growth in the other role.

In this task, then, we have an idealized form of referential communication in which we can look separately at each component of the process: the referent and contrast set, the sender, the receiver, and the transactional patterns between sender and receiver. I am discussing this task in detail for two reasons. First, referential communication is one of the most fundamental and frequent forms of language use. Second, referential communication is one of the most common activities that we employ in language training. We are constantly asking children to name objects or pictures, say utterances that match pictures, choose pictures that match utterances, and so forth. In sum, referential communication is both a training technique and a technique to be trained.

I do not propose that we use the referential communication task described above directly in intervention. There are too many variables to control. If children have difficulty with the task, it is hard to know precisely where the trouble lies. Rather, I suggest that we use the task as a paradigm or framework for approaching the training of words and grammatical structures. It gives us a concrete way to apply the pragmatics model and other ideas from preceding chapters. It explicitly involves concepts, information processing and perception, language, and human exchange. Depending on the child, we can focus on the sender or receiver roles; we can emphasize feedback; we can provide model utterances or let the child decide what to say; we can vary the concepts and the nature of the problem solving; we can enhance the degree to which the task is autotelic and ecologically valid for individual children. Finally, the emphasis on referential communication keeps the focus on options-to-mean, rather than on learning grammatical structures as ends for their own sake. Indeed, most techniques for training vocabulary and grammatical structures can be analyzed within this framework. In the following sections I will exploit this potential more fully. We will look separately at

the roles of the receiver and the sender, and then at the feedback between the two.

EMPHASIS ON COMPREHENSION: THE RECEIVER

In the preceding chapter I described comprehension and expression as different, both in information-processing and relationship factors. These differences led me to conclude that the training of grammatical structures can often be more effective when the focus is on comprehension rather than expression. While there are no convincing data one way or the other regarding language-impaired children, both Winitz and Reeds (1975) and Asher (1977) report that children and adults can be taught foreign languages more efficiently through comprehension. Beyond the differences between comprehension and expression discussed previously, there is a very simple reason for this result: *Language learning depends on input.* Children cannot learn language without taking it in through sensory modalities. Even if a clinician is helping a child with expression, it is first determined that the child knows the items to be expressed—some sort of input is provided. A possible contradiction to this thesis would be in procedures in which a child's vocalizations are progressively shaped toward acceptable utterances. Even here, though, input is present in the shaping stimuli themselves.

While the referential communication task provides a paradigm for comprehension training, the actual techniques used can vary greatly. They may include situations in which specific visual and verbal stimuli are presented, specific responses are required, and specific feedback is provided to the learner. Highly structured comprehension training such as this is exemplified by the programs developed by Winitz and Reeds (1975). On the other hand, talking to a child during play may also be considered comprehension training, this time through what might be called unstructured modeling. Many other variations of comprehension training are possible.

Problem Solving and Language Learning

Obviously, there are always verbal stimuli in comprehension. Frequently, there are also relevant nonverbal stimuli present. The effect of these stimuli is to control the complexity of the problem solving the listener must do. In the classic referential task and in much language training, the emphasis is on concrete concepts with their perceptual attributes. If necessary, core concepts can be made prominent. In teaching grammatical structures, relational concepts become important. Through informal assessment and exploratory teaching, we can determine at what level to begin for each child. Similarly, we can vary the information-processing load for different children.

Let me illustrate some of these ideas with an example. I will teach you a few words from an exotic language called *META*, spoken only by a small but intense group of underground theoreticians. The first word is *ZORK*. Here are some examples of *ZORKS*:

typewriter
rubber band
tree
nail file
block of wood
dishrag
feather
tennis shoe

Now decide what a *ZORK* is. Notice the problem solving you do. Most people run through the list of exemplars several times, looking for common attributes, things that can represent zorkhood. There is no convincing attribute, though, unless we conclude that *ZORK* refers to any object. At this point the only way you can be sure you know what *ZORK* means is to memorize the list of exemplars. This kind of problem solving requires time and effort, mnemonic devices such as rehearsal, and focuses on episodic memory. It is parallel with teaching a child a word by holding a referent for that word in front of a child, repeating the word for the child, and having the child say it over and over: *Here is an apple, Edgar; say "apple"; this is an apple . . .* The cognitive strategies evoked by such teaching are far removed from those in more natural language use and from the performatory acts we hope to encourage in the child's transactions with the environment.

Let me double your vocabulary in *META* now by adding a second word: *FLUDGE*. Here are two examples of *FLUDGES*.

apple
orange

What might *FLUDGE* mean? Now guess what *ZORK* means. Now that I've provided *FLUDGES* as a contrast set, it is easier to provide a meaning for *ZORK*. One might reason that, because both *FLUDGES* are edible, *ZORK* might mean inedible. That would fit all our exemplars. So far, that is. Here is another *ZORK*.

banana

Back to the drawing boards. Notice two things at this point. First, your problem solving is entirely different now that I have provided a contrast set. You are concentrating on categories or concepts, rather than memorization. Second, grant me the analogy that you are engaged in performatory acts. The effect of these acts is to make you aware of the alternatives in the situation. If you thought of both apple and orange as foods, then it made sense to set up the contrast of edible versus nonedible. But the banana destroys that hypothesis, so you must now look for other alternatives. Here are a few more *FLUDGES*.

tennis ball
roll of toilet paper
automobile tire
hard-boiled egg

Compare all *ZORKS* with all *FLUDGES* at this point. Jot them on a piece of paper if necessary. What contrast are you led to? All of the *FLUDGES* are round in at least one dimension. None of the *ZORKS* have this characteristic. Speakers of *META* divide up their world a little differently than we do. A *FLUDGE* is an object that rolls; a *ZORK* is an object that doesn't roll.

I put you through this exercise to illustrate some of the points I discussed earlier. First, language learning is based on input. There is no way you could learn these two words of *META* except through taking in the stimuli I parceled out to you. Second, the stimuli influence the selection of cognitive strategies the learner will employ. Different learning tasks evoke different problem solving. Further, some cognitive strategies are more efficient than others. If you had merely memorized the list of *ZORKS,* you would still have no good way to decide whether additional objects were *ZORKS* or not. Now that you have developed the contrast between *ZORKS* and *FLUDGES,* it would be easy to categorize additional stimuli. Third, stemming from the referential communication paradigm, learning and its associated cognitive strategies are heavily influenced by the feedback the learner receives. Had I been a more

"responsive environment" and given you the banana earlier, along with a wider variety of objects that roll, your problem solving could have been more efficient.

Teaching Grammatical Structures

Contrast sets can also be employed in teaching comprehension of grammatical options. Rather than parroting *is,* a child can learn the contrast between *is* and *was.* The relational concepts represented by these grammatical morphemes are thus highlighted, just as the *ZORKS* and *FLUDGES* were contrasted above. *Is* and *was* become options that mean. There are some complications here, though. As discussed in Chapter 9, perception is incomplete. We look only for those features of a stimulus that we think will be important. As Olson (1970a) suggested, if a child is not already aware of the relevant alternatives in a stimulus, merely observing a model may not illuminate those alternatives. Further, the longer the utterance is, the more likely the child will use analysis by synthesis, thus guaranteeing that perception will be incomplete and grammatical detail possibly ignored. Along the same lines, as discussed in Chapter 3, comprehension seems to be based more on semantics than syntax.

In response to these difficulties, the grammatical contrast you wish to teach must be made as salient as possible. It should reflect the crucial contrast in the referents. For example, one could make a ball of clay and tell the child, *This IS a ball,* then squash the ball flat and say, *This WAS a ball.* Additionally, the target structures can be stressed through vocal inflection. Sometimes they can be placed first in the utterance, such as using questions to teach *is* and *was: IS this a ball?* (Winitz and Reeds 1975). A little exploratory teaching will help in determining how salient the target structures must be for each child. A slow-learning child, for example, may perceive only a fraction of a complex stimulus. It then becomes important to shorten your utterance length and make both the verbal and nonverbal contrasts as obvious as possible.

The referential communication paradigm has the potential for varying the contrasts from very obvious to very subtle. If necessary, one can have only one referent, so that the child cannot help but make the correct choice. Adding items in a contrast set makes the task more difficult, but the discriminations can still be fairly gross. The designs we saw in Figure 9 illustrate this possibility. Each design is markedly different from the others, and the child need only select one design. These discriminations can be made much finer, however. Consider the designs in Figure 10. These designs were prepared for research in the accuracy of referential communication (Baldwin, McFarlane, and Garvey 1971). Each picture varies from the others in a specified number of aspects. A measure is thus provided of the degree to which sender and receiver communicate successfully. In this version of the task, the receiver has a card with all seven pictures on it. The sender has only one of the pictures, and the task is for the receiver to figure out which one it is. It can be seen that the options-to-mean selected by the sender must be fairly precise in order to differentiate among this set of alternatives. Similarly, Whitehurst (1976) used cups that varied in several aspects (size, color, and design) to generate elaborated noun phrases. That is, in certain situations the child would have to select the *big, red, striped cup*. Additional elaborations of the paradigm will be presented later. The point is that we can vary the stimuli in the task to encompass a wide range of language skills.

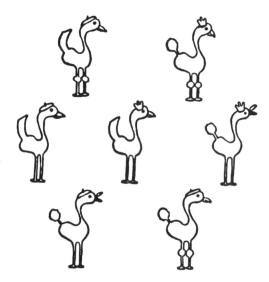

Figure 10. Referential communication designs requiring subtle differentiations. (From Thelma Baldwin, Paul McFarlane, and Catherine Garvey, Children's communication accuracy related to race and socioeconomic status. *Child Development,* 42 [1971], 343–357. Figure 1, p. 350. © by the Society for Research in Child Development, Inc.)

To summarize so far, we are saying things to the child. These utterances contain the grammatical option we wish to teach. The child matches each utterance with a nonverbal stimulus. The utterances and nonverbal stimuli are designed to concentrate the child's decision making on the option we are trying to train. We can vary both the utterances and the nonverbal stimuli according to our teaching goals and the sophistication and interests of the child.

One can carry out this process during play transactions with a child. Sometimes, however, it is desirable to introduce more structure into the interaction by requiring a response from the child. In having the child respond, you evoke problem solving from the child that is relevant to your goals. Otherwise you're not sure what the child is thinking about. Further, you obtain feedback about the success of your teaching. Recall from Chapter 7 the three informal assessment techniques for looking at comprehension: identification, acting out, and formal judgments (Leonard, Prutting, Perozzi, and Berkley 1978). In research with the referential communication tasks, the response is most commonly identification. In clinical applications we may use identification of pictures or objects, acting out, or, occasionally, formal judgments. Additionally, we may ask the child for a verbal response.

Teach, Don't Test

The trick in these procedures is in making sure the children's problem solving is leading to new learning rather than merely testing what they already know. For example, we show a child three pictures, one with a boy holding a lollipop, one with the lollipop in his mouth, and one of him holding the empty stick. We ask, "Which one shows that the boy ate the lollypop?" Much syntax training follows this model, but all we can accomplish with this procedure is to *test what the child already knows.* Similarly, you already know what ZORKS and FLUDGES are; now decide what VETCH means. Vetch is also a word in English. Use that meaning if you'd like . . . I ask you about this word to demonstrate the problem I'm discussing. You cannot learn what a word or grammatical structure means simply by being asked what it means. As with ZORK and FLUDGE, additional input and feedback are required to lead you to decision making that fills gaps in your knowledge. These ideas are summarized neatly in the phrase, "Teach, don't test."[1]

[1] Marcia Campbell, University of Arizona. Personal communication, 1975.

The more this decision making is meaningful for the child, the more powerful the learning should be. It is worth it to search for stimuli that are ecologically valid in each child's life. While this suggestion may seem difficult at first, it simply means that we should select goals and employ activities that are likely to be part of the child's life outside of language training. These activities are likely to include play and other recurring events such as eating and dressing. Learning experiences that have ecological validity emphasize automatic memory over episodic memory, they maximize the chances of generalization, and they are likely to be autotelic for the child.

The Verbal Stimulus

So far I have emphasized the complementarity between verbal and nonverbal stimuli in evoking problem solving in children who are learning language. Let us now focus directly on the verbal stimulus. Anything we say to a child may be considered a model of some aspect of language. Moore (1966), in describing autotelic responsive environments, argued that we should not lead children directly to correct responses because that robs them of chances for problem solving and discovery of relationships on their own. In contrast, though, it could be argued that language-impaired children have not been able to benefit sufficiently from the models naturally available in the environment. Further, there is ample evidence that children can learn grammatical structures that are modeled for them. Bandura and Harris (1966) have shown that normal children's syntactic style can be altered through modeling. Courtright and Courtright (1976, 1979) and Leonard (1974, 1975); Wilcox and Leonard (1978) all demonstrated that language-impaired children can be taught grammatical structures through modeling. Nelson (1977) and Fromberg (1976, 1977) have also illustrated the power of modeling in teaching language to children.

In view of the fundamental importance of input, the question becomes, not whether to provide models in language training, but what form those models should take. There have been debates about at least three different aspects of the verbal input to the child during language training. First, there is the contrast between modeling and expansion. Models are utterances said for a child that would be appropriate for that child to know and say. They are not related in any special way to previous utterances. Expansions, on the other hand, hinge on the child's immediately preceding utterance. An expansion repeats what the child said but expands it to a form that is grammatical for adults (Brown and Bellugi 1964).

A second question concerns the relative merits of modeling and imitation (Courtright and Courtright 1976, 1979). The difference here is that in modeling, no response is required from the child whereas in imitation, the child is to mimic the model immediately after it is presented. As used in this discussion, then, in imitation, the adult's utterance precedes the child's, in expansion, it follows the child's, and in modeling, no utterance is required from the child. At one level, these ideas stem from attempts to punctuate the sequence of events during language learning in linear cause-and-effect fashion. The issue is the order in which things occur.

A third question is about the structure of the clinician's utterances (Duchan and Erickson 1976; MacDonald and Horstmeier 1978). Should they be fully formed by adult standards, or should they employ a telegraphic grammar? If they are fully formed,

they might overtax the child's information-processing skills. If they are telegraphic, on the other hand, the trainer is modeling inappropriate grammar; further, the prosodic cues so important in language use become distorted.

There is another punctuation that could be applied to these questions. Rather than asking which technique is better overall, we could concentrate on how to engage each child most effectively in active problem solving. All of the above techniques then become viable; which to emphasize with a particular child may be decided through exploratory teaching. In this way we can follow Moore's (1966) advice that children be allowed to make their own discoveries. Using the referential communication paradigm as a guide, we can develop interventions that will lead the child's perceptions toward appropriate goals but still allow individual decision making. If a child is learning from relatively unstructured modeling, we can assume that the contrasts implicit in the situation are sufficient to generate appropriate problem solving. For another child, we might want to sharpen that decision making by providing feedback or contrast sets that enhance the salience of the structures or words we are trying to teach. In either case, we can vary the complexity of the situation so as not to exceed the child's information-processing skills. If comprehension is the goal, we can begin with fully formed utterances of appropriate length. If, on the other hand, we are focusing on expression with a preclausal child, we might model telegraphic utterances more exactly paralleling what we hope the child will say.

For modeling to be an efficient training technique, the target structure in the model should be as salient as possible. There are several ways to achieve this goal. Courtright and Courtright (1976, 1979) merely use many models, keeping the target structure the same but varying the content words. A contrast set is implied but not identified. Following Bandura and Harris (1966), Leonard (1974, 1975; Wilcox and Leonard 1978) uses reinforcement and a problem-solving set. He has the child observe someone producing utterances. This individual gets reinforced for certain utterances. Leonard encourages the child to figure out what is common among those utterances that get reinforced. The child's goal is to identify the contrast set. Both Nelson (1977) and Fromberg (1976, 1977) use variations of contrastive modeling, where the contrast set is made clear from the beginning. The target structure is contrasted with some other structure, as in the example earlier of *This IS a ball* and *This WAS a ball*. The child learns the structure and its contrast at the same time, just as you learned ZORK and FLUDGE.

Grammatical Operators

This emphasis on decision making in training comprehension of grammatical structures seems fairly straightforward in teaching vocabulary. It shouldn't be hard to work out contrast sets for *shoe* or *nose* or *apple*. Words such as these are easily associated with core and concrete concepts and are often used in referential fashion. The challenge comes with the relational concepts that underlie grammatical operators. Look at Language Sample 7.

These utterances were excerpted from a longer sample of Joyce's talking. Take a moment, however, and sort out her use of pronouns and BE. As with Language Sample 2 in Chapter 8, there is potential overlap here between nonstandard dialects, normal developmental errors, and language impairment. However, Joyce was growing

---

SAMPLE 7 : Joyce CA = 5-0

1. where him be
2. him a boy
3. him got one of them
4. me be here
5. me press down
6. me see animals
7. here be two
8. what do he be
9. you go faster than this
10. I wanna play with playdough
11. me play that no
12. what be it
13. it a wheel that wind
14. them say Joe in here

---

up in an environment in which only Standard English was spoken. Further, her errors suggest that she is learning the options in *Row B* of the microcosmic matrix. According to Prutting (1979), these areas should be learned by three or three and a half years, with the exception of some of the morphological detail. In any case, they are learned well before five. Joyce's test scores and mean length of utterance were also low. The conclusion is that Joyce does indeed demonstrate language impairment. Given her age and overall level of communicative behavior, intervention began with areas of language other than BE and pronouns. For purposes of illustration, however, let us consider those two options in Joyce's talking. Each has different connections with meaning.

The forms of BE do not generally have any referential function. Their meanings are relational. Therefore they have to be presented in the context of longer utterances, where they can relate subjects to complements. We could begin by teaching contrasts such as *is* and *was*, as mentioned earlier, thus maintaining a focus on meaning and problem solving. Some children may have difficulty with such tasks. If so, we might move to procedures similar to Leonard's, in which, essentially, the child is taught to be aware of when an *is* occurs in an utterance. This approach is based on discrimination learning; we have sacrificed the emphasis on meaning but retained the problem-solving motif. As a child acquires certain forms of BE, we can introduce others, except that we will need to teach pronouns as well.

Pronouns are relational because how they are defined depends on who is talking. It is easier to teach pronouns to small groups of children, so that we have several "referents" to work with. Training could begin with a contrast of two pronouns, using utterances such as, *I am sitting, he is sitting; I am wearing shoes, he is wearing shoes,* along with accompanying gestures at each person referred to. Or the children could be given interesting objects and the clinician could indicate which person has each object in the same manner. Dever (1978) uses another trainer to demonstrate, so that more than one person models *I*. With the help of the gestures, the children should link the verbal stimuli with the contrasts between pronouns. Note that the forms of BE are contrasting as well. Frequently you can work out routines where the children expect this kind of game regularly. Fromberg's (1976, 1977) contrastive modeling is very helpful here. Many aspects of language are based on contrast; she highlights those contrasts in her teaching.

Conclusion

In this section we have been focusing on the child as receiver in the referential communication paradigm. Because language learning always depends on input, the model is a key element in language training. We have seen that we can vary the task to make the target structure more or less salient. In addition, we can vary the specificity and difficulty of the problem solving for the child. In introducing particular contrast sets, we make it clear to the child what decisions to ponder. By requiring a response, we can tell if the child is on target or not.

These variations in how we encourage children to process language models have a further implication. Different types of problem solving lead children to acquire somewhat different knowledge about the model. In a strict imitation task, the child's information processing and decision making are directed toward reproducing the model exactly, with attendant emphasis on episodic memory and restricted cognitive strategies. The child learns an option-to-say. In a task where the child must select among alternatives on the basis of verbal stimuli, the task is more relevant to using language for communication. The child learns an option-to-mean.

With the referential communication paradigm as a guide, we can adjust the intervention strategy to accommodate the child's information-processing skills at least to some degree. If a child has difficulty with short-term memory, the stimuli can be presented so that they remain within that child's span. As the child learns clause types and noun phrases, the chunking inherent in those grammatical relations can be used to enhance span. If a child has problems with intermodal integration, contrasts can be provided that make those integrations clear. Similarly, if it appears that a child needs stimuli to be presented slowly, or requires many repetitions of a model we adjust our procedure accordingly. If a child tends to ignore detail in complex stimuli, we can develop contrasts that make that detail salient.

In short, while the emphasis is on input, our own problem solving leads to different options for different children. Exploratory teaching never stops.

EMPHASIS ON EXPRESSION: THE SENDER

I have emphasized that skill in talking depends on previous input. Comprehension is the main force in building a child's repertoire of options in grammar and vocabulary. Expression, on the other hand, involves selections from that repertoire. Modifications of the repertoire due to expression occur through the feedback that expression generates. The feedback is, of course, additional input.

The importance I have given to comprehension should not imply that expression is unimportant in language intervention. Recall that in expression the child must control all detail in the utterance. There are many decisions to make. It takes practice to make these decisions while talking. Consider Language Sample 8.

Coleen demonstrated adequate comprehension in informal assessment and scored just a few months below age level on standardized language tests. She was the youngest of five children. In the transactional patterns that had developed in her family, she simply didn't need to talk. There was nothing particularly pathological in this situation except that Coleen's expressive language wasn't developing. When we first saw the child, her utterances were mostly one and two words in length. Through individual intervention with the child and working with the parents we made sufficient changes in relationship patterns that Coleen's rate of talking was facilitated. In fact, she began to talk a great deal. Sample 8 was obtained about five weeks after intervention began. At this point she had almost literally sprung into longer utterances. Her lack of practice in structuring so many options at once is clear. Within a couple months her grammatical skill in expression improved dramatically, although we did not focus on syntax training. While other interpretations are possible, my guess is that at the time of this language sample Coleen's main difficulty was that she had had so little practice in putting together longer utterances.

Recall the sender's task in the referential communication paradigm. The speaker must select options-to-mean that will specify a referent in contrast to a set of alternatives. This process is precisely the kind of practice that Coleen needed. In her case, natural interactions with her environment were enough to speed her development along. With other children, more specific models and a responsive environment more finely tuned to language learning may be required.

SAMPLE 8: Coleen CA = 4-4

1. yep boy toys that on sign
2. and come back my school a what
3. now that pink one the big pink cup no pink Jane
4. that one sign
5. put this together again
6. I kick you not my pal again
7. make cake and make with big cup that big cup
8. up big tall on seat
9. no miss me Ed and Betty and Jane
10. come back me and miss me Ed and Betty be mad

Cues for Retrieval

As mentioned earlier, expression involves retrieval. In turn, facility in retrieval revolves around two factors. First, it depends on how well the items to be retrieved are learned. This learning will be based both on the input the child has received and on the amount of practice the child has had with those items. Retrieval also depends on the kinds of cues that are available to the child.

In working with expression we can vary the cues supplied to the child in a number of ways. Consider the techniques for eliciting expression from the assessment chapter. First, there is imitation, which can be immediate or delayed, with some intervening stimuli placed between the clinician's model and the child's response. The cues for retrieval here are very specific, although they may not relate the utterance closely to meaning. Another type of cue is in fill-in procedures, such as, *Today I eat; yesterday I . . .* The cue is still highly specific, but the target structure itself is not modeled. Still less structure is involved in paraphrase tasks, where the trainer tells a story loaded with some grammatical option and then asks the child to tell it back.

Another paraphrase technique mentioned in the assessment chapter involves directing a child to talk to another child or to a puppet (Dever 1978; Chomsky 1969). The directives are designed to elicit particular grammatical options in the target child's responses. For example, if you say to a child, *Tell Grover that you're hungry,* you elicit particular pronoun and BE forms. If you say, *Ask Grover which pencil he wants,* you are likely to elicit some noun phrase elaboration. Similarly, with *Ask Grover when it rained last,* verb phrase detail may be elicited. It takes a little practice before you can ad lib these directives effectively, but they are very helpful in eliciting expression of particular areas of grammar. I know one clinician who has children talk to imaginary friends in this way.

These expression tasks vary in a number of dimensions that have been discussed earlier in the book. First, each evokes different problem solving from the child. Some require more top-down processing and reconstruction from semantic memory, whereas others emphasize bottom-up processing and episodic memory. Following the ecological validity principle, we will choose cues that generate problem solving that is as close as possible to that in natural language use. Perhaps the most natural ways to elicit expression are through normal conversation and discussion of interesting nonverbal stimuli. With some children we may have to compromise the ecological validity principle somewhat in order to get accurate responding. As before, exploratory teaching will be helpful in identifying an appropriate approach for each child.

Introducing Expression

I have argued that learning new words and grammatical options depends primarily on comprehension. Expression provides practice in producing new structures and in using them to convey meaning once they have been learned. Assuming we begin with comprehension training, then, it is natural to ask when intervention should move to expression. There is no universal answer. In a surprising number of cases the child will tell you. As Winitz and Reeds (1975) indicated, after a period of comprehension training, many children will begin to use target structures spontaneously in expression. These children may need no formal work on expression at all. In their research on grammar training, neither Leonard nor Courtright and Courtright waited for spontaneous productions. After a period of comprehension training, they have elicited target structures directly in expression. The Courtrights, in fact, suggested that research is needed to determine the optimal time to switch from comprehension to expression.

There is another matter that clouds the answer to this question. As discussed in previous chapters, expression is an overt interpersonal act. Relationship influences are always involved. Spontaneous production, then, is likely to hinge on two factors. First, as above, the child must have developed sufficient knowledge of the grammatical options in question. Second, the interpersonal context must be appropriate from the child's punctuation.

Let us consider another example at this point. Kitty was a three-year-old child with virtually no expressive language. Assessment through standardized tests was not possible because of the immaturity of much of her behavior. In informal play she provided evidence that she comprehended most of what was said. It appeared that her lack of expression was at least partially tied in with relationship factors. She did not work well in structured training activities. She did participate in various play activities with great enjoyment and enthusiasm, but still produced very little talking. Therefore, the clinician began to model specific utterances for Kitty to say that were related to the activities. The clinician would hold up an object and name it, using iconic signs such as "looking expectant" to indicate that Kitty should name it, too. A contingency was established in which she had to name objects before she could play with them. By now the clinician knew which play objects Kitty liked most, so these contingencies had ecological validity in her play.

At this point the clinician was providing cues for imitation. In addition, however, the models differentiated among the alternatives in the situation, and Kitty was learning a pragmatic function of language in dealing with people. With the combination of the models, the contingencies, and the relationship context in which Kitty and the clinician played together, the child soon began to say words and then preclausal combinations. Before long the models were no longer provided, but the items were held up and expression was cued through the iconic gestures. Within two months Kitty was using many two-word utterances that had not been modeled, and she used them for conversational purposes as well as to obtain play objects. Talking was becoming autotelic for her, and her decision making in using language was broadening beyond what she had been "taught."

Recall Coleen (Sample 7), the child discussed earlier in this chapter, who started out in a similar situation to Kitty's. Both demonstrated sufficient comprehension to conclude that expressive language was possible, but neither exhibited much talking. In Coleen's case, a change in the relationship context was the key to developing expression. She soon began a flood of talking. Her early grammar was bizarre, but before long her syntax improved through her own problem solving. In contrast, Kitty's expressive language did not respond to manipulation of the relationship until she was also provided with specific practice in expressive language through models, contingencies, and nonverbal cues.

Conclusion

While language learning depends ultimately on input, children need practice in expression as they develop skill in sorting out the details of language structure. Some children will undergo this practice on their own as their rates of talking increase. Their own problem solving will carry them faster than we could teach them. Other children will need more specific practice with production, guided by the trainer.

Perhaps one could think of two major levels in working on expression in language-impaired children. First, there is the relationship level, where we are primarily concerned with the child's willingness to talk at all. This is the subject for the next chapter. The second level involves cuing retrieval of vocabulary and grammatical options from the repertoire. A number of different procedures are available, stemming directly from the informal assessment procedures described in Chapter 7. As we have seen, each type of cue puts different information-processing and problem-solving demands on the learner. The tasks also vary in degrees of ecological validity they possess for natural language use by the child. The challenge for us, then, is to find the best compromise between generating efficient practice and focusing on functional language use for each child. These decisions are best made through exploratory teaching.

Returning to the referential communication paradigm, in expression we help the child select appropriate language options to differentiate among the alternatives in the situation. While we may cue utterances in various ways, children ultimately learn about the effectiveness of their utterances through the feedback they receive.

EMPHASIS ON TRANSACTIONAL PATTERNS: THE FEEDBACK SYSTEM

Referential communication tasks generate feedback processes. This fact is of fundamental importance in training language structures. First, it emphasizes that intervention is an interpersonal process. *Success in referential communication depends equally on the contributions of both participants.*

Similarly, achieving goals in language training depends on accommodations between child and teacher. Neither can succeed without the other.

There is a second reason why feedback processes are important. It is through providing feedback to the child that the trainer can function as a responsive environment for the child's attempts at language learning. As we saw in the preceding chapter, feedback may have both motivational properties, as it provides reinforcement, and informational properties, as it provides knowledge of results. It is significant that research in referential communication has demonstrated that feedback is central in the task. Glucksberg and Krauss (1967) found that many young normal children's difficulties with the task were in the area of feedback. As receivers, they didn't ask enough questions, even when the information they had was insufficient. As senders, they didn't respond effectively to the questions they were asked. In another vein, Fishbein and Osborn (1971) found that the feedback provided by the experimenters profoundly affected children's performance on the task. When provided with knowledge of results after each trial, kindergartners performed as well as fifth graders. Similarly, we help language-impaired children in our adaptations of referential communication for language training. In expression, children must learn when their choices of options-to-mean are functioning effectively. In comprehension, they need to know if their selections of alternatives match those of the speaker.

Mahoney (1975) emphasized that children regulate the language models they receive. They indicate which utterances they comprehend and which they don't. If the child is not talking, this regulatory feedback must be accomplished through nonverbal means.

Mahoney suggests that for some language-impaired children, this feedback is distorted or absent.

As the child develops language, there is also the beginning of what Cook-Gumperz (1977) calls negotiated meaning. Through a series of exchanges, parent and child work out what a particular expression is going to mean, for them, in that context. Obviously, this negotiation need not be conscious "metatalk" about how to use words. It evolves naturally out of the problem solving both are engaged in in attempting to communicate effectively. Research in referential communication illustrates an analogue of this process. Krauss and Glucksberg (1977), using designs such as those in Figure 9 note that utterance lengths get shorter in repeated trials with the same stimuli. The first time, one design may be described as *the spider with triangular glasses and wearing an apron;* the next time it may be *the spider with the apron;* the third time it may be only *spider*. These negotiated meanings develop through feedback between both participants. It is through such negotiations that the social codes mentioned in previous chapters develop. Note, by the way, that such negotiated meanings develop in conjunction with increasing top-down processing by both participants.

While the focus of this chapter is on training specific aspects of language, we have gone far beyond any narrow focus on teaching particular vocabulary or grammatical options. We have been exploring the fabric of the transactional patterns in which children learn to communicate. We will pick up this thread again in succeeding chapters.

Returning to the theme of this chapter, the preceding two sections focused on the receiver and sender respectively. You have seen, though, that I couldn't discuss only comprehension and then only expression.

Aspects of each kept cropping up while I was concentrating on the other. This situation reflects the fact that comprehension and expression complement each other. It is the same child making decisions in both processes. Each helps clarify the other in language learning. Therefore, while I still maintain that comprehension is a cornerstone of language teaching, I do not feel that comprehension and expression cannot be dealt with at the same time. The important point is to be clear about what you are trying to accomplish with any particular procedure. Are you teaching? Testing? Providing practice? You can then take advantage of the characteristics of comprehension and expression, and the feedback between the two, to achieve your goal as efficiently as possible.

SENTENCE ELABORATION AND NONREFERENTIAL COMMUNICATION

So far I have emphasized referential communication because it provides a concrete way to tie language options with the communication of meaning. The focus has been on basic options within the microcosmic matrix. With older children, though, we need to move beyond those structures to more subtle uses of language. More elaborated sentences are required for the specificity and detail that is the hallmark of academic learning. In addition, not all language use is referential in the direct sense that the referential communication paradigm implies. In Olson's (1970b) view, speakers are always differentiating among alternatives, and I think this perspective remains helpful in working with older language-impaired children. The alternatives, however, are based more on denotation and sense. When we get beyond the earlier stages, language users function without as many concrete referents. Indeed, many uses of language depend on the communicators being freed from the immediate context. How else could you direct somebody across town, or write a poem, or read this book?

One technique for eliciting nonreferential talking is to ask children to tell stories. Language Sample 9 is a story told by Margaret, who was enrolled in a junior-high class for language-impaired children. She made up the story after looking at a photo from an old horror movie. Read the sample through first to get an idea of the story.

Margaret is certainly able to talk in this nonreferential style. I would say the plot is unique. There is a narrative sequence through the story, although one is not always sure which woman Margaret is talking about in the second half of the story. In all fairness, I must remind you that she was concocting this story on the spot and dictating it into a tape recorder.

Consider her use of grammatical options. All clause types are represented. Margaret uses both noun phrases and verb phrases and combines clauses into longer sentences. While there are some errors of detail, she appears to have most of the microcosmic matrix in her repertoire. Where Margaret's talking suffers most in comparison with her more language-skilled peers is, not in grammar, but in sentence elaboration. Out of twenty utterances, six contain simple coordinated clauses and only three contain subordinating constructions. If we analyzed her verb phrases and noun phrases into columns as in Chapter 8, the lack of elaboration would be apparent in the empty columns. Her verb usage contains no auxiliaries at all except for two instances of the continuum in utterance number 3. While she

---

SAMPLE 9 : Margaret CA = 13–9

1. it was about this man and this woman, and they were married
2. and this man he had another affair with this 'nother woman
3. and the man and the woman that he was married to was laying in bed watching TV
4. and the phone ring on the TV
5. and it was a woman
6. and all the sudden, their telephone ring and they jumped
7. and the wife went up and answered the phone
8. and it was this woman asking for her husband
9. now the woman she gave the phone to her husband and she was pretty mad
10. so um they started talking on the telephone
11. and she said that she wanted to break up and all this stuff
12. he was screaming and hollering
13. and he he put down the phone
14. and all he had on was his underwear
15. and he started running after his wife
16. and that woman she dropped her suitcase and everything flew up
17. and he and he finally caught her
18. and they fell down this big gutter
19. and they were stuck down there for three weeks
20. and they they made up when they were down there

---

uses many noun phrases, the vast majority of them consist only of determiners and nouns. There is one postmodifier and two or three adjectivals.

Clearly, Margaret's grammatical style in this sample was influenced by the context: She was asked to tell a story into a microphone. I don't doubt that she has additional grammatical options in her repertoire. At the same time, in this story she takes little advantage of the options that are available in the language, and the richness, detail, and precision of her communication suffer as a result. Through informal assessment we could find out fairly quickly what other noun phrase and verb phrase options are in her repertoire, but that's only half the story. In line with the pragmatics model from the preceding chapter, she has to decide to use those options in communicating.

Theoretical Issues

The issues involved here are complex. Let us begin with a distinction made by Bruner (1972). He contrasts contextualized and decontextualized speech. Contextualized speech is associated with action, whereas decontextualized speech is divorced from the immediate situation. Asking a waiter for more bread is contextualized; discussing this book while eating that bread is decontextualized. From this perspective, the whole referential communication paradigm I have been developing in this chapter involves the use of contextualized language. It is more convergent than divergent; that is, the child is directed toward a specific response rather than many different responses.

Another distinction of importance here is that made by Bernstein (1970) between restricted codes and elaborated codes. In general, messages in a restricted code contain the minimal information required to accomplish the speaker's purpose, while elaborated messages contain additional detail and subtlety. Imagine that a child is playing noisily near the telephone. The phone rings. As the mother answers it, she says simply to the child, *Quiet*. In contrast, another mother in the same situation might say, *Please keep the noise down while I'm on the phone*. The second message is an ex-

ample of elaborated code. It contains more cognitive stimulation: Requesting and manners through the use of *please;* relativity through *keep the noise down;* and time duration in *while I'm on the phone*. While Bernstein considered these codes in relation to education and social class, they have relevance in the present discussion also. The elaborated code contains the same development of sentences in discourse that we wish our language-impaired children to achieve.

Restricted coding may be encouraged by contextualized speech. One function of the context is to limit the number of interpretations available for an utterance. Consequently, the speaker doesn't need to be as specific because the specificity is supplied by the context. Words such as *thing* and *it* will do if everyone knows what you're talking about. In decontextualized speech, on the other hand, the specificity is in the language itself, requiring more precise selections of options and additional elaboration.

Taking this idea a step further, Ervin-Tripp and Mitchell-Kernan (1977) have pointed out that restricted code usage is related to the idea of negotiated meaning discussed in the preceding section. In continuing interactions we tacitly negotiate what particular utterances will mean, thus eliminating the need for detail. While Bernstein thought of restricted codes primarily as being passed by cultural groups down to their children, one can imagine children eliciting restricted codings from adults as well. A preschool girl asks her father what the moon is. He explains, *It's a giant ball like our earth that's 'way up in the sky*. She says, *Yeah, but what's the moon?* He answers, *It's a big ball in the sky*. Again she asks, *Yeah, but what's the moon?* This time the parent takes the child outside and points to the moon: *That's the moon*. While this example is perhaps a little overstated, there is abundant evidence that through the feedback they provide, children elicit simplified talking from adults. Doubtless, much of that talking involves restricted coding. Thus, this style of decision making in language use may become established in the transactional patterns between parents and child. In the normal course of events this pattern works well for the family at the time, and they move on as the child develops. With some language-disordered children, however, it may become a morphostatic process, one that resists change, and both child and parents become caught in a situation that leads to minimal language growth.

In conclusion, sentence elaboration is not a linear addition to basic language skills. It is a process rather than a set of knowledge. It depends not only on the child's repertoire but also on the communication situation, including the transactional patterns with the listener, the nonverbal context, and the type and topic of discourse. In helping children use more elaborated sentences, then, we need to make sure they possess the repertoire, but that is the easy part. I'm sure Margaret, in Language Sample 9, knows a sufficient grammatical repertoire. We need to provide situations where elaboration is relevant or necessary for successful communication. For example, it was reported in the language-sampling chapter that children's talking contains more elaboration in the home than in the clinic. Why? In the clinic, most of the talking is contextualized. At home, people talk about many aspects of the family's life beyond whatever is in the immediate context.

Intervention Techniques

Sentence elaboration requires increased memory span and other information-processing skills. It also requires sufficient conceptual skills to handle the complexities and interrelations in elaborated utterances. Children with difficulties in any of these areas, then, might be more competent with shorter, simpler utterances, at the cost of less specificity and detail. They may depend more on contextualized and negotiated meanings. At the same time, as I have argued earlier, there is no way to separate cognitive and conceptual skills from language use. We will have to approach all of them together.

Little systematic work has been done with language-impaired children at this end of the continuum. Therefore, the strategy proposed here is highly tentative. We will need to teach whatever aspects of the repertoire the child does not possess. As I have pointed out, though, we also need to encourage children to make richer selections from whatever repertoires they do have. It will be particularly important, then, to provide models, cues for retrieval, and practice. In order to keep language tied with meaning, we could begin by asking children to differentiate among finer and finer sets of alternatives. At this point we would be helping children develop facility with more elaborated language use, but still through contextualized language. Once the child is using a richer set of options, we could then begin to move toward more decontextualized forms of talking.

Communication Tasks

The referential communication paradigm can be adapted toward these goals. As mentioned previously, referents can be provided that encourage the use of elaborated noun phrases for their identification. At first, the clinician can model appropriate noun phrases if necessary. Similar in principle to those in Figure 10, the referents should be the same in overall appearance but also vary in several details. For example, they could all be triangles but vary in combinations of size, thickness, color, and composition. One would then ask for *the thick, blue triangle made of wood, all the plastic triangles,* and so forth. Note that success in these tasks depends not only on language skill but also on perceptual skill. The sender must perceive all the relevant attributes in order to codify them in language. Whitehurst (1976) found that children's difficulty with referential communication was related to their skill in perceiving the contrasts in the stimulus array. In the preceding chapter it was mentioned that there are data indicating that improving children's perceptual skills may enhance their problem-solving skills. While that goal may be beyond our resources, we can begin with fairly simple stimuli and move to more complicated ones, pointing out perceptual attributes where necessary.

Other tasks can be used for more general language elaboration. Any activity in which neither participant has all the information necessary to complete the task can be adapted for our purposes. Chandler, Greenspan, and Barenboim (1974) and Greenspan, Burka, Zlotlow, and Barenboim (1975) discuss a number of referential communication games. They are based on the learning games developed by Furth (1970; Furth and Wachs 1974). Participants can describe different layouts on checkerboards to each other; one can direct another in how to build something with blocks; each can have a copy of a map—one directs the other to get to a certain place on the map.

The common ingredients of these activities are that they provide experience in the precise use of language toward accomplishing some goal and they provide feedback regarding the effectiveness of the

messages children develop. One cannot simply put two language-disordered children together playing such games and be done with it, however. The level of difficulty must be monitored carefully because it is important that each child achieve a large measure of success in communicating in these tasks. Frequently the clinician will take either the sender's or receiver's role, in order to provide models, cues, and feedback tailored to individual children's needs. The relationship aspects of these activities must also be monitored closely. While different activities will vary in how autotelic they are for individual children, it is important that children generally enjoy communicating with other human beings through these tasks.

Contrastive Modeling

Another technique that can be used, and one that is particularly helpful in encouraging decontextualized talking, is the contrastive modeling described earlier. Fromberg (1976) uses this procedure in a turn-about fashion, where the teacher provides a model and then the child responds. There are contrasts both in the model and also between the teacher's utterance and the child's utterance. Once the children have learned the routine, the dialogue in a small group might go like this.

Teacher: *I can buckle my belt or hang it in the closet.*
First child: *I can tie my shoe or let it fall off.*
Second child: *I can button my shirt or let it flop open.*

This sequence focuses on coordination. Others can be developed around subordination.

I go home when the bell rings.
I eat lunch when my stomach's empty.

More elaborate sequences can be included.

*When I leave the house, I lock the door
so we won't get robbed.*
*After I leave school, I wait on the side-
walk so I can see my friends.*

Many other variations are possible. While
Fromberg discusses these techniques in conjunction with young children, older age
groups also enjoy them. In fact, with practice and a positive interpersonal atmosphere,
they lead to increasingly more intricate
dialogues. One must be careful not to
overtax the participants' language skills so
that they become embarrassed. Generally,
though, they see the task as a talking game
and focus on the content. The clinician can
provide models, cues, and feedback as appropriate.

The techniques described above illustrate
a progression from teaching the repertoire,
to using elaborated talking in referential
speech, and finally to decontextualized
situations. They are merely suggestions,
however. Individual clinicians will need to
develop methods for moving in these directions that are consonant with their own ways
of working. Where possible, it is very useful
to know something about each child's
language habits. Around what topics and
what situations does the child talk the most?
Similarly, what talking situations generate
the most involvement and enthusiasm?
Labov (1972a) found that these situations
are likely to elicit more elaborated talking
than most teaching or clinical situations. It
shouldn't be too hard, for example, to find
some communication situations with great
ecological validity for Margaret. Situations
such as these could provide a bridge between
our interventions and the child's most competent experiences in talking.

240

Conclusions

Difficulties with sentence elaboration in
children are not well understood. Historically, lack of elaborated language in talking
has not received much attention except in
relation to social class, where it has
generated much controversy. In terms of
language disorders, it is hard to define just
what an impairment in sentence elaboration
is. Some readers may not feel that Margaret
shows a true language impairment. In fact,
that is why I chose her for an example,
rather than a more clear-cut case. Lack of
elaborative talking could be related to
information-processing or conceptual difficulties; it could be related to transactional
patterns within the family; it could be
related to peer values; it could be related to
general learning difficulties; it could be
related to the specific context, or even to
sheer boredom. Probably more than one of
these factors is often involved.

However, the meager data available suggest that difficulties with sentence elaboration are related to poor language skills.
(Hass and Wepman 1974; Loban 1968;
Naremore and Dever 1975). We can assume
that language-impaired children, once they
have acquired a basic repertoire, will
evidence problems in this area. Intervention
must involve helping children express ideas
more effectively through language. Teaching
grammatical skills alone will not evoke the
combination of metarules and problem-
solving strategies necessary for more
elaborated language use. Naremore and
Dever suggest that the ". . . emphasis [be]
put on fluent oral communication in connected discourse, rather on linguistic drill"
(1975, p. 94). While their discussion is
limited to educable retarded children, I
think their recommendation is relevant to
most language-impaired children who are
functioning at the clausal level, and is par-

ticularly important with those at older age levels.

CULTURALLY DIFFERENT CHILDREN

The principles that have been explored in this chapter apply to intervention with language-disordered children from any background. The picture is more complicated, however, when the child punctuates things from a set of cultural values different from those of the clinician, and it may be still more complicated when that child lives in a bilingual or nonstandard dialect environment. As emphasized in previous chapters, the fundamental distinction to make is between disorder and difference, whether that difference be due to dialect or bilingualism. As we have seen, this distinction must be based on as full assessment of the child's skills as possible, but never on the basis of a language sample only. For our purposes, the fundamental contrast between the two is that most nonstandard dialect and bilingual children do have adequate knowledge of language appropriate for their culture, whereas language-disordered children do not possess normal language skill in any language or dialect. Only the second group show an "impairment" in language skill, and it is only with that group that we possess any special expertise.

Language Disorder in the Context of Cultural Difference

Let us consider first the child who is both language disordered and culturally different. Our goal remains the same as for any other language-impaired child. We want to enhance the child's effectiveness as a com-municator. In terms of overall strategy, the beginning focus will be on relationship factors. We need to define a relationship that will be productive for both child and clinician, and especially one in which the child can grow as a communicator. Because of cultural differences, this process may take longer than it otherwise would (Cazden 1970). Similarly, early language-training goals will be broad. We will want to encourage as much spontaneous talking as possible and help each child develop basic options-to-mean.

Here we face a dilemma. Recall that language learning is based on input. What input is appropriate for a language-impaired child who is from a nonstandard dialect or bilingual background? Should we emphasize the language patterns of the child's own culture or the Standard English of the classroom and middle-class culture? In answering these questions we have to begin with a realistic appraisal of what is possible for us to accomplish successfully. For many of us that will mean working in Standard English. Rarely can a language clinician do a competent job except in a language and dialect with which that clinician is very familiar.

Beyond the matter of clinician skill, the question of which language or dialect to emphasize becomes a value judgment. Much ink and emotion have been expended regarding bilingual and bicultural children, compensatory education, and so forth. These value judgments are complex. One should keep very clearly in mind that our primary focus is on language *disorders,* albeit embedded in bicultural contexts. In working through assessment and exploratory teaching we attempt to define intervention goals for each child. As we will see in Chapter 13, defining goals is essentially a process of value judgment. Therefore, it is important to consult with the child if appropriate, and certainly with the parents. Once the goals are defined, we can then decide what language emphasis might accomplish those goals best. For example, if the goal is to help the child develop sufficient language skill to succeed in school, then the language of instruction in the child's school will have to be emphasized in intervention.

If it is decided that Standard English should not be the vehicle of intervention, then that intervention will have to be carried out by someone who speaks the appropriate dialect or language. In situations where the clinician speaks only Standard English, it may be possible to find an aid or volunteer who has the necessary language skill. In selecting this person it is highly desirable to seek an individual who is flexible enough to adopt the different interpersonal styles that various children may require. Merely being bidialectal or bilingual is not enough, because language disorders are never only linguistic.

Standard English as a Second Language

Let us now consider children who are not language disordered but who speak a nonstandard dialect of English or some language other than English. The situation here is very different, because these children usually do have adequate command of language. A specialized field has developed for teaching English as a second language (ESL). The techniques for teaching ESL have been refined by professionals in that field. While these procedures were developed for adults, they have been employed with schoolchildren, both nonstandard dialect and non-English speakers. In contrast to work with language-disordered children, ESL techniques are based on the

assumption that the learner already knows a language. Teaching focuses on contrasts between the student's native language and Standard English. Through pattern drills somewhat reminiscent of Fromberg's (1977) contrastive modeling, the student learns these areas of contrast. Of course, many other techniques are also used. The point is that ESL teaching takes for granted that the learner is already a competent language user, a far different view from that in the field of children's language disorders.

In spite of these differences, language clinicians in the schools do get referrals for nonstandard speakers. From the teacher's point of view, the child is a poor language user in the classroom—or perhaps unintelligible. If there is no ESL teacher available, the language clinician is a logical choice for working with nonstandard dialect and non–English-speaking children. Individual clinicians must evaluate their own competencies and decide whether or not it is appropriate for them to accept these referrals. Should you decide to work with bilingual or nonstandard English speakers, the following guidelines may be of help. First, remember again that these children present differences, not disorders. There are two levels at which to make this distinction. Obviously we should not regard such differences as representing impoverished language unless we can convincingly demonstrate that a language disorder is present. Further, though, at a more subtle level, we should not approach these differences as "errors." Unfortunately this view is well ingrained in our training, as it relates to both language and articulation. This observation leads to the second guideline. If we are going to work in this area, we should become familiar with ESL teaching techniques. In so doing we not only learn efficient teaching procedures but also we leave behind the "disorder" or "deficiency" perspective. K. Johnson (1970) gives some introductory examples of ESL procedures for speakers of Black English Vernacular.

The third guideline is the most problematic. Teaching a culturally different child Standard English implies a value judgment about the way the child already talks. That is why the emphasis has been on teaching Standard English as a *second* language or a *second* dialect. The hope is to minimize the value comparison between the child's language use and the prestige dialect. There is more involved than this comparison, however. As noted in Chapter 5, language use is a powerful means of identification with a cultural group. Further, the dominant cultural group for children is the peer group, and peer pressure can be powerful indeed. By teaching a child Standard English we may be placing that child in a situation laden with conflict unless the child is able to switch codes in different interpersonal contexts. This situation exemplifies how the variable rules discussed in Chapter 8 are realized through the pragmatics model of Chapter 9. Children decide how to talk according to the situation.

These observations lead to a final conclusion. In teaching Standard English as a second language or dialect, the student's motivation is all-important. From the child's point of view there may be little reason to learn Standard English other than that the teacher requires it. Peer values may be opposed to doing what the teacher says in the first place, much less learning the Standard English that teachers favor. Consequently, motivation for learning Standard English may be very low in some culturally different children. Teaching attempts might better be delayed until the child is old enough to appreciate the usefulness of Standard English in various occupational and educational pursuits and mature enough to realize that one can learn new skills without necessarily abandoning one's cultural identification.

CONCLUSIONS

In 1799 Itard wrote about his attempts to teach language and social behavior to the Wild Boy of Aveyron, a boy who was discovered living without human contact in the forest (Itard 1962). It is remarkable that Itard used the same general techniques that we use today! We've certainly gathered a lot of data since then, but Itard was faced with the same kind of problem solving then that we face today in working with language-disordered children. What can we do to teach language? Ultimately, we can provide stimuli or input, we can encourage responses, and we can provide feedback, which is, of course, additional input. Literally billions of children have learned to talk through these mechanisms. The details and the content vary with different cultures and smaller groups, right down to individual families. Similarly, in the language disorders field, they vary with different practitioners and theoretical perspectives. Given all this variety, there cannot be one set of procedures that is best.

Consequently, the goal of this chapter has not been to specify a set of techniques for teaching vocabulary items and grammatical structures. Not all language-impaired children need that specific training. Further, when they are used, specific procedures will vary from child to child.

Rather, the goal of this chapter is to describe a framework in which intervention procedures can be devised and evaluated. There are two parts to this framework. First, there are the general principles which were summarized at the beginning of the chapter: ecological validity, transactional model, problem solving, autotelic environments, responsive environments, and exploratory teaching. These principles form the groundwork from which we develop intervention strategies for individual children. To make our consideration of language teaching more specific, however, I added a second level to the framework: the referential communication paradigm.

I find this paradigm useful because referential communication is fundamental in everyone's use of language. It is a significant component of the transactional patterns that develop in families with language-learning children. In fact, Dickson, Hess, Miyake, and Azuma (1979) found that skill in referential communication between mother and child predicts later cognitive development in the child. These observations suggest the theoretical importance of the referential communication paradigm for language intervention. It is also valuable for practical reasons. First, it is very flexible. As noted earlier, different types of feedback dramatically affect children's success in the task. Further, Whitehurst (1976) demonstrated that young children's performance in the task can be greatly enhanced by modeling ways for the children to participate. In sum, not only is referential communication important in language use, but the paradigm is flexible enough that it can be altered in various ways to increase children's skills in communicative problem solving.

The focus of the referential communication paradigm is not on the individual, but on the transactional patterns between the participants. I have used these patterns to illustrate how various themes from previous portions of the book might be applied. We have seen how problem solving, grammar as options-to-mean, and meaning as differen-

tiating among alternatives come together in the child's functioning as receiver or sender. Through the paradigm we hope to make grammatical structures as discrete, discursive, and linear as possible. Because of its referential nature, much training focuses on contextualized meaning. It is fitting to me that early training rest on that concrete basis. At the same time, if we are to help children use language normally, we must help them develop decontextualized speech as well, where the alternatives of meaning are present only in the language system, or perhaps I should say only in the mind.

We have seen that a number of the debates regarding clinical training, such as whether to emphasize comprehension or expression, modeling or imitation, and telegraphic or complete utterances, become nonquestions. We cannot answer these issues for all children. Rather, through exploratory teaching, we ask how we can best serve each child's needs. Following in the footsteps of Itard, we engage in problem solving anew with each child.

Winitz and Reeds (1975) suggested that syntax training be based on the child's problem solving. Learning grammar is the product of that problem solving. Snyder and McLean (1977) and Snyder-McLean and McLean (1978) suggest that we go a step further and focus directly on the child's language-learning strategies, the problem solving itself, rather than the syntax. Through the referential communication paradigm, we can manipulate that problem solving in many ways, but the child is always making decisions that are relevant to language use in communication. Hopefully, we can thus instill a "problem-solving set" in children as language users, involving both comprehension and expression. At least we can heighten their perceptions of the options in language and how they function in communication. It seems to me that these emphases are a key to what Bateson (1972) called "deuterolearning," or learning to learn. Through problem solving in ecologically valid communication situations, the child learns how to learn about language. The referential communication paradigm provides a framework for developing just such performatory acts.

I have stressed comprehension as an efficient way to make children aware of grammatical options. Comprehension training also forces you, the trainer, to deal with meaning somehow. I have emphasized the importance of expression in facilitating retrieval of grammatical structures the child has already encountered and in providing practice in combining grammatical options. Throughout the chapter we have focused on the conceptual-semantic decision making from the pragmatics model in the previous chapter. By its very nature, however, expression is also at the heart of using language to deal with people. This observation brings us to the relationship decisions in the pragmatics model. This area of decision making is the topic for the next chapter.

11

INTERVENTION:
LANGUAGE
AS AN INTERPERSONAL
PHENOMENON

At the end of Chapter 5, I concluded that the most powerful interventions would be those that focus on language in human relationship contexts that are significant in the child's life. As we have seen, language use is profoundly affected by the relationships in which it occurs. Similarly, human relationships are affected by language use. If we are to work effectively with children's language disorders, then, we will have to deal with human relationships as well.

In the previous chapter we concentrated on one particular relationship context, exemplified by the referential communication paradigm. It was implied that the child cooperated willingly, and we focused on teaching language *qua* language. That is, we assumed an appropriate or constructive relationship context in which we could work. From the perspective of the pragmatics model, this assumption allowed us to focus only on the conceptual-semantic decisions underlying the use of specific options-to-mean.

The pragmatics model, however, reminds us that language use involves relationship decisions as well. It is now time to expand our view of the child's meaning potential accordingly. In the language-sampling chapter I pointed out that relationship factors affect language decisions in, for example, choice of clause variations. Use of a particular clause structure frequently structures the relationship as well. In uttering an imperative you may imply that you are one-up. Conversely, it is in relationships in which you are one-up that you are most likely to use imperatives. The reciprocity between language use and human relationships is much more pervasive than that, however, as illustrated in the chapter on principles of intervention. The rule hierarchy for expression involves relationship decisions ranging from very obvious, as in deciding whether or not

to talk to a stranger, to very subtle, as in selecting vocabulary items to match a particular listener.

Further, as pointed out in Chapter 5, relationship communication involves not only language but also nonverbal behavior. Again, we must expand our concept of the child's meaning potential to include communication of this type. In sum, we are interested not only in how children use language but in how they use language and nonverbal communication to deal with other people.

It might be argued that human relationships and nonverbal communication are beyond our purview as language specialists. In terms of the pragmatics model, however, this argument limits us to teaching only the repertoire. If we are concerned with language use, then we are by definition involved in human relationships. Moreover, if we are involved in human relationships, we are also concerned with nonverbal communication.

HUMAN RELATIONSHIPS AND ACTIVE LEARNING

Each child grows in a particular set of environments. Both environment and child change over time. The interactions between child and environment may be characterized as a set of transactional patterns. That is, the environment and the child develop consistent ways of behaving toward each other. These transactional patterns involve a mix of metarules and decision making. Or, using a different metaphor, they evolve around a set of negotiated meanings. All participants know how they are expected to behave toward one another, but each instance of behavior involves individual decisions about how to function within these guidelines, or whether indeed to break some of the rules.

Through learning and negotiating transactional patterns with significant individuals, each child develops consistent ways of dealing with other people. So have we, and so do we continue to develop, both as human beings in general and in our special role as teachers and clinicians. It is our hope to define and negotiate clinical relationships in ways that will maximize the processes of language development in each child.

Language-Learning Strategies

Snyder and McLean suggested that intervention "... focus less on the products of language development and more on the processes, or strategies, critical to such development" (1977, p. 341). Along these lines, a goal to be hoped for in the techniques described in the preceding chapter is to foster a problem-solving set in the child's use of language, so that further language development occurs through performatory acts. We cannot focus just on these processes in the child, however, because they can only occur in the context of human relationships. In fact, they become significant components of the transactional patterns between child and family. Let us see what some of these processes might be.

Snyder and McLean (1977) and Snyder-McLean and McLean (1978) described several possible language-learning strategies. First, parents and children work out ways to establish shared reference, so that both are focusing on the same stimuli. It is through this process that language options become related to the child's perceptual world. Second, children become selective listeners, developing sensitivity about which utterances are relevant to their world and which aren't. Third, children provide feedback to their parents regarding whether or not they comprehend utterances spoken to them. Fourth, children can imitate utterances or parts of utterances they hear. Fifth, children elicit additional information about language through their utterances. They may ask questions or evoke responses in other ways. To this list I would add that expression, both imitative and spontaneous, provides practice in retrieving and combining grammatical options. With this exception, it is noteworthy that most of these processes are based on obtaining or clarifying input from the environment, again emphasizing the interactional nature of these language-learning strategies. Note also that the relative success of these information-gathering strategies depends largely on the degree to which more mature speakers in the environment function as responsive environments. In this capacity one must not only provide appropriate feedback and allow the child to discover relationships, one must also allow the child considerable freedom in acting on the environment.

Writing from an ecological perspective, Bronfenbrenner described three aspects of relationships that are of particular importance in fostering development in children: "The developmental impact of a dyad increases as a direct function of the level of reciprocity, mutuality of positive feeling, and a gradual shift of balance of power in favor of the developing person" (1979, p. 59). The first two of these need no further comment at present. The third emphasizes the child's role as an active learner and the importance of self-esteem. Bronfenbrenner further suggests that learning is enhanced when both members of the dyad see themselves as doing something together. There is a parallel here with the emphasis in the preceding chapter on child and clinician together involved in communication tasks.

Finally, Bronfenbrenner also emphasizes the importance of ". . . the participation of the developing person in progressively more complex patterns of reciprocal activity with someone with whom that person has developed a strong and enduring emotional attachment . . ." (1979, p. 60). Again the relation between problem solving and transactional patterns is maintained. These views will provide a perspective for considering the relationship aspects of language intervention in this chapter. They will be even more important in the next chapter, when we will consider family relationships.

Interpersonal Contexts That Encourage Language Use

I have conjured up another tall order. How can we establish human relationships that will embody all the ideas in the preceding section? Let us begin with a more modest goal and consider contexts that will encourage as much language use as possible in children. The evidence is scarce regarding comprehension, but we can follow some of the principles summarized at the beginning of the preceding chapter. Comprehension requires attending. Therefore we will need situations where the language input has ecological validity for the child. The problem here is that we cannot declare what will be ecologically valid for an individual child. We will have to check with that child somehow. Further, the situation should be as autotelic as possible, both in terms of the topic of discussion and the broader affective qualities of the relationship—Bronfenbrenner's "mutuality of positive feeling" quoted above. In addition, the language structures employed will have to be appropriate for the child's level of comprehension.

The same principles apply with expression, but we can develop a more specific focus. Two factors are particularly important in influencing expression. Both have been discussed in earlier chapters but require mention here because of their relevance to relationships.

First, Cazden's (1970) review suggests that children talk more when the topic of discussion is of immediate interest to them. A moment's reflection will indicate that this assertion is generally true of children of all ages—and of us as well! Ask me about my banjo sometime or if I like to write textbooks. This idea is innocent enough until you realize what it implies about the relationship between trainer and child. If increased expression is a goal, *the child should select the topics of discussion*. This conclusion follows Bronfenbrenner's suggestion regarding a shift in the balance of power. In so doing it illustrates the second factor influencing expression, namely, the relationship context. This factor derives from what Labov (1972a) termed the power relations between child and listener. A child's output is likely to be enhanced when that child is one-up vis-à-vis the listener. As Cazden (1970) notes, children may be more willing to talk to younger children or even animals than to older, more powerful children or adults. Labov (1972a) vividly illustrated in his studies of language use in black youths that power relations affect not only the amount of output but also the quality and complexity of children's utterances.

At a practical level these power relations can be approached through the concept of constraint. Broadly, a constraint is any interruption or limit on the child's ongoing activity (Bayles 1974; Hubbell 1977). Constraints, then, include physical factors, such as not having enough room to complete an activity or running out of glue. More important here, they include attempts by adults to change or guide children's behavior. Questions and commands are frequently more constraining than statements. There is considerable evidence that the degree of constraint present in a situation directly influences the way both normal and language-impaired children talk (Hubbell 1977).

In sum, children's talking is most enhanced when they are talking about topics of immediate interest to them and when the situation contains a minimal amount of constraint. Both of these factors are clearly components of the relationship between child and listener, rather than aspects of language structure *per se*. Further, these two relationship factors are fundamental components of responsive environments as described in Chapter 9. In fact, Moore (1966) argued that adults should not even be present if an environment is to be truly responsive for a child. We have an overwhelming tendency to direct children, rather than allowing them to make their own decisions and discoveries. I will return to this problem. In any case, it is something of an eye-opener to view conventional grammar-training techniques from this point of view. In teaching syntactic structures the trainer typically supplies the topic, often from a set of pictures. Further, the trainer maintains a one-up position over the child, directing the child's activity heavily. Such teaching strategies do not enhance children's problem-solving efforts in learning language, either by encouraging as much talking and practice as possible or by providing a responsive environment for that talking.

The contrast between relationship factors that enhance talking and structured language-teaching procedures is dramatized starkly in attempts to reinforce children for talking. Imagine that you went into a lunchroom and ordered a piece of pie and a cup of coffee. Now imagine that the waitress

answered you with, *GOOD TALKING!* While this example illustrates the situation in simplistic form, the problems here are complex and important.

The "Be Spontaneous" Paradox

We find ourselves in a bit of a paradox, then. If we attempt to teach aspects of language in a straightforward manner, we run the risk of structuring a relationship that discourages talking in the child. We met this problem before in the pragmatics model from Chapter 9. It is another example of the contrast between focusing on the repertoire and focusing on the child's decision making in using language for communication. From the perspective I am developing in this chapter, it is related to a more general phenomenon in human relationships, which Watzlawick, Beavin, and Jackson (1967) call the "be spontaneous" paradox. Their classic example goes as follows. Suppose someone tells you to do something spontaneous. You literally cannot comply with this directive. Obviously, if you don't respond, you're not complying because you're not doing something. On the other hand, if you do something, it's not really spontaneous; you're doing it because you were told to. Thus, you are caught in a paradox.

The language clinician is caught in a similar paradox. We want children to want to talk. But as soon as we elicit talking from them, they're not talking because they want to, but because we got them to talk. I might call this situation the "want to talk" paradox. Often we can encourage, cajole, reinforce, or in other ways get many children to talk, but we cannot get them to *want* to talk. Similarly, we cannot get them to want to engage in the problem solving associated with language learning. These decisions are private to each child. It is for these reasons that I stress ecological validity and autotelic communication in language intervention. In past chapters these ideas have been related primarily to the types of stimuli and activities offered the child. Now it can be seen that they are also related to the larger context of the human relationships in which language learning and use occur.

It may take you some time to appreciate the power of the "want to talk" paradox. In my case, I had read Watzlawick, Beavin, and Jackson (1967), nodded wisely, and set their ideas on a back burner. Sometime later I was working with a language-delayed boy named Dennis. He demonstrated adequate comprehension to support at least moderate development of expression, but he spoke not a single word. After a period of time, I happened to meet the child on the sidewalk outside the clinic. Dennis talked in phrases! Following that instance, he still would not talk in the clinic. Dennis taught me the importance of the "be spontaneous" paradox. There was simply nothing I could do that would make Dennis want to talk. We could think of this situation in terms of attitudes in the boy's head: He was stubborn, or resistant, or not motivated. However, it is instructive to view his behavior (or lack of it) in terms of his relationship with me. Dennis had me outfoxed either way. If I pressed him to talk, he remained silent, and I failed. If I didn't attempt to elicit talking, he remained silent, and I failed. Questions of whether he was aware of this situation or if he was following a purposive strategy are irrelevant. The point is that I was truly caught in the paradox. While I don't know what he was thinking, it seemed that Dennis was also caught in a paradox. It was obvious that he was uncomfortable no matter how I tried to elicit talking from him. At the same time, for whatever reason, he was unwilling to talk and thus escape his discomfort. Dennis

didn't have a way out any more than I did. We were caught in a circular trap similar to those Laing (1970) illustrated so powerfully in his book *Knots*.

When I realized how intractable the situation was, my first thought was to shift to teaching comprehension. Dennis cooperated with me as long as his responses could be nonverbal. It quickly turned out, however, that his comprehension was at age level. Therefore, I took a third tack, employing contingency management techniques to develop expression. In this process I became even more constraining than before. Eventually he began to produce imitative and "fill-in" responses. At this point, it would be hard to decide whether or not he wanted to talk. On the one hand, he was making verbal responses; he must have wanted to talk in some way, one assumes, because of the positive consequences. On the other hand, I obtained zero generalization. He never talked when reinforcers weren't in the offing. My attempts to fade the reinforcement were unsuccessful. After some months Dennis became eligible for clinical services through the public schools, and he stopped attending the clinic. I lost track of him, but about a year later I ran into the whole family in a supermarket. When he recognized me, he turned his back to me and remained that way until I left.

There are several lessons to learn from Dennis. I may not have had sufficient skills in contingency management. More important in the present discussion, he illustrates the importance of relationship factors in language delay. Not only was his talking related to the relationship context, but Dennis and I quickly became caught in a reciprocal set of relationship tactics in which neither of us could succeed and in which change became increasingly difficult. Further, it would be risky to assume that one of us was at fault. He did talk in other situations, which suggests that he should receive the blame; but I pressed him to talk and I worked with him in a clinic with a somewhat impersonal atmosphere, suggesting that I was to blame. In any case, our relationship contained none of the components mentioned earlier in this chapter that enhance children's development; nor were we acting in a relationship in which performatory acts were complemented by a responsive environment. One can easily imagine how a similar transactional pattern in a family could have considerable impact on a child's development as a communicator. In sum, my work with Dennis illustrates the "want to talk" paradox in concrete form. Indeed, it is not merely another abstraction, but a clinical reality. Nor is it limited to expression. We face a similar paradox when we want children to want to attend to the stimuli we present.

First-Order Change and Second-Order Change

We can look at my problems in working with Dennis in another way. My attempts to change his behavior were not successful. Perhaps the difficulty was in how I viewed trying to change him. Watzlawick, Weakland, and Fisch (1974) describe efforts to change people as occurring at two levels. First-order change involves our typical "common sense" methods of working with children. It is illustrated by my attempts to change Dennis's communicative behavior through employing different activities and stimuli, asking questions, directing him to talk, providing incentives, and so forth. Similarly, I tried being friendly, stern, and playful at various times. While there is considerable variety among these techniques, at a more abstract level they are all the same.

They all stem from my punctuation of the relationship, which remained unchanged even as I tried various approaches. I was The Clinician, and my job was to help Dennis develop better language skills. I saw myself as one-up and so did he, and I took responsibility for changing his behavior. As long as I viewed the situation this way, the "want to talk" paradox had me over a barrel, and I didn't know it.

Second-order change requires a change in punctuation, in how we view the whole situation. It requires bringing an entirely new perspective to the situation. For example, what would Dennis have done if I had stopped attempting to teach or elicit talking from him? The "want to talk" paradox would become irrelevant, because no one would be asking him to talk. The relationship context would be very different.

Second-order change can be difficult to achieve, especially at first. Generally, we are limited by our perceptions, our construction of reality, so that it does not occur to us that other punctuations exist for a problem. Thus, we continue trying different things, but all within the same frame of reference. Watzlawick, Weakland, and Fisch (1974) refer to these attempts at change as "more of the same." In working with Dennis I saw myself as trying a variety of approaches, but at a higher level they were all the same, because they all stemmed from my view of myself as the teacher or elicitor. Reinforcement techniques provide another example of first-order, more-of-the-same, attempts at change. One might begin with social praise as a consequence. If that is not effective, tangible objects can be used, such as tokens. If these consequences don't affect change, food can be introduced. If change is still not forthcoming, the child can be deprived of food for some time before each training session. Each of these consequences is different, and yet each is clearly more of the same.

Some other observations about contingency management as relationship communication may be useful here. While it is usually recognized that reinforcement influences are reciprocal, the typical punctuation is that the trainer is one-up. Generally it is important that trainers see themselves as maintaining stimulus control over their clients or subjects. This punctuation of the relationship emphasizes linear cause-and-effect relationships rather than reciprocity. In the view I am developing here, the child's behavior changes because of the ecological validity of the consequences, but the relationship tactics of both child and trainer remain the same. It may be for this reason that generalization in language training has been so difficult to achieve when the focus has been on training the repertoire. When the relationship context changes (that is, when reinforcement is removed), the child continues to employ the same relationship tactics (means of communication) that were present before training. The metarules remain unchanged.

It seems to me that most contingency managers view communicative behavior within the larger framework of behavior modification. I would rather view behavior modification within the larger framework of communicative behavior. Reinforcers can then be seen as iconic relationship messages that are defined through negotiated meaning. Behavior modification gets its power through defining relationships on a discrete, discursive, and linear basis, rather than on one that is more continuous, nondiscursive, and intuitive. When used well, it is an effective means of first-order change.

Returning to second-order change, it can be particularly elusive in approaching the relationship side of the pragmatics model. There are three reasons for this problem. To begin with, as mentioned earlier, it is hard to change our perceptual set in the first place. Second, stemming from this difficulty, we frequently do not view behavior in terms of its function in relationships. Following the linear model, we are inclined to see it as representing mental states in the child, such as shyness or anger. Alternatively, we may not interpret it all, but just "stick to the behaviors." The third problem is that relationship communication does not follow the linear logic of the classical models of science on which we were raised. As pointed out in Chapter 5, it is based on intuitive logic.

Conclusions

A major theme of this book is that language learning depends on the child's problem-solving activity. This idea has appeared in different forms as I have discussed cognitive strategies, decision making, performatory acts, and so on. In the preceding chapter I applied this assumption directly by looking at language training and learning through the referential communication paradigm. In the present chapter I described some language-learning strategies that underlie this problem solving. Just as performatory acts require a responsive environment to be most effective, so these strategies require an appropriate relationship context for their success. Beyond any language-learning strategies, then, children's interpersonal behavior itself also derives from problem solving, but now the problems are couched in the intuitive logic of relationships. The metarules for these decisions evolve through each child's transactional history. Children's relationship decisions profoundly affect their opportunities and strategies for learning the nuts and bolts of language.

For some language-impaired children, intervention based on some form of first-order change will be sufficient. With other children, the "be spontaneous" paradox will remain a problem. Some of these children may learn new language options but not elect to use them, a difficulty with metarules as discussed in earlier chapters. Training specific grammatical options requires that the child's behavior be constrained so that the structures of interest can be emphasized. Is it possible, in this constraining context, to get children to use their newly learned structures on their own? In the preceding chapter I suggested that we meet this challenge by teaching language options in the service of communication, thus increasing the chances that new metarules will develop.

There are some children, however, whose relationship tactics are such that communicative functioning is impaired or distorted. Consequently, such children may not use the language repertoires they possess effectively, nor the language learning strategies described earlier in this chapter. For these children, a second-order change may be the most powerful intervention.

In discussing exploratory teaching in Chapter 7, I quoted Dearborn's phrase: "If you want to understand something, try to change it." The perspective of second-order change takes this idea to another level. We change how we attempt to make change. In the case of children's language disorders, one such change would be to focus directly on relationship tactics, avoiding direct attention to language options. We change our metarules for intervention in order to change the child's metarules for communicative behavior. The assumption is that, if children develop more constructive ways of relating with others, they can then take better advantage of the language-learning strategies and skills that they possess. Similarly, they can make more efficient use of whatever responsiveness there is in the en-

vironment. Let us consider more directly now how we might approach making such second-order changes.

RELATIONSHIP STRATEGIES

We begin with two principles from Chapter 5. First, interpret children's behavior as relationship communication, whatever else it might be. Ask yourself, what effect does that behavior by that child have on our relationship? How does it affect my behavior? Thus, a child with short attention span effectively controls your teaching strategies; a tantrum simply cancels your lesson plan. Similarly, children who do not talk significantly affect how other people interact with them. As discussed in Chapter 5, there is no way to tell whether such behaviors represent states within the child or are relationship tactics. In either case, they define the relationship in certain ways. In the present context, they are possible targets for intervention. The second principle derives from the reciprocity of human relationships. Recall that all behavior contributes toward defining the relationship between two people. If you want to change the child's relationship behavior, then change your own. Thus, you communicate directly in the intuitive logic of relationships. I will present examples as we go along that will help clarify this point. While you may feel that second-order change is somewhat mysterious at present, it can be very simple, as we will see in the next section.

Facilitative Play

Instead of designing a strategy for "teaching" language, let us think about designing a human relationship context that might maximize the chances of children's developing language through their own active learning strategies. A good place to begin would be with the two factors noted earlier in the chapter that encourage children's language use. The situation should be one in which the topics of discussion are of immediate interest to the child and there is a minimum of constraint supplied by the adult. As pointed out earlier, these factors are aspects of the relationship between child and clinician; they are not language-teaching techniques.

A relationship context incorporating these principles could be established through a procedure I call facilitative play. This approach is based around the following guidelines.

1. Follow the child's lead in play. I would select several play activities and have appropriate materials present in the room. These activities will represent your best guesses of what might be appealing to the child you are working with, although it may take a few sessions before you know what is autotelic for that child. With young children I would begin with a variety of activities, such as clay, blocks, a dollhouse, a play kitchen, and some puzzles and books. One of my favorites is water play with funnels, cups, bowls, eggbeaters, and so on, and some water containing enough detergent to produce lots of bubbles. Whatever activities are used, they should be freely accessible so that children can select among them on their own. Some clinicians prefer to join in the child's play; others observe and participate less actively.

2. Talk about what the child is doing.[1] Whatever the child selects, the clinician provides verbal input about that activity. If the

child changes frequently from one thing to another, your line of talking changes as well. The form of this talking depends partly on you and partly on the child. Some clinicians provide essentially a narrative of what is happening. Others participate in more direct interaction with the child, either talking about the activity or taking on play roles themselves. There is no one best way to provide this input; you will have to sense what seems appropriate for each child and what you are comfortable with. Whatever style you take, however, it must fit within the third guideline.

3. Minimize the constraints on the child. It is important that you not direct the child, either in selecting activities or in establishing details of how the child carries those activities out. Avoid the temptation to use many commands and questions. Especially, one should refrain from attempts to elicit talking. Paradoxically, those attempts provide a heavy constraint that decreases spontaneous talking. I should note that minimizing constraint does not mean giving children totally free rein in the situation. It is perfectly legitimate and necessary to establish limits. I would not let a child kick me in the shins or mash clay into the carpet. You will have to establish boundaries that are practical in your situation and, again, that you are comfortable with. What is important is that you not assume the active role of trainer or teacher, directing the child's behavior and eliciting responding.

We can think of the clinician's repertoire as including both facilitative behaviors, such as following the child's lead and talking about the child's activities, and constraining behaviors, such as commands, questions, and other forms of direction. As illustrated with the "good talking" example earlier in the chapter, even praise may function as a constraint (Patterson and Cobb 1971). What we are attempting in facilitative play, then,

---

[1] The first two guidelines together describe the same procedure that Van Riper discussed years ago as "parallel talking." As life goes on, I become increasingly convinced that there are very few new ideas, if any. Accordingly, perhaps creativity should be defined as providing new rationales for old ideas.

is a situation in which the ratio of facilitation to constraint favors facilitative behaviors, rather than the typical teaching situation, where constraint is dominant (Hubbell 1977). A similar strategy has been developed in the reactive language-teaching project directed by Rita Weiss at the University of Colorado. In the same vein, Seitz and Marcus (1976) stress the responsiveness of the parent with language-impaired children.

It has been my experience that facilitative play frequently increases language-delayed children's rates of talking. It incorporates both of the factors described earlier as encouraging expression. The topic is of immediate interest to the child because the child selects the activities. The clinician merely follows the child's lead. In minimizing constraint and following the child's lead, the clinician alters the power relation with the child. Beyond enforcing some basic limits, the clinician allows the child to be one-up.

The "be spontaneous" paradox does not become a trap for child or clinician because the child is not directed to perform. Haley (1963) suggested that people resist being told what to do. Any such resistance will heighten the effects of the paradox. In an earlier chapter I gave examples of children who were clearly resisting interventions that were highly constraining in nature. While some respond with lack of attention, poor cooperation, or anger, my favorite was the child who told the clinician, *NO MORE PICTURES!* Paradoxically, many of these same children talk willingly during facilitative play. I urge you to experience this phenomenon yourself by working with a few language-delayed children in a constraining manner and then switching to facilitative play.

We can also consider the play materials and the clinician together as a responsive environment. Children learn about the play activities, and also about language use, through their own decision making. They have a relatively free hand to explore the use of language on their own, with the adult merely providing models and responses to their utterances. As mentioned earlier, Moore (1966) recommended that no adult be present if a situation is intended to be a responsive environment for children's learning. This view, however, would emphasize only the conceptual-semantic side of language learning. Because language also involves relationship decisions, other individuals must be present so that children can experiment with this second set of decisions. As we will see in the next section, play is well adapted to this endeavor.

Play and Language Learning

I have been discussing facilitative play as an intervention technique aimed at establishing a relationship context that is likely to enhance language development. In fact, the potential of play in language learning goes far beyond anything I have said so far. Let us take a more general look at play. I will draw primarily from Bruner, Jolly, and Sylva (1976). These authors did not write from a perspective emphasizing language intervention. What they have to say, however, makes a compelling case for the importance of play in language development.

First, play represents a special relationship context, one in which the normal consequences of behavior are suspended (Bruner, Jolly, and Sylva 1976). It provides a somewhat sheltered atmosphere in which children have opportunities to practice and explore many behavior patterns in the culture, including, of course, those related to language and communication. In some ways the interpersonal risks of talking discussed in Chapter 9 are lessened in play. In pretending to be an adult, for example, a child can experiment with various forms of verbal directives without suffering the full consequences. It is, after all, only play. Of course, some interpersonal risk is present; feelings do get bruised. What is important, though, is that the metarules of play provide a relationship context in which the sanctions of everyday life are altered.

Beyond its relationship quality, a second aspect of play is that it is based on real aspects of the culture. It is not entirely fanciful, but involves components of "serious," or nonplayful, activity. Bruner, Jolly, and Sylva (1976) refer to these components as subroutines upon which more complex skills are built. They enter the child's repertoire through observation. Bruner and his colleagues further note that play involves using, modifying, combining, recombining, sequencing, and in other ways exploring these components of behavior. Through play, then, children become familiar with and competent in using and manipulating these subroutines. Weir (1962) provided the classic example regarding language, in which she described a child's bedtime soliloquies. This child literally practiced combining and recombining grammatical options, all by himself. Bruner, Jolly, and Sylva stress the ". . . extraordinary combinatorial push behind play, its working out of variations" (1976, p. 19). Similarly, children explore the uses of language in dealing with people through enacting parent-child dialogues, telephone conversations, tea parties, and so on. Play provides an excellent vehicle, then, for children's performatory acts in exploring the alternatives in language and its use.

So far, there is striking parallel between play and a great deal of language intervention. Both provide special contexts in which the normal connections between language behavior and its functions are suspended; children quickly recognize what is "real"

and what isn't. In addition, both increase awareness and skill in combining and using the options that make up language. In addition, however, play is autotelic. It has affective qualities that beckon children and adults alike. Recall from Chapter 9 Allen's (1965) goal of combining learning with enjoyment in autotelic activities. Children have been making similar combinations since the dawn of play.

In summary, play has an abstract quality to it. Its definition as "not real" is something that even very young children can sense. Consequently, it seems quite natural to associate play with the use of symbols and therefore with the development of language. Many authors have done so (Piaget and Inhelder 1969; Bruner 1975; Miller and Yoder 1974). This symbolic quality, coupled with play's emphasis on combining and recombining culturally relevant sequences of behavior, its autotelic nature, and its apartness from the real consequences of life, make it a highly desirable format for language learning. With young or immature children it provides a direct entry into the world of symbols. With older children, it provides a bridge between mechanical drill and functional use of language in daily life. For all children it provides a context to explore and practice language use without the sanctions of the real world.

In view of these observations, questions of whether or not play is appropriate in language intervention miss the point. As with some other intervention issues discussed previously, we should be asking when it is appropriate, with which children, and toward what goals. The answers to these questions hinge on the characteristics of play, which have been illustrated above. In intervention, play may consist of structured games, such as ones based on the referential communication paradigm. Similarly, Fromberg's (1977) contrastive modeling is an excellent example of play involving the combination and recombination of language options. Play may also be unstructured, as in facilitative play or in helping parents play with their children in ways that foster language development (Levenstein 1970).

I began by describing facilitative play as a technique focusing on relationship aspects of language use. We can see now that it capitalizes on the more general function of play in isolating behavior from its real-life consequences. It should be clear that this function is enhanced when the clinician follows the child's lead and minimizes constraints on the child. At the same time, by modeling talking and providing utterances that are relevant to the child's play, the clinician heightens the language learning and practice. Thus, we hope to take advantage of the interaction between the characteristics of play and the language-learning strategies described earlier. Facilitative play maximizes shared reference, because the clinician attends to whatever the child is attending to. The child's feedback and information-gathering strategies (Snyder and McLean 1977) are also able to operate with some efficiency, because the clinician's job is to be as responsive an environment as possible. Finally, in the course of play the child has increased opportunities for practice and decision making in expression.

Facilitative Play and Training Based on Referential Communication

Let us compare facilitative play with intervention based on the referential communication paradigm described in the previous chapter. The play regimen is indeed a second-order change, albeit perhaps a mild one, because it involves quite a different perspective: We are no longer attempting to

teach specific language options. I don't think the question of whether one approach is better than the other will be fruitful to explore. As before, it will be more productive to ask what each involves and what each can accomplish. Training based on the referential communication paradigm is highly constraining. This fact allows the teacher to make the alternatives clear and the learning specific. The child's responding is convergent. Everything is designed to marshal problem solving and behavior in a narrow area. Spontaneous behavior is thus discouraged. Facilitative play is just the opposite. The degree of constraint is low. As a result, the language learning is not specific, and the alternatives range from vague to clear. As a matter of fact, the children decide what alternatives they will focus on; sometimes we know what they are and sometimes we don't. The children's decision making and responding can be very divergent, depending on the child and the situation. Spontaneous behavior is the goal.

Facilitative play can be modified slightly in hopes of encouraging the development of certain language options in the child's talking. On the basis of preliminary language sampling, the clinician can select certain structures as likely candidates for the child to develop and then model those structures heavily while talking. These structures can be made even more salient through contrastive modeling. The problem here is that there is an almost overwhelming tendency to begin teaching at this point, with the result that the relationship context will become more constraining and less facilitative.

Conclusions

I do not see facilitative play as appropriate for all language-impaired children. While you will have to experiment with it yourself, I have found it particularly useful in three situations. First, it is an excellent way to collect language samples. What we want in language sampling is plenty of output, as little constraint as possible, and autotelic talking by the child. All of these conditions are met in facilitative play. While the technique has been described as it applies with young children, the principles fit what has been said earlier about eliciting talking from older children as well.

A second application of facilitative play is as one option for intervention with young language-delayed children. It encourages language-related problem solving in an ecologically valid context, namely play, and it facilitates the use of language as a way to deal with people. Seitz (1975) used similar techniques with retarded children. Facilitative play lends itself easily to working with small groups of children as well.

I have also found facilitative play useful with some young children who demonstrate frequent negative behavior or resistance, such as crying or tantrums. It is here that facilitative play functions most clearly as second-order change. Frequently negative behavior can be interpreted as a message expressing resistance to constraint the clinician is introducing into the relationship. In facilitative play there is very little constraint, and consequently very little for the child to resist. I mentioned in an earlier chapter a child who cried frequently during structured training. After the intervention was switched to facilitative play, the child ceased crying except occasionally when it was time to go home. We will explore this phenomenon further in the next section.

One should not read an "either-or" connotation into my comparisons of facilitative play and more structured interventions. In fact, a combination of the two might be rather efficient with many children. Certain language structures could be trained through some adaptation of the referential communication paradigm, perhaps emphasizing comprehension. Generalization of these structures, as well as more general language development, could be facilitated in play sessions. The structured training could be done on a one-to-one basis, while the play might take place in a small group.

There is a problem in combining these approaches, however. If children see you as a "constrainer" during structured training, they may continue to perceive you in that way during your attempts at facilitative play. You can shift roles, but the children may not appreciate that the metarules of the situation have changed. Therefore it is necessary to make the two situations as clearly distinct for the children as possible. Ideally, they can be conducted in different rooms with different clinicians. At least they can be done in different parts of the room, using different materials. Sometimes a specific symbol can be used, such as a big, decorated "star box," which is always present during structured work but physically removed from the room during facilitative play. Use whatever techniques you want to distinguish between the two, but each will be more effective if the children know which "game" they are playing.

I have not given any extensive examples of facilitative play because I have found that each clinician goes about it somewhat differently. Ultimately, perhaps it is more of an attitude than a technique. We provide an atmosphere and watch children grow, rather than engineering the details of that growth. To become skillful at facilitative play is to learn to be responsive to children, to read their cues, to follow their logic and interests, to "tune in" to them. It is a way to learn to make our behavior complement theirs. For this reason alone it is worth experimenting with. Similarly, as we will see in the next chapter, it can be helpful to encourage parents to develop skill in facilitative play.

Reframing Relationship Messages

In discussing facilitative play, I emphasized the relationship meaning of the clinician's behavior. By altering our perceptions of our role (a second-order change) we can behave in ways that facilitate children's own growth mechanisms, rather than making that growth dependent on our own teachings. Through our behavior we structure a relationship that maximizes the child's growth potential. Let us now concentrate on the relationship meaning of the child's behavior.

Relationship Tactics

We can define relationship tactics as consistent ways of dealing with other people on a relationship level. Relationships are defined and maintained through these iconic signs. They include both talking and nonverbal behavior. Relationship tactics develop through the child's participation in transactional patterns with significant other people, particularly family members. The meanings of relationships tactics, then, are negotiated over time. These meanings are likely to be more intuitive than linear. Further, they may be beyond the conscious awareness of the people concerned, that is, those individuals may not interpret certain kinds of behavior as relationship communication.

I once knew a language-delayed preschooler named Kathy. She was difficult to manage in individual language-training sessions. Her cooperation was poor. Especially, she rarely responded appropriately, either verbally or nonverbally, to the clinician's directives. In a play group Kathy's behavior would have to be called independent, particularly in situations where she

was expected to respond in some way. For example, we had a large cardboard box that had been decorated to represent a television set. It had a hole cut out for a screen, and children would enter the box one at a time and show puppets through this hole. When Kathy was in the box, she would lie on the floor completely out of sight. No amount of coaxing would cause her to appear behind the screen. Her mother reported that Kathy would frequently cry and complain at home but would never indicate what was the matter or what she wanted. In sum, one of Kathy's relationship tactics was to hold out on adults. She frequently refrained from responding in situations where a response was required.

These behaviors illustrate what is meant by a relationship tactic. Holding out was a consistent way in which Kathy dealt with other people and, in fact, exercised power over them. Whether or not this tactic represented some state in her mind, such as fear, cannot be known. In any case, it affected the relationships in which she participated. Further, it was part of a larger transactional pattern. When it was appropriate for her to respond, she would refuse; other individuals would then attempt various relationship tactics of their own, such as begging, cajoling, punishing, threatening, or whatever; she would continue to refuse, and on and on in cyclical fashion. Parenthetically, we can note again the presence of the "be spontaneous" paradox, and that the adults' tactics were first-order, more-of-the-same attempts to deal with the situation.

It is not always so easy to interpret children's behavior as relationship communication. A few years ago I did a series of demonstration sessions with a young language-delayed boy. Many of these sessions were videotaped. I worked with the child in a small clinic room. The clinic was equipped with one-way mirrors and sound equipment so that any room could be used to observe and listen to the next room. Consequently, each room had a microphone, a speaker, and knobs to control them. This little boy was rather distractible, and he played with these knobs among other things. He soon discovered that he could adjust the two knobs together to produce an electronic feedback noise of piercing intensity. He went through this activity on an irregular but fairly frequent basis. I suspected that it was related to something I was doing, but for the life of me I couldn't figure out what. Some time later I was reviewing all the videotapes, and it struck me. He only produced that squeal when I pressed him too hard. I had evolved an intervention strategy with this boy involving intensive work with both comprehension and expression in the context of autotelic play activities. When the pressure became too great, he turned to the knobs. It was an effective relationship tactic. I couldn't continue as long as that noise was going on. At the same time, I never comprehended the meaning of these iconic messages during my direct contacts with the boy. It was only when I had a more objective attitude while watching the videotapes that I could see the pattern.

As these two examples illustrate, many relationship tactics are nonverbal in nature. Consequently, they may seem somewhat far afield from our interests in language intervention. It might be argued that such behaviors are important in terms of general clinical management, but only because they should be controlled so that training can be as efficient as possible. In my view, these nonverbal behaviors have a much more central role than that. The pragmatics model includes both conceptual-semantic and relationship aspects of language use. Nonverbal behavior is a primary way in which relationships are negotiated and maintained. As noted in Chapter 5, nonverbal communica-

tion and language complement each other in the child's dealings with other people. With at least some children, therefore, it will be necessary to focus directly on these relationship tactics.

We will be particularly interested in relationship tactics that are maladaptive as communication strategies or that tend to make the child's language learning and use less effective. A definitive list of these tactics would not be possible because we must evaluate each child separately. Certainly we will include behaviors such as crying, tantrums, hitting, refusal, and resistance. Other aspects of behavior are of interest as well, such as short attention span, distractibility, hyperactivity, lack of interest or motivation, and echolalia. Areas of behavior such as these are usually not thought of as relationship tactics, probably because of our tendency to punctuate them through the linear cause-and-effect model. However, a moment's reflection will reveal that they have profound effects on relationships. How can you converse with someone whose responses are echolalic or who attends to only a little of what you say? Further, as such behaviors become incorporated and maintained in significant transactional patterns in the child's life, they could indeed inhibit language growth. They tend to be morphostatic processes; they resist change and development. Indeed, then, with some language-impaired children, nonverbal tactics may be an even more important area of intervention than language itself.

Reframing

We have only one means of dealing with children's relationship tactics, and that is our own relationship tactics. We can, however, view these tactics in terms of first-order and second-order change. In first-order change there is generally little attention to the relationship *per se.* Rather, the focus is directly on the child's behavior. Within this perspective there are a number of techniques to choose from. One can get stern with a child, search for activities that are more appealing, or apply systematic behavior modification procedures. For many language-impaired children, techniques such as these will suffice. As suggested above, however, some language-disordered children's relationship tactics seem particularly maladaptive in the child's development as a communicator. While first-order changes can be attempted with these children, it may be useful to consider the possibilities of second-order change.

As stated earlier, second-order change requires that we develop a different perspective on the situation. Our understanding of another person is based on our perceptions of that person, but, as noted in Chapter 1, those perceptions are our own personal construction or interpretation of the person; they are not an objective view of reality. In Chapter 6 the term "punctuation" was introduced to refer to perceptions of human relationships and causality. We cannot avoid punctuating different situations; we must see them from some point of view. The problem is that any particular punctuation is likely to limit the number of alternatives or options we see in the situation. This is the reason that attempts at first-order change can often be described as more of the same. Children are similarly restricted by their own punctuations, which helps explain why they are likely to maintain the same relationship tactics even if they are maladaptive.

In second-order change we try to enlarge our perceptions, to see the situation from a different level, so that new and different options become available. In first-order change relationship tactics such as those listed above are viewed as undesirable behaviors to be changed. One second-order change would

be to try to understand how those behaviors function in the child's participation in relationships, and then attempt to change the relationship so that that function is no longer maintained. In facilitative play, for example, resistance or refusal becomes irrelevant because the child is not being directed. The child is thus led to experiment with other options.

Watzlawick, Weakland, and Fisch (1974) describe another approach to second-order change, which they call "reframing." Recall from Chapter 5 that there is no truth or falsity to a relationship message. Its import depends only on whether or not the receiver believes the message. Typically, language trainers and other adults "believe" children's relationship messages, that is, they accept those behaviors at face value. Again, the result is more of the same in the adult's attempts to change the child. In reframing, the receiver doesn't believe the message. In fact, the clinician changes the interpretation or perspective so that the behavior cannot mean the same thing that it did previously. The perceptual "frame" in which it occurs is changed.

Some examples will help illustrate these ideas. A clinician is working with a first grader on basic academic concepts. The clinician draws different shapes, such as squares and circles, on pieces of paper and asks the child to name them. (Note that this is testing, not teaching.) The child resists by grabbing each piece of paper, crumpling it up, and throwing it in a corner. Soon the clinician draws a quick rectangle, hands it to the child and says, "Make it into a ball and throw it away." The child does. The clinician repeats the maneuver with another piece of paper, this time asking the child to crumple it as small as possible. Again the child complies. The clinician repeats the sequence still again. This time the child doesn't crumple the paper and, in fact, works cooperatively through the rest of the session. Notice what happened here. The child was resisting through the tactic of crumpling and throwing the paper. The clinician reframed this behavior by asking the child to do it. Hence, it could no longer be a tactic of resistance but was, in fact, an act of cooperation. Since the behavior had lost its power as a relationship tactic, the child stopped employing it and moved to other tactics in his repertoire.

Another child, another clinician. The child refuses to enter the clinic room but hangs on the doorknob and cries. All children who use tactics such as this have experienced many first-order attempts to change them, such as coaxing, pleading, and punishment. Instead, the clinician says, "Keep the door open for me while I go in and play." The clinician enters and plays alone for the entire session. When done, the clinician thanks the child and the session is over. The next time, the clinician gives the same instruction, but the child enters the room and begins to play.

For a third example, recall Dennis, the child who refused to talk in the clinic. After having gained some acquaintance with reframing, I encountered a similar child. It took a few sessions to realize what his game was. Once I had decided that his lack of talking was primarily a relationship tactic, I sat him down and concentrated entirely on input. I read, explained toys, described pictures, and so on. At the same time, I gave the child frequent admonitions to listen carefully and pay attention. Shortly after I had begun the third session of this treatment, the child suddenly burst into song! It was entirely unintelligible, but it was definitely singing. There are two postscripts to this anecdote. First, it is interesting that he still wasn't talking for me. Even with these fancy techniques, one wonders who's in charge. Second, I tried a similar technique

on a third child but with no success. This child finally began to talk after about a month of facilitative play.

I rush to point out that none of these examples were instant cures. The first child, the paper crumpler, soon attempted other disruptive tactics. All three children continued in the clinic for some time. What is important is that each of these instances was a turning point in the course of intervention. In all three cases different transactional patterns between clinician and child developed after these events. In my judgment these new patterns were more productive. Children and clinicians both began using a wider range of options in how they communicated with each other.

Conclusions

Reframing assumes a phenomenological view of reality. That is, the focus is on the individual's perceptions of reality, on the meanings of behavior, rather than on an objective view of behavior itself. It is the perceptions and meanings that are changed through reframing. The effect is to change the function of various relationship tactics. The goal is to decrease maladaptive relationship behaviors so that more constructive communicative tactics and language-learning strategies can come into play.

The examples I have given all represent noncompliance in fairly obvious forms. It may take different tactics by the clinician to deal with behaviors such as hyperactivity, distractibility, and short attention span. In Chapter 2 it was pointed out that behaviors such as these are influenced by the context. At that time the focus was on content, on whether or not the materials or activities were appealing to the child. We now see that behaviors of this type are also dependent on the larger relationship context. Children who demonstrate hyperactivity and similar difficulties illustrate nicely the problems in deciding whether such behaviors are "state" or "tactic." Recall the hyperactive child described in an earlier chapter who would sit absolutely still for an hour at a time before the television set, or the child with memory difficulties who, when switched into a game routine, was soon reminding the clinician what the rules of the game were. It is fine to say that a child is highly distractible, but that does not explain whatever problems are present. I urge you to experiment with different contexts for such children and see for yourself the differences in their responding. Only in a few cases will you end up suspecting the presence of some neurological state underlying the disorder.

Reframing and the general idea of second-order change might seem to be unusual topics for a book on children's language disorders. In my view, however, they follow directly from taking the pragmatics model seriously. If we are concerned with language use, not simply training the repertoire, then we have no choice but to grapple with relationship factors somehow. I find the work of Watzlawick and his colleagues particularly appealing because it attempts to deal with behavior in terms of its meaning in relationships. I need hardly point out that the business of language is also to communicate meaning in human relationships. Thus we have a toehold in our climb toward a more comprehensive understanding of language-disordered children.

I find the perspectives of second-order change and reframing appealing for other reasons as well. First, they illustrate the intuitive, sometimes nondiscursive nature of relationship communication. It is not the same as the linear, discursive communication that is emphasized in our technological culture. In attempting to institute second-order change, we respond to the child's relationship tactics with intuitive, iconic signs of our own. Second, I have had some success with the facilitative play and reframing strategies that have been described above. They add another level to exploratory teaching as well as intervention itself. Again, they are not cure-alls, but they are useful ways of dealing with relationship factors in the context of language intervention. Finally, I can't resist pointing out that the idea of second-order change is itself a second-order change (a metachange). As Haley (1977) suggests, it requires taking a gamelike perspective in approaching human behavior, although the behavior itself and its effects are anything but a game.

A Note on Ethics. Reframing is a very powerful technique. Once I worked with a first-grade girl who cried a lot. This crying appeared particularly when she didn't like what was going on. In order to reframe this tactic, I began to admire her ability to cry. Indeed, she was a master, from subdued, tear-infused blubbers to heartrending shrieks. I told her so and encouraged more salvos; I told her to let me know how she felt through the crying.[2] Suddenly, there was a change in her facial expression and in the tone of her crying. At least for the moment, I had destroyed one of her major control tactics. She began to change to another level of anger, one of much more depth and intensity. I backed off immediately. She simply didn't have the resources to handle the powerful techniques I was using. It was a long time before this girl trusted me again.

We face a real question of professional ethics, then. Is it appropriate for a language clinician to employ relationship tactics such as these? Your answer will depend partly on

---

[2] It was important that this admiration be genuine, and it was. Had I spoken to her in sarcasm, it would have remained an attempt at first-order change, and the effect would probably have been quite different.

your own background and skills. As we have seen, language intervention requires expertise in a multitude of areas. At the same time, we cannot be all things to all people. Clinicians, teachers, and trainers must evaluate their own competencies and skills and operate accordingly. On the other hand, there is no reason why you can't acquire new competencies and seek out additional training if necessary.

In my own view, the strategies described above are appropriate for language clinicians to employ, or I wouldn't have included them in the book. We are, after all, working with communicative behavior. Further, reframing isn't any more "powerful" than behavior modification techniques. Just as with behavior modification, however, it is important that you develop your skills carefully and thoroughly. In using any clinical technique, plan your interventions thoughtfully, rather than acting on impulse. Similarly, it is essential that you watch the results closely. In the case of reframing, change should occur fairly quickly. In particular, watch for extreme responses such as those of the girl I described two paragraphs ago.

In sum, if you are interested in techniques such as these, go out and learn about them. As with language-sample analysis, contingency management, and a host of other techniques, they will enrich your work with language-disordered children, but they do not come free.

CONCLUSIONS

The challenge is to find links between language development and human relationships, links that will be useful departure points for intervention. The pragmatics model from Chapter 9 shows the conceptual-semantic area and the relationship area as parallel and equally important. So they are, but at the same time they are very different. Conceptual-semantic decisions center around symbols, relationship decisions around iconic signs. The symbols associated with conceptual-semantic decisions tend to be more discrete, discursive, and linear, while the iconic signs so important in relationship communication are more continuous, nondiscursive, and intuitive. There is plenty of overlap between the two areas, but each is unique in its own way.

To me the issue is not how to "teach pragmatics" in some way. I have already argued that English has more grammatical options than we can conveniently teach, and certainly more vocabulary items than we can possibly teach. Multiply these options by some unknown but large factor called pragmatics or the social code, and the job becomes literally overwhelming. In addition, pragmatics is not a single set of processes, as noted above. Pragmatics is not the goal of language training any more than semantics or syntax is. However, the pragmatics model underscores the importance of bringing together the conceptual-semantic and relationship areas as productively as possible.

I certainly cannot propose a solution to this problem, but a perspective for approaching it has evolved through the course of this book. Begin with the assumption that children participate in their own learning, that they actively apply whatever language-learning strategies they possess in acquiring the ability to communicate through words. Now note that language learning requires input; these strategies can only come to fruition in interactions with other people. The question then becomes, what kinds of human relationships will foster the development of such language-learning strategies and maximize their use and effectiveness?

We are asking fundamental questions

about human development; answers will vary with one's views on that subject. At the very least there are three factors involved. First, children must have opportunities to use and hear language. They must explore and experiment with language as communication in order to implement their language-learning strategies. Second, they must participate in communicative situations that provide sufficient input and feedback; some degree of responsive environment is required. Third, they must have the ability and opportunity to participate in human relationships in what might be called a constructive manner. Maladaptive relationship tactics cannot be so dominant as to impair the strategies and situations just mentioned.

I must stress again that all three of these qualities are embodied in human relationships; they are not factors within the child, nor, for that matter, in the environment. Our goal, then, is to establish transactional patterns based on these qualities, so that language development and use can proceed to optimal levels for each child. These transactional patterns should provide contexts that foster the development of successful communication in language-impaired children, both at linguistic and cognitive levels and at affective, relationship levels. This communication will allow the child to take advantage of language-learning strategies such as shared reference, selective listening, feedback processes, and practice with expression. While I have not always pointed out the connections explicitly, these patterns also incorporate the Guiding Principles from the preceding chapter. They are based on ecological validity, the transactional model, problem solving, autotelic activities, responsive environments, and exploratory teaching.

The focus of this chapter has been on relationship tactics, but I have not empha-

sized the decision making that is associated with these processes. Indeed, however, the entire chapter has been about decision making. The strategies I described for changing children's unproductive or maladaptive relationship tactics are based on removing the power in those tactics rather than confronting them directly. Children who find their tactics don't work anymore become aware of other alternatives in the situation because they cannot *not* behave. They must do *something*. The child's decision making is fundamental in this process, although the problems to be solved may be more intuitive than linear. Relationship communication involves selection from a repertoire just as much as content communication does.

Relationship strategies have a relevance beyond that specifically discussed in this chapter. Work with culturally different children requires special sensitivity to interpersonal factors. One must begin with the assumption that the child's cultural values may differ from those of the clinician. Consequently, child and clinician will punctuate the same situations differently. Similarly, the sentence elaboration discussed in the preceding chapter is influenced heavily by the relationship context. Children talk more freely, and get more involved in their talking, in some situations than in others. These ideas come together in disadvantaged children who demonstrate minimal language use in the schools.

The second-order change in which certain relationship tactics are reframed or redefined so that they cannot have the same meaning they had previously suggests an intriguing possibility. Consider a child with functional language delay whose relationship communication is primarily maladaptive. If we turn around those relationship tactics so that the child's participation in relationships is positive and constructive, would language then develop "spontaneously" without intensive training?

Work in other fields will shed some light on this question. Having left the linear cause-and-effect model, communication-oriented psychotherapists are finding that a number of human problems dissipate with a change in the interpersonal context. The whole family-therapy enterprise is based on this assumption. Both Whitaker and Pittman illustrate how other people can turn on and turn off dysfunctional behavior in a disturbed individual (Haley and Hoffman 1967). Minuchin, Rosman, and Baker (1978) describe how anorexia nervosa (refusal to eat) and certain diabetes and asthma crises are also related to interpersonal contexts. Bronfenbrenner (1979) summarized evidence demonstrating that behaviors such as distractibility and short attention span are related to interpersonal factors.

If disorders such as these are inseparable from the communicative contexts in which they occur, how can it not also be true of language impairments, where the disorder itself is literally in the area of communica-tion? I do not mean to imply that human relationships are the "key" to language disorders any more than that minimal brain dysfunctions are. I simply wish to say that relationship factors are a part of the equation that cannot be left out.

In Chapter 10 we concentrated on transactional patterns that might enhance children's learning of specific grammatical options. The emphasis was on conceptual-semantic decisions. As discussed in Chapter 9, however, relationships embody metarules that govern when and how linguistic decisions will be made. Therefore, in the present chapter the focus was enlarged to consider those relationship decisions and to look for qualities that might make a relationship conducive to language learning. Both chapters centered on the relationship between child and clinician. With this background regarding both the conceptual-semantic and the relationship aspects of transactional patterns that foster language growth, we are now ready to move to a much more important set of transactional patterns, those between child and family.

12

INTERVENTION: LANGUAGE AS A FAMILY PHENOMENON

It is in the context of the family that we all begin our careers as communicators. Everyone—great orators, language-disordered children, even clinicians—first learns about language in a family or family substitute. In the past two chapters we've considered both the representational and the interpersonal functions of language. The emphasis has generally been on how these functions can be manipulated in exchanges between child and clinician. Ever since introducing the transactional model in Chapter 6, however, I have been suggesting that the ultimate target of intervention is the transactions between child and environment. It is time, then, to look at how the representational and interpersonal aspects of language come together with the transactional patterns between children and their families.

We will begin with some basic principles of family theory. These principles provide an excellent framework for looking at the process of language acquisition. With these ideas in hand we can then consider children's language disorders in the context of the family. Finally, I will make some suggestions regarding intervention.

THE FAMILY SYSTEM

The basic tenet of family theory is that the family is a social system, a unit with an identity and properties of its own. Many of the ideas that underlie this view were presented in earlier chapters. Permit me to bring them together in summary form. In Chapter 5 we saw that human relationships are defined through many exchanges. Gradually a set of metarules develops, regulating what may happen in particular relationships. In well-established relationships, the behavior of any individual is often predictable because of these metarules. Families are perhaps the

quintessence of such enduring relationships. Interpersonal behavior patterns become highly entrenched and yet so subtle that family members are often unaware of them. Relationship tactics develop and are maintained through negotiated meaning. The overall impression is one of consistency in how family members behave toward each other and in what they expect from each other. The whole process consists of communication, which makes family theory doubly important for us in working with language disorders.

Social systems were defined in more abstract terms in Chapter 6, where some principles of general systems theory were presented. Families are open systems, that is, they are influenced by events occurring in the larger environment. Families exhibit wholeness. Change in one family member causes changes in others. Equifinality is also a component of family systems. Different beginnings can ultimately produce the same result, and similar beginnings can lead to different outcomes. Finally, the family system incorporates both morphostatic and morphogenic processes. There are influences both toward maintaining the status quo and toward initiating change. All of these processes, too, depend on communication of various sorts. Now let us begin to flesh out these ideas.

Family Homeostasis

One of the central concepts in family theory is family homeostasis (Jackson 1965). The term is borrowed from biology, where it refers to the tendency of any organism to maintain a balance among its functions. For example, humans maintain approximately the same body temperature in spite of fluctuations in environmental temperatures. Homeostatic systems are essentially feedback mechanisms, that is, they are regulated by their own output. For example, you set the thermostat in your home at a certain temperature. The furnace comes on and runs until the room is slightly warmer than the setting you've selected. Then the furnace goes off until the temperature is slightly lower than that setting, and so on. The furnace-thermostat system is thus regulated by its own output. What causes the furnace to go off is the fact that it's been putting out heat.

The proposition is, then, that a similar mechanism operates in families. (I'm not referring to heat, but to feedback.) Family homeostasis is a morphostatic process. Families tend to maintain a balance in their functioning. They resist deviant behavior in any family member and tend to bring that person back into line. "Deviant" here means behaving in ways that are not typical for that family; it is not necessarily the same as deviant as defined by the larger culture. In a talkative family, if one family member is quiet on some occasion, others may try to bring that person out; in a family in which strong expressions of emotion are avoided and the atmosphere is generally low-key, family members are likely to attempt to calm a person who has an emotional outburst. You can probably think of similar patterns in your own family.

Family homeostasis also incorporates the principle of wholeness. If one member changes, others will too. Again, a balance is maintained. Language development provides a good example. As a child acquires language skill, other family members change the ways they communicate with that child. Other changes in behavior also require accommodations.

Bronfenbrenner (1979) emphasized the importance of primary dyads, such as parent-child, in children's development. In the preceding chapter I listed three characteristics of such dyads that he thinks are particularly important. Family homeostasis provides a good framework in which to appreciate those characteristics. They include reciprocity, mutual positive feeling, and a gradual shift of power to the child. All three suggest balance and accommodation.

Family homeostasis is important in considering language disorders because it underscores the reciprocity of behavior in families and the consistency of functioning that I have represented in earlier chapters with the metaphor of metarules. Language-impaired children are not independent of their family communication systems. Family homeostasis also suggests that many families resist change. They may not accept the suggestions that we cheerfully offer.

Cohesion and Adaptability

As work with families has developed, a need has arisen for more precise characterizations of family functioning than that provided by the concept of family homeostasis. Olson, Sprenkle, and Russell (1979) described the family system in terms that lend themselves more directly to empirical applications. These authors see families as varying around two major dimensions: "cohesion" and "adaptability."

Cohesion refers to the closeness between family members. From the opposite side of the coin, it represents the degree of separateness or autonomy in each family member's functioning. Cohesion ranges on a continuum. On one end there is almost completely independent activity by each person in the family, while at the other pole family members are so absorbed in each other that they have almost no individuality at all. Minuchin (1974) calls these extremes disengagement and enmeshment, respectively. Olson, Sprenkle, and Russell (1979) believe that, in our culture, normal families tend somewhere toward the middle of this continuum, while dysfunctional families are likely to appear at either extreme. Cohesion also varies with the developmental level of the family. One would expect more independence in families with high-school-aged members than those with preschoolers.

Adaptability is concerned with the family's ability to change its ways of behaving, to alter its metarules. It is also distributed along a continuum from an extreme resistance to change and an adherence to the status quo, to almost continual change and lack of consistency. Olson, Sprenkle, and Russell (1979) label families at these two poles as rigid and chaotic, respectively. Again, in our society, successfully functioning families tend toward the middle of this spread.

As with the more general concept of family homeostasis, these two dimensions will be useful in considering families with language-disordered children. A child who is enmeshed with a parent may have difficulty dealing with other people and, at least at a young age, may have little need for language at all. A child who is disengaged may have little opportunity to learn language. Similarly, a child who is learning language is changing rapidly. A rigid family may be unable to accommodate that change. A chaotic family may be unable to guide and respond to the child in a consistent manner.

Support and Creativity

Olson, Sprenkle, and Russell (1979) base their description of family systems on cohesion and adaptability. However, there are two other factors that they consider important as well, namely support and creativity. Cohesion and adaptability are aspects of the family system itself. Support and creativity are more related to how the family functions within the system that they have developed. Support refers to praise, recognition, encouragement, and other ways in which family members enhance each other's self esteem; it is the positive affect in a family. Creativity is related to how a family approaches the problems that it encounters, both big and small. A highly creative family generates a number and variety of solutions and courses of action in these situations. Creativity is the term Olson and his colleagues use at the family level for the problem solving and decision making that I have discussed at the individual level. Whereas optimal levels for cohesion and adaptability appear to be somewhere around the middle, high levels of both support and creativity are associated with well-functioning families (Russell 1979).

Perhaps I should note that I am not recommending that we go into the family-diagnosis business. As a matter of fact, family therapists have as much or perhaps even more trouble than language clinicians do with diagnosis. Similarly, I do not wish to stereotype families, especially before I've met them. At the same time, I am searching for a perspective that will be useful in approaching families of language-impaired youngsters. Concepts such as cohesion, adaptability, support, and creativity will contribute as much to that perspective as some of our more traditional concerns, such as amount of language stimulation in the home.

Family Structure

Each family develops characteristic behavior patterns that involve levels of both cohesion and adaptability. Murrell and Stachowiak (1965) referred to these patterns as family structure, the regular, predictable aspects of a family's functioning. They described three areas of family structure, all of which have relevance to children's language use.

Style

One component of family structure is what Murrell and Stachowiak call family style. Individual families develop consistent ways of relating and communicating together. One family may joke much of the time; in another, family members frequently yell at one another; in still another, the style is to intellectualize everything, with little expression of feeling; one family may be very verbal while another is taciturn; one may enjoy a lot of physical contact, another not, and so on through an infinite number of variations. Family style is extremely important in language development, because it is the model of how people communicate with which the child grows up. If you live in an environment where you get your head bitten off for saying the wrong thing, you become cautious in how you talk. If you grow up in a family where people rarely talk to each other, you may not talk much either, especially now that we live in an age where the screen is queen. Conversely, if you live in a home where people enjoy using language to deal with each other and to talk about the world, you pick up similar attitudes about communication.

Let me cite a brief example of family style. Kevin was a four-year-old language-delayed boy. His behavior was unusual in other ways as well. In fact, he was a classic case of a child who could be "diagnosed" as retarded, disturbed, or aphasoid. A clinician visited the home for an hour and a half. Kevin was on the floor playing and watching television. The parents were preparing dinner. No one said a word. When dinner was

ready, the father silently picked up his son, carried him to the table, sat him on his chair, and placed his fork in his hand. These actions were performed gently and lovingly. The parents were not cold, but absolute silence prevailed during the entire visit. Of course, there is a lot more we need to know about this family, particularly about talking in other situations. While it might be tempting to criticize the parents at this point, we don't know what history of transactions has led to this situation. In any case, to the extent that this situation is typical of this family, it is certainly a family style that is profoundly related to language development.

Patterns of Interaction

Murrell and Stachowiak (1965) describe patterns of interactions as a second component of family structure. The emphasis here is on the sequence and frequency of events, with little attention to the content of those events. For example, a pattern might develop in which the child does something, one parent then praises the child, and then the other parent undercuts that praise, providing a negative evaluation of either the child or the first parent. Note that this pattern could occur in many different situations.

Patterns of interaction are very much related to language development. The exchanges described by Brown and Bellugi (1964), in which mothers frequently use imitation with expansion and children use imitation with reduction, are an example. Similarly, the peekaboo games described by Bruner (Bruner, Jolly, and Sylva 1976), the feedback processes emphasized by Mahoney (1975), the parental language-teaching strategies discussed by Moerk (1976), all are examples of patterns of interaction. I mentioned in an earlier chapter a child who would sit on the floor in the middle of the room and whine. The mother would rush about, trying to guess what the child wanted. In discussing the "be spontaneous" paradox, I described a pattern in which the adult presses the child to talk, but the child refuses. These, too, are patterns of interaction, but ones which do not enhance language development. Note that in all of these examples, the content can vary. It is the sequence and frequency of events that forms the pattern. Ironically, the participants in such patterns are often unaware that they are playing parts in a sequence that occurs over and over. Further, such patterns can only encourage "more of the same."

Power Hierarchies

The third aspect of family structure is what Murrell and Stachowiak (1965) refer to as the power hierarchy. The questions now are about who makes the decisions in the family and who provides the sanctions. In a pure systems view, it might be argued that power is an inappropriate metaphor because all behavior is multiply determined and interdependent (Keeney 1979). In our day-to-day punctuations of life, however, indeed, some individuals do appear to exercise more power than others. In normal families, children have less power than parents, although as Bronfenbrenner (1979) notes, increasing power gradually accrues to the developing child. In some families, however, the children may wield disproportionate power. For example, the child's behavior may be so wild that the parents can never hire a baby-sitter and consequently never get any time to themselves. It is here that some of the maladaptive relationship tactics described in the previous chapter become particularly important. Their effect is to upset the typical hierarchy in the family so

that the children manifest great power. Communication, and perhaps most of living, is bound to be strained in families such as this.

An Example

In sum, all families demonstrate styles, interaction patterns, and power hierarchies. Of course, these three areas overlap and intermingle. They are avenues through which the more general variables of cohesion and adaptability are developed and maintained. Let us consider an example of family interaction. In Sample 10 (page 274) both parents have been asked to help their daughter work on some small jigsaw puzzles. In addition to the puzzle pieces, there is a picture of each completed puzzle available. The child's name is Marie, and she is five years, seven months old.

This excerpt is much too short to characterize this family. It will, however, illustrate some of the aspects of family systems that I have been discussing. First, note that active decision making occurs in both the referential communication and problem solving associated with the task, and also in the relationship negotiations between Marie and her father. Regarding conceptual-semantic decisions, puzzles are interesting because all of the alternatives are available but none of them are identified. As father and daughter work on the puzzle, some pieces are differentiated verbally (door, bottom) whereas others are referred to only as a "piece" and are differentiated visually as they are combined with other pieces on the table. Further, one can see the fundamental importance of joint reference as Marie and her father work with the puzzle pieces. Without such shared meaning, both ordinary communication and language learning are severely hampered.

Father: Which one would you like, Marie, the face or the horse or the car or the person?

Marie: The car

Father: Here we are. Now do you want the picture of what's on it or you want to just make it?

Marie: I want the car

Father: Uhuh. Here are the pieces. Now which part are you gonna try an' put first?

Father: Can you see any of the pieces?

Father: Tell daddy what you're doing.

Father: How 'bout starting with this piece?

Marie: (whispers)

Father: No, I don't think . . . Now look, let's start with the piece that's got the—

Mother: Why do you start with the hardest one; why don't you start with an easy one?

Father: We start with another one? No, we'll do this one.

Marie: (whispers)

Father: OK. Well look, there's . . . there's a start.

Mother: You can talk, you don't have to whisper.

Marie: OK.

Father: Marie, see which piece that is? That's that door. See, with the handle?

Marie: Yeah.

Father: Now, what're you gonna do now?

Marie: I might top it. Goes down there probably. Doesn't . . . That's gotta be the bottom of the car

(They continue working on the puzzle, with the father alternating between asking questions and giving suggestions. Marie makes brief remarks, and her mother watches quietly. After a while Marie makes a bid for more independence.)

Father: How 'bout try that like that?

Marie: Don't wantcha to help me.

Mother: Why don'tcha want daddy to help you?

Marie: 'Cause I don't want him to help me. That's why I don't want him to help me.

Mother: Does Miss Anderson help you at school?

Marie: No.

Father: (whispered) I can see where that piece goes now.

Marie: Can you?

Father: Yeah. Daddy help?

Marie: No.

Father: No, I'll tell you if you're warm or cold. You ask daddy and I'll tell you.

Marie: 'M I warm?

Father: Fairly warm. (pause) Colder.

Marie: (sigh) Is this the right piece?

(They continue in this fashion until the puzzle is completed.)

In the course of this referential communication, father and daughter are also negotiating their relationship. The puzzle is difficult, and Marie is not having an easy time with it. The father directs her heavily at first. Later Marie asks to redefine their relationship so that she can work without his direction. The father then negotiates a compromise with her, so that she can make her own decisions but he can still help her. In this way he can operate as a responsive environment without compromising her performatory acts too severely. Note that while Marie can verbalize her request to alter the relationship, she does not give her mother a good explanation of why she wants the change. For heuristic purposes, I'll consider that an example of the difficulty in communicating with linear logic about the intuitive nature of relationships.

With regard to the family system concepts discussed above, it is impossible to make a judgment about cohesion from these excerpts. From the longer tape, it is clear that all are participating and share a closeness in working together. Adaptability and creativity appear in the father's negotiations with Marie. Both parents support Marie's efforts to complete the puzzle. On a larger scale, all three support each other through tone of voice and other expressions of positive affect. Family style is also hard to capture in so brief a sample. On the tape there is considerable laughter and warmth and an enthusiasm in talking about the puzzle. The patterns of interaction can be approached on more than one level. First, there are the frequent exchanges between father and daughter where the father provides information and the daughter responds. Second, the number of utterances by the father far outnumber those by his wife and Marie. The third level also involves Marie's mother. While the father's remarks are task oriented, all four of the mother's remarks deal with affective or relationship matters. Again, further data would be needed to conclude that these observations represent consistent patterns. Finally, regarding the power hierarchy, the father maintains a position as one-up, although he is able to give Marie at least a feeling of more autonomy when she requests it.

I do not propose that we take Marie's family as a model of a normal family system or of a language-learning environment. Marie has good command of language, but many other children do as well, although they live in very different families. I have presented this example only to illustrate family systems and to show the interrelations between language, conceptual-semantic decisions, relationship decisions, and family processes.

Transactional Patterns

I have used the term transactional pattern frequently since introducing the transactional model in Chapter 6. However, the term has special significance in family theory. Minuchin (1974) regards transactional patterns as a cornerstone of the family system. They are the regular ways that family members deal with each other. They are established and maintained over time, and they embody all the family processes that have been discussed on the previous pages. The idea of transactional patterns is a powerful metaphor in conceptualizing family functioning, because it is through these patterns that families express their degrees of cohesion and adaptability, their style, interaction patterns, and power hierarchies, and other aspects of their functioning. Transactional patterns are based on shared reference and negotiated meaning. The development of transactional patterns is synonymous with the definition of relationships and the development of metarules in the family system.

When we watch parent-child dyads interact together, what we "see" are transactional patterns. Minuchin (1974) argues that a major goal of family therapy is to change dysfunctional transactional patterns. Similarly, when a language trainer teaches parents techniques for encouraging talking or teaching vocabulary, the result is an alteration in the transactional patterns between parent and child.

As emphasized in earlier discussions of human relationships and of the transactional model, transactional patterns are developed and maintained by all participants. Our goal in working with parents, then, is not to teach the parent to teach the child. Rather, it is to establish transactional patterns between child and parents that maximize the opportunities for language growth in the child. On some occasions other family members may be involved as well. The characteristics of such transactional patterns have been described in previous chapters. Ideally, they provide a responsive environment in which the child's language-learning strategies can flourish in a human relationship emphasizing growth and reciprocity. From what has been said about family processes, it should be clear that there is no one form that these patterns should take. Language can flower in a wide variety of family systems. In the next section we will look at language learning in the context of the family.

Language Learning as a Family Process

Seitz and Marcus (1976) point out that parent-child interaction is the foundation for language development. In developing the transactional model in Chapter 6, I illustrated the reciprocal nature of this process, so I will only briefly summarize it now. Language acquisition depends on matching between child and parent (Nelson 1973). Included are both cognitive matches, such as shared reference, and modifications in the parents' talking style. The input provided by parents is simplifed and selective (Broen 1972; Snow 1972; Phillips 1973; Siegel 1967). Children influence the forms this input will take through the utterances they produce and through their comprehension (Bohannon and Marquis 1977). Mahoney (1975) stressed the importance of feedback processes as the child provides cues to the parent regarding what is comprehended and what is not. In this way children regulate the input they receive and hence the language models that they learn from. Zlatin and Phelps (1975) demonstrated that the resultant matches in communicative behavior between parent and child can be quite subtle and very specific to the child's levels and styles of functioning.

From the family perspective, these reciprocal processes contain all the requirements for transactional patterns: They involve both participants, they are feedback controlled, they last over time, and they contain both morphostatic and morphogenic processes. Here, then, is a fundamental link between language acquisition and family theory. Indeed, language acquisition is a family process.

Nelson (1973) also emphasized parental selection strategies in language learning. Parents select which of the child's utterances to respond to and the content and form of those responses. Moerk's (1976) study of language teaching in parent-child interaction illustrates how these selections contribute to the child's language learning. As mentioned in Chapter 6, Moerk analyzed interactions between mothers and young children. Four conclusions from his data are particularly important in the present discussion. First, mothers do engage in language teaching, sometimes of an intensive nature. Second, this teaching can be analyzed as a feedback system between mother and child. In fact, Moerk illustrates several transactional patterns related to language teaching that occurred regularly in the mother-child dyads he studied. These patterns always involve sequences between parent and child. For example, a mother may direct an utterance toward her child. The child responds and the mother evaluates that response. She may then provide either corrective feedback or confirmation as appropriate. In the case of corrective feedback, the child responds again as a new cycle is initiated. A third conclusion is that the nature of these transactional patterns varies with the child's age and mean length of utterance. The teaching was different for children at different levels. Finally, there were great individual differences among the twenty mother-child dyads studied. During one-hour interactions, the number of language-teaching exchanges varied from one to sixty-two. There are many possible reasons for these differences. Partially, they must reflect the levels of cohesion and adaptability in different families. They are also related to family style, for example, in the total numbers of utterances produced by each dyad in a sixty-minute period. The variety and success of the language-teaching transactional patterns employed also depends on the creativity of the mother and of the family in general. The relation between frequency of teaching exchanges and the child's language level was not specifically explored. Moerk's data on individual dyads do not indicate that less teaching was paralleled by lower language levels, however.

In any case, the language-information-gathering strategies (Snyder and McLean 1977; Snyder-McLean and McLean 1978) described in the preceding chapter do not occur in a vacuum. Moerk (1976) demonstrated conclusively that mothers are actively involved in language teaching. In ideal situations, then, we have a combination of the child's performatory acts and a parental responsive environment. It should be emphasized that these language-teaching transactional patterns occur both during attempts by mother and child to communicate and in more conscious efforts by the mother to instruct her child in the ways of language.

We can also relate language learning to broader perspectives on growth in families. Both Briggs (1970) and Satir (1967) stress the importance of self-esteem in child development. Indeed, self-esteem is one of the most powerful influences on human behavior. According to Satir, self-esteem is associated with mastery. Masterful people are individuals who can do for themselves. Of course, mastery is relative to age. Language is important here because it is a set of skills to be mastered, but in addition it is a means to mastery in many other areas. Self-

esteem and mastery are related to the support each family member receives. The term Satir (1967) uses is "validation." Older family members validate growth in younger members. In order to validate growth, parents must first recognize that it is occurring. Then they must communicate this recognition to the child somehow and provide opportunities for the child to practice and develop further in this new area of mastery. Validation is not simply praise, then. It is noticing and encouraging growth and allowing the child to express new areas of mastery and develop them further.

In conclusion, language learning and teaching occur in a broader context of transactional patterns in the family. Consequently, they are related to the cohesion and adaptability with which the family functions. They include style, patterns of interaction, power hierarchies, and other family processes. Similarly, they involve the reciprocity emphasized by Bronfenbrenner (1979). Mutual positive feeling and increased independence on the part of the child, the other qualities stressed by Bronfenbrenner, are amplified by Satir's concepts of self-esteem, mastery, and validation in the family.

Conclusions

The view of family processes that I have been developing is a direct extension of the ideas in Chapter 5. People establish and maintain relationships through communication. The ideas of human relationship and communication are synonymous. In families these relationships achieve a special character because of the frequency and intimacy of human contact. This depth is the source of the joy and fulfillment of family relationships, and also of the pain they may involve. Because of the enduring nature of family relationships, they are fittingly described with systems terms, such as morphostasis and morphogenesis. The transactional model is directly reflected in both the stability and change of family life.

A family is often described as being more than the sum of its parts. While each member is unique, the relationships that are negotiated in a family transcend many of these individual characteristics. Thus, we can talk about a family as having a particular style, or maintaining a certain amount of cohesion, or providing some level of support for its members. Following Minuchin (1974), I have taken the transactional pattern as a metaphor for summarizing the various aspects of family functioning. Transactional patterns involve all of these processes and provide a means for us to approach them concretely.

Language learning occurs in the context of the transactional patterns of each family. Various patterns are negotiated between child and parent that relate directly to language acquisition. Both content and relationship communication are simultaneously involved. A match or balance of some sort develops between the child's language acquisition strategies and the parents' teaching strategies, all in the service of communication. While both sets of strategies have been described separately (Snyder and McLean 1977; Snyder-McLean and McLean 1978; Moerk 1976), in a larger perspective they are parts of the same process. Finally, we note the importance of self-esteem and validation for both parent and child. Parents validate their child's progressive mastery of communication skills at the same time that children validate their parents as caregivers and teachers. Let us now consider children's

language impairments from this family perspective.

CHILDREN'S LANGUAGE DISORDERS IN THE FAMILY SYSTEM

Family members must communicate. They have no choice because all behavior has message character. Further, people living in the same household must deal with each other to some degree. It does not matter, then, whether a child uses language or not. Communication with other family members will develop. These assumptions form a base for the transactional model. From a more practical standpoint, parents must communicate with their children. They have to get them clothed, bathed, off to school, fed, and a host of other things. Again, children cannot not respond, whatever their degree of language skill. Consequently, transactional patterns will develop between parents and language-impaired children just as with any other children.

The question, then, is about the quality of the transactional patterns in which language-impaired children participate. If a child's use of language is minimal, the family will develop a style, pattern of interaction, and power hierarchy in their dealings with that child that does not require much talking by the child. On one level, this accommodation might seem unproductive because it does not encourage language growth. In fact, it can incorporate a self-fulfilling prophecy that the child will not talk and harden into a morphostatic process of considerable power. On the other hand, such transactional patterns have a productive side because they allow some means for conducting the business of daily life, and they may allow the parents a mechanism for validating the child's growth in areas other than language.

Family-Oriented Research on Language Delay

There are few studies of children's language disorders as family processes. The studies that are available concentrate on language delay. Cramblit and Siegel (1977) studied one language-delayed four-year-old boy. They found that his father, mother, and a high-school–aged baby-sitter all talked to him in ways that would normally be used to talk to younger children. This finding is parallel with studies of adults interacting with retarded children. Farber (1960) noted that families treat a retarded child as the "baby" of the family. More directly related to language, Marshall, Hegrenes, and Goldstein (1973) and Buium, Rynders, and Turnure (1974) describe the tendency of adults to simplify their language use when interacting with retarded individuals. Unfortunately, while these studies focus on verbal interaction, they confound language level with retardation. Earlier studies by Siegel (Siegel 1963a, 1963b; Siegel and Harkins 1963), however, employed retarded individuals with different levels of language skill. Again, adults adjusted their talking according to the language level of the person they were talking with. It has also been found that language-impaired youngsters elicit simplified talking from peers (Guralnick and Paul-Brown 1977). It seems safe to assume, then, that much of the talking that is directed to language-delayed children may be simplified in form. From the family systems perspective, this process may be considered a homeostatic mechanism and illustrates some adaptability in families of language-delayed children.

Observations of the Home Environment

The above studies concentrated directly on verbal interaction. Some studies have focused on home environments in which language development occurs, using the HOME (Home Observation for Measurement of the Environment) inventory (Caldwell 1978). This instrument has six subscales: Emotional and Verbal Responsivity of Mother, Avoidance of Restriction and Punishment, Organization of Physical and Temporal Environment, Provision of Appropriate Play Materials, Maternal Involvement with Child, and Opportunities for Variety in Daily Stimulation. The inventory is administered in a home visit that includes both an interview with the mother and observations of the home and natural interaction between mother and child during the visit.

Jordan (1978) evaluated the influences of several variables on vocabulary development. This research was part of a larger prospective study of children from birth to five years. Along with eight other measures, the HOME scale was administered at each birthday to 181 children. Vocabulary was assessed with the *Wechsler Preschool and Primary Scale of Intelligence*. HOME scores were found to be the prime predictor of vocabulary scores at age five. The HOME scores, in turn, were found to be related to the mothers' educational levels.

In another study, Elardo, Bradley, and Caldwell (1977) looked at the relations between the HOME subscales and scores on the *Illinois Test of Psycholinguistic Ability* (ITPA). In this prospective study, the HOME inventory was administered to seventy-four mothers when the child was six months and again at twenty-four months. The ITPA was administered at approximately thirty-seven months of age. As would be expected, correlations between the ITPA scores and the twenty-four-month HOME scores were stronger than those with the six-month HOME scores. The correlation between the overall scores on the ITPA and twenty-four-month HOME was .65, a substantial correlation considering the time span between administrations and the many factors affecting both home environments and language skills. The three ITPA subtests showing the strongest relations were all in the area of auditory-vocal language rather than visual or gestural skills. The three subscales of HOME that predicted overall ITPA scores most successfully were Emotional and Verbal Responsivity of Mother, Provision of Appropriate Play Materials, and Maternal Involvement with Child. Elardo, Bradley, and Caldwell (1977) concluded that there is a strong relationship between the home environment and language development, but that some factors in the environment are more prominent than others.

In another study, HOME was used to assess the home environments of language-delayed children. Wulbert, Inglis, Kriegsmann, and Mills (1975) studied twenty functional language-delayed children, twenty matched normal controls, and twenty preschool Down's syndrome children. Language skills were assessed with a variety of techniques, both standardized and informal.

The HOME inventory results for the normals and Down's syndrome children were very similar. In comparison with these groups, the language-delayed group scored significantly lower on three of the HOME scales. One was Emotional and Verbal Responsiveness of Mother, which involves how the mother talks to the child and responds to the child's communications and how the mother talks about the child to the interviewer. In terms of family systems, a low score on this subscale suggests moderately low cohesion and support between mother and child. The second category was Avoidance of Restriction and Punishment. Mothers of language-delayed children were more likely to restrict and punish their children verbally or physically, rather than using more positive strategies such as reasoning or redirecting the child's attention. This result, coupled with the lack of positive affect from the preceding subscale, suggests that there may be little mutuality of positive feeling in these families. Rather, the children were constrained heavily. As we have seen, constraint does not encourage talking. The largest difference between the other two groups and the language-delayed group was in another category, Maternal Involvement with Child. The parents of the language-delayed children interacted much less with their children than did those in the control and Down's syndrome groups. In family terms, this result suggests behavior toward the disengagement pole in cohesion. It appears that there was little reciprocity and minimum interaction between these mothers and children.

One could argue that the presence of a handicap of any sort in the child might cause mothers to behave in the ways described above, but the data on the Down's syndrome children eliminates this possibility. Recall that the HOME scores for the latter group were not significantly different from those of the normals. It is also noteworthy that these results appeared regardless of social class as measured with the Hollingshead Two-Factor Index. Social class was not a factor in language delay.

This study by Wulbert, Inglis, Kriegsmann, and Mills (1975) is suggestive of strong links between language delay and family processes. Taking the three subscales on which the language-delayed group's scores were low, one could conclude that there was little opportunity in these families for language-enhancing transactional patterns such as those discussed earlier, to develop or flourish. It is noteworthy that two of those subscales, Emotional and Verbal Responsivity of Mother and Maternal Involvement with Child, were among the three with strong relations to ITPA scores in the Elardo, Bradley, and Caldwell (1977) study. It is also possible to overinterpret these results. As Wulbert and her associates point out, their study suggests that certain types of parent-child interaction may be present in families with functional language-delayed children, but the data tell us nothing about causation or even about directions of influence. At the same time, the study gives us some good leads regarding transactional patterns that may be important in families with language-delayed children.

Conclusions

Research in other areas has also shed light on the relations between family processes and language skills. As mentioned earlier, Bronfenbrenner (1979) summarized evidence from several studies showing a relation between divorced parents and difficulties in children with information-processing skills such as attention, memory span, and distractibility. These studies, however, do not lead to simple conclusions about the relation between divorce and learning difficulties in children. In those divorces in which the

parents were still able to communicate and cooperate in managing their children, difficulties with memory and attention were no greater than in the general population. It was only when communication and parenting remained strained after the divorce that increases in these difficulties were found.

It is in working with families that we can see most directly how a theory of causation, the transactional model, becomes a framework for intervention. Both center around the transactional patterns between child and family. Rutter (1979) provides additional perspective here. He poses an infrequently asked question: Why do some children who are at risk for developmental problems *not* end up with any such difficulties? First, he notes that there are various factors whose effect is to foster normal development even in the presence of at-risk conditions. For example, even in a dysfunctional family full of pain and discord, a good relationship with one parent in the home may "protect" the child, thus allowing normal development.

Rutter (1979) also suggests that, in a transactional view, the combined effects of different at-risk conditions are not merely additive. Rather, the child's chances of developing problems of some sort are heightened dramatically. For one thing, the presence of one at-risk condition increases the chances that other conditions will also be present. For example, low socioeconomic status may be associated with poor medical and educational services. In addition, Rutter describes a transactional effect in which one condition exacerbates another. For example, consider a family in which the parents tend to be very critical. A child with adverse temperamental characteristics such as negative mood is twice as likely as other children in the family to be the recipient of criticism from such parents (Rutter 1979). While the research has not been done, we can imagine similar unfortunate combinations relating to language impairments.

In summary, there are three lines of evidence regarding language delay as a family process. The first is in the area of family style. Family members simplify their talking when interacting with language-delayed children. Second, based on one study only, it may be that language delay is related to more pervasive differences in family functioning, resulting in transactional patterns that are not conducive to language development. Finally, there is evidence from studies in other areas of developmental disturbance that normal development is related to family functioning in complex ways and that outcome is dependent on transactions between various factors in the child, family, and the larger environment.

Some Examples

Sandy

Let us enrich these theoretical and research-oriented views with some examples of interaction in families with language-impaired children. The first child, Sandy, is a five-year-old Down's syndrome child who is severely delayed in language development. She and her mother had been asked to play together. The tape recording was made in their home. Most of Sandy's unintelligible remarks were one-syllable utterances. Some appeared to be attempts at words, while others were grunts or other nonlinguistic sounds.

We may note first that there is a high degree of reciprocity in that mother and child regularly respond to each other, although, of course, they may have felt they had no other choice with the clinician's tape recorder in view. As in our previous excerpt, it is clear that both conceptual-semantic and

SAMPLE 11: Sandy and Mother CA = 5-1

Mother: You want a yellow one?
Sandy: Yeah. That
Mother: Yeah.
Sandy: (unintelligible)
Mother: Oh, don't bang it down so loud.
Sandy: (unintelligible)
Mother: Oh, you turkey.
Sandy: (unintelligible)
Mother: What color is that one?
Sandy: (unintelligible)
Mother: No, what color is this?
Sandy: (unintelligible)
Mother: You're a turkey.
Sandy: Blue.
Mother: No, what color is it?
Sandy: Red.
Mother: What color?
Sandy: (unintelligible)
Mother: I can't hear you when you're laughing.
Mother: What color is that?
Sandy: Red.
Mother: I don't know, I think I'll throw you away.
Mother: Can I throw you out the door?
Sandy: (unintelligible) No.
Mother: Shhhhhh.
Sandy: (unintelligible)
Mother: You're being silly.
Sandy: (unintelligible)
Mother: Hey, not so loud.
Sandy: (unintelligible)
Mother: You're being bad now.
Sandy: (unintelligible)
Mother: Settle down.
Sandy: (unintelligible)
Mother: Settle down.
Mother: What color is this one?
Sandy: (unintelligible)
Mother: No, that's—
Sandy: (unintelligible)
Mother: No, green.

Sandy: (unintelligible)
Mother: Can you say green?
Sandy: (unintelligible)
Mother: Green.
Sandy: Green. (unintelligible)
Mother: Shhhh.
Sandy: (unintelligible)
Mother: Hurry up, put the green one on.

---

relationship decisions are governing the talking between Sandy and her mother. The task is referential, but much of the talking involves relationship negotiations.

The vast majority of the mother's remarks are constraining. She is testing rather than teaching. Sandy resists by being silly and occasionally a little naughty. It makes sense to say that Sandy elicits much of this constraint through her poor responding and lack of cooperation, especially with the tape recorder present. At the same time, one could say that her mother elicits those behaviors through testing without sufficient modeling and pressing Sandy to respond. The behavior of each, then, complements the other in a transactional pattern that continues over and over.

Regarding language learning, they do establish shared reference. The mother simplifies her utterances as we would expect. At the same time, she provides little input that Sandy can utilize in increasing her vocabulary. By constraining heavily, the mother minimizes her effectiveness as a responsive environment and concurrently allows Sandy little room to experiment with language. Recall that constraint is effective when the focus is on specific items to be learned. In this exchange between Sandy and her mother, we have the constraint and a specific focus (colors), but insufficient modeling. The result is that there are few opportunities for Sandy to get validated for

mastery, nor, for that matter, is there much validation available for her mother. Note that when the mother does provide a model at the end of the transcript, Sandy does respond appropriately. However, because of her immediately following unintelligible remark and the mother's subsequent "Shhh," Sandy gets no payoff for her correct response.

Note again the metalevel of relationship communication over referential communication. When Sandy gets silly enough (an iconic sign that she does not want to play her mother's game), the mother's attempts at referential communication simply stop. Regarding the mother's high rates of commands and questions and Sandy's low rate of appropriate responding, Seitz (1975) cites data that compliance generally increases when the number of commands decreases. Similarly, Lobitz and Johnson (1975) demonstrated that a high level of constraint by parents generates negative behavior in the child. Finally, both Sandy and her mother are caught in a no-win, morphostatic system. Sandy isn't learning much language; further, she isn't enjoying the situation very much, as evidenced by her resistance. Her mother isn't pleased either, as demonstrated by her attempts to get Sandy to cooperate, her gentle name-calling ("Turkey"), and her poignant suggestion that she throw Sandy away.

Linda

The first example illustrates a rather specific transactional pattern. We don't know much else about Sandy and her mother. Consider now an example of a larger family pattern. Linda was a three-year-old child with a severe delay in expression and a mild deficit in comprehension. Assessment revealed intellectual develop-

283

ment within normal limits. No evidence of hearing loss or organic pathology could be found. Linda was a very social child; she loved to play with both children and adults, but with virtually no talking.

Linda lived with her mother and a seven-year-old sister. Her mother was recently divorced and lived on the same block as her parents, who also had a twelve-year-old daughter at home. There was a high degree of cohesion among all three generations, perhaps bordering on enmeshment. In addition, there was a great deal of support all through this extended family. The result was that Linda's grandmother, grandfather, twelve-year-old aunt, mother, and older sister all waited on her, anticipated her needs, babied her, and generally took care of her. After all, she'd just experienced the divorce of her parents. This transactional pattern is on a much larger scale than in the previous example. It's almost as if there were a "conspiracy" to keep Linda immature. She was bathed in support but had few opportunities to develop new masteries. While there was tremendous reciprocity in the system, there was little change in the direction of gradually giving Linda more independence.

The family was full of behaviors such as that described by family therapists as "spokesmanship," where other people would speak for Linda. Of course, she maintained many of these behaviors through her own positive affect and cuteness. As in the previous example, the result was a morphostatic system that impeded language growth. In both of these cases it must be stressed that there was nothing deeply pathological in the family members' behavior. They were positively motivated and doing their best to help their children. At the same time, their interactions with those children

evolved into transactional patterns that militated against change.

Carol

Let us look at a third example. This family consisted of mother, father, and two girls, one three and the other seven months. When first seen in the clinic, Carol, the three-year-old, demonstrated a severe language impairment. She used virtually no expressive language and evidenced very little comprehension. Standardized testing was impossible. In addition, she employed some unusual behaviors, such as high-pitched whining, recurrent hand-flapping, and a "distant" gaze. Through free-field testing and play audiometry, it was established that she had adequate hearing for language development.

For reasons beyond anybody's control she was not enrolled in an intervention program until several months later. At that time the whining, flapping, and gazing had diminished considerably. On occasion, though, she would cover her ears tightly, sometimes acting almost as if she were in pain. No environmental stimuli, auditory or otherwise, could be identified that brought on this behavior.

The clinician visited the home to administer the HOME inventory (Caldwell 1978) and to gain additional general impressions. All four family members were present. Carol's mother and father sat on a couch, the baby was on a blanket in front of the couch, and Carol was in and out of the living room and an adjoining patio. Consistent with the Wulbert, et al (1975) study discussed earlier, the mother's responses to HOME were low on two subscales, Emotional and Verbal Responsivity of Mother and Maternal Involvement with Child.

As Carol went in and out of the house,

her mother paid no attention to her at all, never glancing to see where she was or what she was doing. At one point Carol climbed up on a footstool in front of the couch, put her arms out, and half-fell, half-dove toward her mother. She fell short, her face hitting directly on the floor. During this entire sequence her mother never looked at Carol or reached for her, even when she fell. In contrast, the mother looked and smiled frequently at the baby. Similarly, in talking to the clinician, she became more animated and warmer in tone when discussing the baby, while she remained relatively flat in affect while talking about Carol. In a brief tour of the house it was noted that the baby's room was alive and bright and full of toys and pictures. Carol's, on the other hand, was absolutely plain except for one poster, which was on the back of the door, so that one had to enter the room and then close the door before it could be seen. The baby's toys were prominently displayed in their own box. Carol's were kept in her closet. As part of the intervention program, Carol participated in a nursery school group in which frequent craft projects were made and sent home. All of the other mothers had these collages, junk sculptures, macaroni necklaces, and whatnot plastered all over their refrigerators. Carol's were not anywhere to be found.

In short, there was considerable evidence of a transactional pattern in this family in which the baby was treated as one might expect in a middle-American family, while the existence of the other child was virtually ignored or even denied. The father was warmer toward Carol but relatively inactive during the visit, so we don't know what part he plays in this pattern. Carol, with her strange iconic signs and her lack of language development, is also part of this system.

You may have already related this situation to some of the family processes discussed earlier. There is almost no reciprocity between Carol and her mother. Their relationship could be called disengaged, whereas other relationships in the family appear within the normal range of cohesion. Carol surely has plenty of independence, but she receives no validation for skill mastery or for her own identity as a person. It is almost redundant to say that Carol has little opportunity to participate in transactional patterns conducive to language growth.

The Validity of Home Observations

All three of these examples rest on clinical observations. It is appropriate to ask about the validity of these situations. Do they really represent what these families are like? This question is particularly germane because of the presence in the homes of observers who were known to be ''speech experts.'' Patterson and his associates have studied the validity of home observations empirically (summarized in Patterson and Cobb 1971, 1973). They employed an extensive observation code that covers a wide range of behaviors that occur in family interaction. It could be reasoned that an observer is a novel stimulus and that after a while family members would adapt to the observer's presence. Using their observation code, however, they found little evidence of such adaptation across ten observations in a number of families. In another study they trained mothers to use the same observation code that the visiting observers used. Following this training, the mothers surreptitiously took data on their own families on some occasions, and visiting observers took data on other occasions. A comparison of the two sets of data showed differences in the absolute frequencies of various behaviors for the two conditions. However, the same relations between different behavior categories were obtained in both cases. That is, if a father used more positive remarks than negative remarks toward his son, that pattern occurred both when his wife was taking data and when the outside observer was present.

Lobitz and Johnson (1975) took quite a different approach to studying the validity of home observations. They purposely attempted to bias the data. In twelve families they asked parents to make the child look as "good" as possible, while in another twelve parents were to make their child look as "bad" as possible. Both groups included families with a child who had behavior problems and families with children without such problems. Lobitz and Johnson (1975) found that parents could make their children look worse than they typically were, but they couldn't make children look better than usual. As an aside relating to the preceding chapter, the techniques parents used to make their children look bad could be summarized with one word: constraint.

These studies suggest that there is some validity to home observations and that whatever bias is present is likely to be in a negative direction. On more intuitive grounds one could argue that people get conservative when they are being evaluated. Being observed is not the time to stick your neck out. Thus, while families may "dress up" for outside visitors, they will wear that dressing on well-established transactional patterns that are consistent with their everyday behavior.

There is another perspective that can also apply to home visits. The validity of our observations is related to what we do with the information obtained. If the purpose is to make pronouncements or diagnoses of what the "true" family is like, then our data must be representative. However, one can argue that we can never know the "true" family. Whatever we see is partly a product of the situation, because families do not occur except in situations. Many family therapists take this notion a step further and act on the assumption that the observer is part of the system rather than external to it (for example, Keeney 1979). This view is exactly parallel with the idea presented in the preceding chapter that the child's behavior cannot be understood except in relation to the clinician's. The question of whether or not what you saw during a home visit is "true" or representative, then, becomes moot. What is important is what you're going to do about what you saw. The parallel with Chapter 11 continues. If you are working with a child and that child is distractible or naughty, normally you do not ask if that behavior is typical; rather, you ask what it means at the moment and how you should respond to it. We can adapt this same strategy in working with families.

Regarding validity, home observation is similar to language sampling. We face what Labov calls the observer's paradox. We want to observe how people behave when we aren't observing them. What I am suggesting in the preceding paragraph is a reframing of this situation so that the paradox is no longer relevant.

Conclusions

Empirical studies of children's language disorders as family phenomena are rare. Nevertheless, what evidence we do have supports such a view, at least for language-delayed children. Level of language skill is an important contributor to the transactional patterns between parent and child, and those transactional patterns are an important contributor to language skill. Transactional patterns develop and change through constant negotiation among family members. I do not mean conscious, purposeful negotiation here, but rather the definition of relationships through participation in relationships as described in Chapter 5. In this sense, to behave toward someone is to negotiate. However a language disorder may begin, perhaps as the result of an unhappy combination of at-risk factors, it becomes part and product of the transactional patterns in which the child is living and growing.

Obviously this view underscores the potential of working with parents as one aspect of intervention. The transactional model, however, does not imply that we must always work with parents. Recall that changing a child will change the transactional patterns in which that child participates. At the same time, I would argue that home interventions would be useful in families such as the three examples described above.

HOME INTERVENTION

As in working with children directly, home intervention involves problem solving by the clinician. In the remainder of the chapter I will discuss some principles to guide that decision making. These principles will provide a framework in which to develop specific interventions for individual families.

Changing Transactional Patterns as the Goal

If we enhance the family's effectiveness as a language-learning system, the result should be increased rate of learning by the child. As we develop skill in this endeavor, many children should be able to learn language faster than we could teach it to them in conventional clinical interventions. But enhancing the family's effectiveness does not mean making family members into "little clinicians." It means taking the ways they already communicate, their transactional patterns, and helping alter those patterns so that language learning can be more efficient. There are many avenues toward accomplishing this goal, including both structured training and more global interventions. More specific interventions will be discussed later in the chapter. At present, let us consider some other principles from which we can build constructive home interventions.

Supporting the Parent's Role as Child-Rearing Agent

I try to approach parents with an attitude of "How can I help you?" rather than, "Here's what I want you to do for me." It is easy to express the first attitude in words to parents. It can be difficult, however, to organize our approach to parents around this principle, to punctuate our relationships with parents in this way. Much of our work with language-disordered children involves teaching, and it is natural, therefore, to approach parents either with the idea of teaching them as well or with the intention of using them as aides to extend our teaching.

Operating with the goal of helping parents has advantages. First, it is realistic. It forces us to act on the fact that parents have more influence on their children's development than we do. Second, it implies that parents have talents and skills and that they can be influential in fostering language growth. The effect, again, is to validate the parents as competent people.

Consider the parent functioning as an aide or assistant in language intervention.

The clinician designs the program and instructs the parent regarding what to do. In so doing, the clinician takes full responsibility for effecting change in the child. The parent may not even know the larger goals of the program. The clinician provides weekly instructions and materials for the parent to take home and evaluates the child's progress. There is no appreciation of the parent's role as a change agent, and in fact the parent is maintained in a dependency relationship with the clinician.

A home intervention such as that just described ignores the family system even though it utilizes parents. In another view, some parent programs may undermine parents' roles in child rearing. Typically, this effect does not come about through teachers' or clinicians' acting negatively toward parents. Rather, it occurs when we take over certain parenting functions, when we usurp the parents' responsibilities for teaching and raising their children. The evidence comes mostly from programs related to Head Start. Bronfenbrenner (1979) cites data demonstrating that programs in which such transfer of authority takes place do not have as powerful effects as those in which parents' perceptions of themselves as primary influences on their children's lives are maintained and enhanced. There is a difference between programs in which parents assist the teachers and programs in which teachers assist the parents. One of the most successful Head Start–related interventions consisted entirely of home visits during which mothers were taught to play and interact with their preschoolers in ways that would foster language and cognitive development (Levenstein 1970).

This perspective presents a real challenge in designing interventions for language-impaired youngsters. It is customary for us to work individually with each child in school or clinic. Placing the major emphasis on parents would indeed be a second-order change for us. A combined program, including both home and clinic, might be a solution, but the problem again would be to maintain the parents as the major change agents.

Developing a Problem-Solving Attitude

I have used problem solving a number of times as a metaphor for the decision making that underlies intervention. In working with parents, I suggest that we focus literally on problem solving, rather than emphasizing disabilities or pathologies (Haley 1976). A problem needs a solution; a pathology requires a cure. Of course, neat solutions do not exist for many of the problems associated with language disorders. The point is that we can identify specific problems, define them carefully, and set to work on them. This process is one to which parents can contribute meaningfully. Indeed, it requires their participation to be successful.

Emphasizing pathologies leads to an interesting "perceptual problem." If you look hard enough for pathologies in people, you are bound to find them. No one is without at least one quirk, suspicious history, attitude, behavior pattern, or other sign that could represent pathology. Not only is there a danger of finding pathologies that don't exist; once identified, such pathologies easily become reified into explanatory principles, for example, "What do you expect from a child with parents like that?" I am not arguing that we should ignore the possibilities of psychopathology any more than those of neuropathology. Clearly, we should make referrals when conditions warrant. I am suggesting, however, that the search for pathologies does not lead directly to intervention strategies.

This problem-solving framework is also related to the preceding principle of maintaining the parents' responsibilities as parents and to the medical model. If we define a situation as a disability in the child, then that child should be enrolled for treatment. The parents' responsibility is thus reduced to bringing the child to us. Consequently, their roles as change agents are not recognized and they are much less actively engaged in the intervention. This is frequently the case with language-impaired children in the public schools. As we will see later, there is an implicit contract between parents and clinician, one in which the clinician takes responsibility for changing the child.

In sum, we can define the child's situation in terms of problems that are directly accessible to intervention. As much as possible, the parents should be involved in both the identification of such problem areas, and in working toward solutions. If the focus of home intervention is to be on problem solving, then those problems must be clearly defined, which brings us to our next principle.

Keeping the Focus on Behavior Change

Parents of language-disordered children are likely to experience a number of emotions regarding their situation. They may fear that the child has other problems as well. They may feel some combination of anger and guilt: anger and frustration because the child is not developing on schedule, and guilt because of the possibility that part of the problem is the parents' fault somehow. And always there is the worry about what the child will be like in the future.

I knew a father and mother who purchased a sound movie camera to film their child's first words. Two years later the camera was still unused. The mother of another language-delayed boy told me that the child had been talking normally, but at about two years of age he tipped a pan of hot water onto himself from the stove. His mother was absolutely convinced that this incident caused the language delay and blamed herself for allowing it to happen. Still another family, after their language-delayed child had been enrolled in the clinic for several months, had to move out of state. They wrote me later that the child was now imitating the dog perfectly and that they hoped that eventually she would use human speech as well. We know from anecdotes such as these, as well as direct expressions from parents, that the presence of a language-impaired child generates a host of emotions. It is appropriate for us to respond to these feelings and provide support (Webster 1966, 1976).

At the same time, I am inclined to believe that concentrating on emotions may not be a very efficient means of effecting change. These feelings are likely to be focused on the past, on what might have happened and what could have been. The transactional model, however, suggests that emphasizing the past is not likely to be productive, because only the transactional patterns that are occurring now are amenable to intervention. In addition, strong emotions are not likely to lead to problem solving. Rather, they are reactions to problems, and they tend to maintain attempts at first-order change or feelings of helplessness.

For these reasons I suggest that parents be encouraged to focus on the present, where they can take action and where there is potential for change. Dwelling on the past or on fear and guilt is simply not constructive. Rarely is it effective to make such a statement to parents, however. It may be more helpful to direct their attention to the present and immediate future, and involve them in decision making and intervention as soon as possible. Hence, we engage their help in defining the problems that will be the goals of intervention. These problems are best described in behavioral terms. As behaviorists have been telling us for years, such descriptions help clarify understandings of just what needs to be done. Further, their very concreteness tends to diminish emphasis on emotions.

Haley (1976) suggests another advantage of emphasizing behavior change. He notes that people frequently do not benefit from good advice. He is talking about clinic families, ones that are caught in dysfunctional transactional patterns, but the same is true of most of us. The world is full of good advice about how to be tolerant and patient in raising children, how to provide good models in a serene atmosphere. However, as Haley suggests, ask a parent sometime, "If I were to give you some good advice, what would I say?" (1976, p. 54). Parents will then recite to you the good advice that you had in mind. As Haley notes, giving good advice is based on the assumption that people have rational control of their actions. As we have seen, however, behavior in relationships is controlled by intuitive processes. Decisions in this area of behavior, then, are not likely to be influenced by the linear logic underlying good advice. Consequently, the clinician may be better off working more directly for behavior changes in the parents, rather than relying primarily on talking and making suggestions.

I do not mean to imply that all parents resist change: far from it. Many are actively seeking help. However, transactional patterns do evolve which discourage language growth in children and may in addition trap the participants in no-win situations. Further, because of the tendency for individuals to punctuate relationships from their own perspectives, parents may not be aware of the reciprocal nature of these patterns or that there are other alternatives possible.

Establishing a Contract

Once you have assessed the situation, it is helpful to make an agreement with parents regarding what the home intervention will entail. Such contracts should include what the parents' responsibilities will be, what the clinician will do, and specify the duration of time during which the agreement will be in force. This contract need not be a legal document at all. It can be a very informal verbal agreement. In fact, any time you agree to work with a child, you imply a contract, whether you are aware of it or not.

The idea in establishing a contract is that everyone knows what to expect. The parents are clear about what they are committed to do, and they should be equally clear about how the clinician will behave. This arrangement minimizes fear of the unknown because the parents know what to expect. Further, it underscores their commitment because they have agreed on how they will participate. At the same time, it allows a way out for both parents and clinician because the contract is only for a specified period of time.

It is helpful to set a relatively short time commitment when first establishing a contract, perhaps one month. At the end of that month parents and clinician can evaluate progress and procedures together and decide what to do next. It should be made explicit that either parents or clinician may decide to terminate participation at the end of the contract, but all parties are committed to give their full cooperation and support until that time. If the intervention plan is appropriate, however, parents rarely drop out. Rather, a new contract is arranged, usually for a longer time period.

Some clinicians and teachers may feel uncomfortable in establishing the duration of intervention in advance. Who can tell how long it will take for a child to improve in language skill? On the other hand, working in this manner brings a little extra discipline to our work. We choose to make changes that seem probable in a given time period rather than the traditional open-ended interventions for which there is often no end in sight. Further, and most important, it is not necessary to contract or "guarantee" what results will be produced. Rather, the contract establishes what the parents and clinician will do, and both parties evaluate the results together.

Historically, contracts have rarely been negotiated between parents and language trainers in the public schools. As already mentioned, however, a contract is implicit in public school language programs, one in which the trainer takes responsibility for change in the child. Federal laws now require that we meet with the parents of each handicapped child to discuss and agree on what the child needs and what should be done. This situation presents us with a challenging opportunity to negotiate contracts that involve more meaningful participation by parents, at least for some language-impaired youngsters.

Maintaining Contact with Parents

My emphasis in the preceding sections has been on changing parent-child transactional patterns by working directly with the parents. In effect, we have a two-stage intervention. First, establish transactional patterns in the home that are conducive to language growth. This stage the clinician does directly. In the second stage the child develops greater language skills because of these changes in transactional patterns. The clinician's influence on the child in this stage is indirect; it is through changes in the parents' behavior.

At one time I thought this approach would be very efficient because parents could be trained relatively quickly, and from there on things would take care of themselves. As usual, life turned out to be more complicated than my perceptions of it were. For example, one clinician trained two mothers to engage in facilitative play with their language-delayed children. Prior to training both mothers were highly constraining in how they approached their children. After nine sessions of facilitative play in the homes, both children were talking more, and the mothers were very pleased. The clinician made a follow-up visit in each home about two months after completion of the project. Neither parent had engaged in a single play session during that time period. They dropped the play sessions in spite of the fact that both mothers said they enjoyed the sessions and believed their children had improved as a result of those sessions. This situation illustrates the power of morphostatic processes within the family system.

This lack of generalization could be easily explained through the tenets of family therapy: We should have worked with both fathers and mothers together. Beyond family system factors, however, there is another variable operating in home programs. Whether we choose to work with one parent or both, we may be able to train parents quickly in the first stage mentioned earlier.

Stage two, however, is likely to take some time because it depends on the child's practice and learning. Therefore, we need to maintain the parents' new behaviors long enough for them to have a real impact on the children's language use. It is here that the importance of continued home contacts becomes vital. Even rapid language development is a relatively slow process. Parents may need considerable encouragement and support during this period.

Accordingly, provisions should be included in home intervention contracts for regular contacts between trainer and parents. These contacts may involve home visits or meetings in school or clinic. Once the intervention program is moving, contacts can frequently be handled over the telephone. In any case, they should be regularly scheduled in order to reinforce the mutual commitment between parents and clinician. In addition to providing support and maintaining the effects of intervention, regular contacts have other advantages. Obviously, they provide a means for the clinician to monitor progress and the course of events in general. In addition, they provide parents with consistent access to the clinician for asking questions, discussing problems, and so forth.

Implementing Home Intervention

Home interventions may take different forms. Just as with individual intervention, they vary in degree of structure and in goals. Let us consider a few examples from the literature. MacDonald and his colleagues (MacDonald and Blott 1974; MacDonald, Blott, Gordon, Spiegel, and Hartmann 1974; MacDonald and Horstmeier 1978) developed a program for parents of young retarded children. The program focuses on preclausal structures. Parents learn specific language-teaching procedures that they carry out in the home. They use materials and situations that are present in their homes. The methods for training parents are direct and structured. In contrast, Seitz (1975; Seitz and Hoekenga 1974; Seitz and Riedell, 1974) teaches parents of retarded children to engage in facilitative play with their children. The parent training is low in structure. Parents observe models (clinicians) playing with the children. It has been demonstrated, however, that different observers may find different aspects of a model's behavior appealing. Further, one parent might identify better with one clinician, and another with another. Therefore, Sietz and Hoekenga (1974) had mothers observe different clinicians modeling play behaviors. Each mother then adopted those behaviors that seemed most appropriate to her. The training, then, was unstructured in that different parents "learned" somewhat different techniques.

Levenstein (1970; Madden, Levenstein, and Levenstein 1976) designed a home intervention program that is somewhere in between the two just described. It is intended for disadvantaged families rather than language-impaired children. The focus, however, is on language, conceptual development, and mother-child interaction, and consequently it may be of value for families with language-delayed children. Levenstein teaches mothers to play with their children in ways that encourage language and conceptual development. Each week a "toy demonstrator" visits the home, bringing a gift for the child and mother. The toy demonstrator then models for the mother how she can foster growth in the child through play utilizing these gifts. The techniques include describing things and activities, engaging the child in verbal interaction, encouraging reflection by discussing consequences and alternatives, providing praise, and so forth. The resulting transactional patterns between parent and child will have much in common with Moerk's (1976) parental language-teaching strategies mentioned earlier.

In the above interventions the clinicians decided in advance what general areas would be trained. In still another approach Whitehurst, Novak, and Zorn (1972) observed interaction between a parent and a language-delayed child during mealtimes. On the basis of these observations they decided how they should intervene. The mother was encouraged to provide more models of utterances for her child to say and to increase her general level of talking. This intervention was based on behavior modification methodology, with baseline, intervention, extinction, and reinstatement phases.

In all of the approaches just described, the authors report language growth as a result of their interventions. We can conclude, then, that there is no one strategy for home intervention. It can be structured or unstructured. It can focus on specific language options, or on relationships and more global communication. However, while the above programs are quite different, they also have important similarities. First, the effect is to enhance language development in the child by altering the transactional patterns between child and parent. Second, the language learning in these programs revolves around stimuli and events that are parts of the child's daily life; it is high in ecological validity. Third, all four programs focus on behavior change. Finally, they all emphasize the parent as the change agent. The parent does not aid the clinician; rather, it is the other way around. The whole focus is on helping the parents to enhance their children's language use.

Matching Interventions with Families

Given the variety of home interventions possible, we have the opportunity to select interventions that will match families, at least to some extent. Let me illustrate by citing two examples of "mismatches." The first was a family with a severely impaired girl who had been variously diagnosed as autistic and retarded. She demonstrated both language and behavior problems. She was placed in a contingency management program in the clinic, in which the clinician fed her breakfast. Her parents brought her in the morning, with her breakfast in a lunch box (I suppose I should say a breakfast box). The clinician then used the food, bite at a time, as a reinforcer. The child responded well in this regimen, and so we decided to expand the behavior modification techniques into the home. There were three older siblings in addition to the parents. The family was one of the most loving, caring groups of people I have ever met. Indeed, I was deeply moved by these qualities in their home. It was important to them that their daughter be accepted and loved, that she be validated as a human being and a member of the family. Consequently, they were not interested in taking observational data for us and certainly not in applying contingency management principles at home. That was our job. In retrospect, in encouraging them to use behavior modification techniques we did not appreciate the power of their family style. We were asking them to do things that were quite apart from that style.

Consider a second example of such a mismatch. I once worked with a family in which the father was a very successful salesman. He had in abundance the drive, ambition, and energy associated with the business of selling. Both he and his wife could be described as upper middle class, educated and highly motivated. The mother had an older sister who was retarded and resided in an institution. There was great concern, then, when their child was delayed in talking. As a result of all these factors, there was considerable pressure on the child to talk. I thought it would be helpful to reduce this pressure, so I began to teach facilitative play to the parents. They learned the technique readily, but the pressure remained in more subtle forms. A game became a race, an activity became a contest, all still with the implication that the child should participate verbally. I might have been more successful if I had helped the parents focus on teaching comprehension, but with only nonverbal responses by the child. This child could then have had the benefits of the parents' tremendous enthusiasm and talent, but without as much pressure to talk. One might say that my error was in how I approached their family style. I asked a "high-key" family to interact in a "low-key" fashion.

Cultural Differences

Home visits are a good means for enlarging one's perspective about both language-delayed children and their families. One such visit took place during dinnertime. It happened that the father's brother and his family were also present. All together, there were the four adults and five or six children. The meal looked and smelled absolutely delicious, especially in view of the fact that the clinician's job was to observe, not to join in dinner. Just as they were about to begin, the father's brother slapped a dollar bill on the table and said, "The first kid who's done gets the dollar." Before the clinician had time to think about what this behavior might mean, the father stood up and removed his belt. It was dark leather

with a brass buckle and his name tooled across the back. He laid it across the end of the table, saying sternly, "The first kid who makes any noise gets the belt." It took some time for the clinician to recover her objectivity after these two assaults on her middle-class values. Then she noticed that the children were enjoying themselves quietly and that they weren't stuffing themselves rapidly to win the dollar. No trauma appeared to have occurred, and the meal proceeded pleasantly. In retrospect, this family belonged to a cultural group within the United States in which family patterns are structured quite differently from the way they are in middle-class culture. It took considerable discipline on the clinician's part to avoid judging behavior in these two families in terms of her own middle-class values.

Cultural differences add an additional challenge in developing home interventions for language-delayed children. We are inclined to think that all families ought to operate the way ours do. Consequently, we are likely to evaluate families from different cultural backgrounds in terms of our own punctuations. For example, in my case, I expect children to be talkative around adults; I consider parental tactics such as those described above as being too heavy-handed. Caution is the watchword, however, in making such cross-cultural comparisons. Sluzki (1979) describes some of these contrasts in family functioning. As he notes, middle-class families are egalitarian in how they function, whereas many Chinese and Latino families are autocratic. Similarly, middle-class families emphasize long-term planning and a future orientation, in contrast to the short-term orientation that lower socio-economic groups have found adaptive. Again, Sluzki (1979) points out, independence is important in the members of middle-class families. Some other cultures, such as Arabs, Chinese, and southern Italians, favor mutual dependence, associating it with loyalty.

The family traditions in different cultures represent the wisdom of those cultures regarding childrearing, among other things. In consonance with the principle of equifinality, children become communicators in many different cultural environments. Nevertheless, the general principles of language learning still apply. Children must experience shared reference somehow; they must receive input and feedback; they must engage in some sort of performatory acts while the family provides a sufficiently responsive environment for language learning to occur. The point is that these processes will occur in ways that fit each family's cultural values, ways that are consonant with that family's construction of reality.

Return now to the idea of a "match" between a family and the type of intervention that is offered. There are two levels at which a certain type of intervention may not match a particular family's patterns and style. The intervention may run contrary to values that the individual family holds, as in the two examples cited earlier. On the other hand, an intervention may conflict with cultural patterns that are influential in the family's functioning. There is a good likelihood that such interventions will fail because they conflict with fundamental family values.

These situations require considerable skill on the clinician's part. You may not know which patterns are specific to a particular family and which represent cultural values. Building on Sluzki's (1979) ideas, the clinician should communicate that there are different ways to raise children, with none of them necessarily being right or wrong. Consequently, it does not seem appropriate for the clinician to come in with a "grand plan"

for all culturally different families. As with any family, the clinician's task is to help the family develop transactional patterns that will foster language growth, but these patterns will have to be valid in the cultural heritage of each family. The goal is for family members to encourage and accommodate the child's language-learning strategies in ways that are consonant with their values and construction of reality.

Another Example

Let us consider one more transcript now, to see how ideas for intervention can stem from observation of family interaction. The child, Hortense, is four and a half. She has very little expression and scored at the one-and-a-half to two-year level on tests of comprehension. The family lives in the country, where they run a small farm. They would best be described as lower middle class. In this transcript, the parents have been asked to help their daughter put a puzzle of a car together. See Sample 12 (page 296).

I was struck immediately in watching this family that the parents were having difficulty establishing joint reference with the child. They land on the car, but that's about all. It should be added that Hortense isn't helping much; she doesn't attend very well, and some of her responses are irrelevant. In addition, the parents frequently use an unproductive tactic: They ask questions that the child cannot answer. Hortense is using a few single words, and not always appropriately, and she is being asked what a car does and what she does in town. As in previous examples, the result is a transactional pattern that does not foster language development and does not appear very satisfying to anyone involved. During the session from which this sample was excerpted, the pattern of interactions is one in which the parents

Father: C'mere and see what Dad's got. In here.

Father: Get up on the chair. What is that? Huh?

Hortense: Chair.

Father: Chair. Look here. What's that?

Hortense: Cah [car].

Father: Car? What's a car do? Huh?

Father: What does a car do? Couldja tell Daddy?

Mother: Wh- what were you doin' in there? (gestures to another room)

Hortense: Cah [car].

Mother: Huh?

Hortense: Cah [car].

Mother: What were you doin' in the other room?

Hortense: (unintelligible)

Mother: Monkey? [There was no monkey in the other room.]

Hortense: Yeah.

Mother: Was there a monkey in there?

Mother: What was he doin?

Father: What is that?

Hortense: Cah [car].

Father: Car?

Hortense: Yeah.

Father: What does a car do? Huh?

Father: What does a car do? Do you know?

Hortense: Yeah.

Father: What's it do? Does it take you to town?

Hortense: Mhm.

Father: What do you do in town? Huh?

Hortense: (unintelligible)

Father: Huh?

Mother: Hortense.

Hortense: Hm.

Mother: What do you buy when you go to town?

Hortense: (unintelligible)

Mother: Huh?

Hortense: Tau [town].

Mother: Town. What d'you buy in town?

Hortense: Uy.

Mother: Why?

Hortense: Hm.

(A minute or so later, the father finishes the puzzle.)

Father: Lookit here. I got the car together.

Hortense: Ah.

Father: What is that?

Hortense: Cah [car].

Father: Car. What does a car do? Huh?

Hortense: Wowee.

Father: What kind of noise does a car make?

take turns trying to elicit talking from their daughter, with little continuity between them. One has the impression that the parents haven't had much practice in talking to children. Indeed, that turned out to be the case with this little girl. Both parents worked hard on the farm and didn't spend a lot of time with her.

A number of interventions could be fruitful here. The first goal we chose was to help Hortense and her parents develop means to establish joint reference more readily. In a related vein, it seemed important to help the parents become more responsive to the child, more sensitive to her communicative needs. These two goals were selected because they would contribute both to enhancing communication between parents and child and to developing transactional patterns that would accelerate Hortense's language learning. Facilitative play could accomplish both of these goals. Consequently, a contract was arranged with the parents in which we would teach them to engage in facilitative play with Hortense. The problem was defined to the parents as one in which they were having difficulty communicating with Hortense, a punctuation with which they readily agreed. Because of their busy life on the farm and their taciturn family style, we agreed that they would have only four play sessions at home per week. They learned the technique in a few days and had play sessions faithfully. Their talking in the sessions we observed was at times a little cumbersome, but the result was impressive. Hortense soon began to use a great many more words and occasional two-word combinations. As the parents discovered the power of modeling, they began to provide models at other times, such as meals and dressing. Hortense's vocabulary began to grow in those areas. A new contract was arranged in which the parents were to explore various "real-life" situations in which they could provide models regularly. A nice transactional pattern developed in which Hortense and her parents were able to validate each other as their communication expanded. Much of the day, however, Hortense was still alone. After a few months she was enrolled in kindergarten. She was soon identified as retarded and placed in a special education program emphasizing language. We lost contact with the family shortly afterward.

The above example is not intended to illustrate an ideal home intervention. It does show an intervention that is consonant with family theory and one that involves a mix of referential and relationship factors. Communication and language learning each enhanced the other. Other interventions would certainly have been possible. I invite you now to go back to Sandy, Linda, and Carol, the three examples presented earlier in this chapter, and speculate on what interventions might be most appropriate for those families.

Ethics Again

It should be clear that language trainers are not family therapists. If you feel the situation warrants it, make a referral. I recall a family with a language-delayed child who also had behavior problems. I asked to talk with the parents. They entered my office at the appointed time. Within sixty seconds they were in a bitter battle with each other. I tried to bring the topic back to their son, but they used my remarks as ammunition to hurl blame at each other. This situation was clearly outside the competence of a language clinician.

Other situations present other kinds of problems. Another language-delayed boy lived as follows. His mother brought him to the clinic. Along with the father, who was unemployed, they lived in a deteriorating trailer house in a rather unsavory neighborhood. Another couple, friends of the father, also lived there. Both of these individuals were heroin users. The mother, who had not received much education, worked two jobs to provide enough income to support the whole crew from month to month. Home intervention was simply not in the cards for this child. In fact, it was impressive that his mother brought him to the clinic at all.

One final example. This child, five years old and using single words only, had an intense attachment to her mother. Their relationship was one of enmeshment. The mother was very concerned about the child, but the father would have no contact with the clinic. He wouldn't even talk to me on the phone. According to the mother, he denied or ignored the whole problem. The child was very immature and untestable. As we got acquainted with her, we noticed that she was clumsy and had difficulty with fine motor coordination. We recommended a complete physical, including a neurological exam, but the parents refused. After literally twelve months of prodding, a medical evaluation was finally obtained. It turned out that the girl had cataracts in both eyes. Happily, her sight was restored through medical procedures. At the same time the attachment between mother and daughter lessened, and the child began to flower in school.

I do not describe these cases because of their emotional appeal, although there is much drama to be found in them. I cite them for two reasons. First, they illustrate that no child exists alone. It is of direct clinical importance to understand as much as we can about the family systems in which language-impaired children are learning to communicate. Second, in cases like the first one, we are ethically bound not to intervene in the marriage dispute. In cases like the other two, we may feel ethically bound to intervene, but we are restrained for other reasons. We cannot be all things to all people.

Conclusions

There is tremendous variety in how families operate. In fact, family theorists and researchers have been unable to define what a normal family is. This variety is nicely portrayed in the title of the book by Lewis, Beavers, Gossett, and Phillips (1976), *No Single Thread.* Add now the differences among language-impaired children and also the variations in how different clinicians operate. It must be concluded that there is no one way to work with parents. Consequently, I have described a set of general principles around which various home interventions can be built. These principles provide a framework for intervention that is consonant with what is known about how families function and that is complementary

with the principles for individual intervention discussed in earlier chapters.

The view of the clinician as problem solver is central here. Ideally, you will generate interventions that are tailored to each child and family. You may wish to begin by adapting strategies from the published literature. Eventually you will work out your own style. As you might predict, I recommend that you develop a broad perspective. Of course, you will be interested in improving specific aspects of each child's language skill. At the same time, though, focus on communication, both clear communication between you and the parents and also effective communication between parents and child. The latter means that we are dealing with transactional patterns, but not in some mysterious way. Rather, the attempt is to change the behavior of parents, child, or both, so that the result will be enhanced communication and language learning. Finally, I must underscore again the importance of self-esteem. Home intervention should build competence in both child and parents, and it should recognize parents as responsible change agents for their children.

CONCLUSIONS

There is a close relationship between this chapter and earlier portions of the book. Family theory is akin to relationship communication, iconic signs, negotiated meaning, punctuation, decision making, second-order change, and the like. It provides a framework for applying the transactional model in approaching language-impaired children. Language acquisition is truly a family process, in which the child's language-learning strategies and the parents' language-teaching strategies are melded together in reciprocal transactional patterns. There is direct evidence for the importance of these patterns in language delay. We may assume that family processes are related to the more subtle language impairments of older children, although this question has received little study.

Our focus in approaching families is on the transactional patterns involving the language-impaired child, although, of course, these patterns are inseparable from other aspects of the family system. We seek out these patterns, not with the intention of assigning blame, but because they will be the locus of intervention in the family. It therefore becomes important to observe family interaction, or at least that between parents and language-delayed children. Tape recording, verbatim transcripts, and videotaping are all useful here. At the same time, there is some danger of overinterpreting what you see and hear. A clinician cannot observe a family. A clinician can only observe a family-with-clinician. Just as with individual children, part of the family's behavior is in response to the clinician's presence. We can take this situation in stride, however, because it is only in the same family-with-clinician context that we can offer an intervention.

It is interesting, but not always necessary, to make home visits. There is good evidence that people do behave differently at home (Bronfenbrenner 1979), but beyond these empirical contrasts, there is a qualitative difference between home and the clinician's workplace. In the clinic or school we are in our fortress, and the parents and child come to us. Frequently we are surrounded by long hallways, waiting rooms, impersonal clinic rooms, and perhaps even institutional green paint. In the home we are in their fortress. A home is an expression of the people who live in it (Ruesch and Kees 1956); the clinician is

the outsider. So while we may see the parents and child differently in their own home, in addition, we may get a little of the feel they have in coming to our clinics and classrooms.

It is useful to try to understand the situation as the parents see it. For example, I have come to believe that many parents of language-delayed children view language as talking. They do not make the technical distinction between language and speech that we take for granted. Consequently, they may punctuate their role as one of eliciting talking from the child. The result is likely to be a high degree of constraint without much modeling. We have seen this pattern in some of the examples in this chapter. The parents are testing rather than teaching. Language learning, however, is like a savings account: you have to make a lot of deposits before you get any interest back. Therefore, I often teach parents facilitative play techniques, with the emphasis on modeling and input.

Just as with children, parents should be approached as active learners and decision makers. Given half an opportunity, they will frequently work out their own solutions. However, as illustrated in the preceding paragraph, they may not see that they have other alternatives available. In this they are no different from clinicians and teachers, except that we have the advantages of special training and an "objective" attitude. Parents may be trapped in transactional patterns that do not enhance language growth. They may not be aware of the possibilities of second-order change. Here it is worth considering Dearborn's advice again: If we want to understand these transactional patterns, we may have to intervene in them.

As we have seen, home intervention can take many forms. Most frequently it involves helping the parents in being responsive to the child's communicative efforts and in providing appropriate input to the child. Frequently, the parent training can be relatively brief, but it may take some time before the child begins to respond. Sharf (1972) concluded that one must follow a child for at least six months in order to be sure that that child's language skills are changing. Our intervention, then, may take on the flavor of Haley's (1976) good advice. Parents may accept it but not follow through, either because they don't see change in the child or because of other morphostatic processes in the family. Hopefully, of course, our interventions will be powerful enough that change will begin reasonably soon, but it is nevertheless important to maintain regular contact with parents and to monitor change in the child.

Home intervention is only appropriate when two conditions are met. First, the clinician should have a clear suspicion that something concrete can be accomplished in each family that is offered a home program. Home intervention should not be recommended routinely to all families just on general principles, any more than aspirin should be prescribed for all headaches. Second, if the family seems to have problems beyond those of language learning in a child, our language intervention by itself is not likely to be effective. We almost cannot avoid being drawn into larger family issues.

Virginia Satir, a noted family therapist, said once that she conducts each session with a family as if it were the last one. This perspective may be quite novel to us, with our background of working month after month with the same clients. However, it has much to offer. In adopting this punctuation, one minimizes the tendency to establish the parent in a dependency relationship under the clinician. Instead, the clinician must depend on the parents' own problem-solving skills. The parents are thus validated as competent people. In this view, our job becomes one of setting up some sort of second-order change, establishing a different transactional pattern between parents and child, and then letting them work out the details. Our follow-up contacts are more directed toward encouragement than continued instruction.

It should be clear that our understanding of children's language disorders as family phenomena is just beginning. Our interventions, too, then, must be tentative. I can only say, in my own case, that having begun working with families of language-impaired children, I will never go back to closeting myself with the children alone.

13

CONCLUSION: DESIGNS FOR INTERVENTION

I learned the word "metalog" from the writing of Gregory Bateson (1972). A metalog is a discussion of some problematic topic in which both the form of the discussion and its content carry a message about the topic. For example, consider a dialogue about how logical arguments disintegrate as they go along. This argument would itself become splintered and disorganized progressively through the dialogue, so that at the end it had indeed disintegrated. The form makes the same point as the content. It is my intention that this entire book be at least a mild form of metalog. Each chapter makes the most sense in the context of the other chapters, paralleling the message in the content that children's language disorders are best understood through an integration of the topics in the separate chapters. To the extent that this book really is a metalog, one should be able to take any chapter and weave a thread connecting it with all the other chapters. I leave that as an exercise for you to engage in the next time you are vacationing at the seashore or in the mountains.

I have argued that children's language, both normal and disordered, is based on interactions among four areas:

1. Concepts and rules, that is, knowledge of the world.
2. Information processing and perception, through which we gain knowledge of the world, including language, and through which we use that knowledge in communication.
3. Language, its structure and function, and its relationships with knowledge and communication.
4. Human relationships, which ultimately are defined as communication, but which also form the context for the development of language and communication; human relationships include child-clinician dyads, family systems, and other interpersonal situations.

For our purposes, the focal point of the reciprocal influences among these factors is intervention. We may still wonder, however, how to integrate these many factors together in a coherent fashion. One theme that runs through all of them is choice. Call it decision making, problem solving, cognitive strategies or whatever, language use always involves choice. Consequently, I have emphasized the child's active role in language learning and use. I have also alluded to the clinician as a problem solver, and in the preceding chapter I suggested a specific focus on problem solving. Let us now take a more careful look at intervention as a process based on problem solving by the clinician. My discussion will draw heavily from the work of Rubinstein (1975).

THE CLINICIAN AS PROBLEM SOLVER

In his masterful book Rubinstein (1975) discusses problem solving as it applies to many disciplines and areas of human functioning. While most of the book is relevant to intervention, at least in an abstract way, we will concentrate only on some of his general guidelines for problem solving.

We can begin with a common difficulty in problem solving. People may not use all the information they have available in solving a problem. This view may be a little novel to language trainers because we are used to thinking of ourselves as not knowing enough about the children we work with. Rubinstein suggests two ways in which we may not take advantage of available information. First, there may simply be more information than can be dealt with at one time. We are certainly familiar with this situation, with the many areas that are related to children's language impairments.

The second difficulty in using available information Rubinstein refers to as the ". . . introduction of unnecessary constraints" (1975, p. 10). We may limit our field of view, usually without awareness that we are doing so. We have met this problem before also. Recall that perception of reality is a subjective matter. Individuals develop their own constructions of reality, their own punctuations. These individual punctuations then guide further perceptions and actions. To break these constraints is to achieve second-order change, that is, to develop a different perspective. Rubinstein illustrates that such unnecessary constraints can be situational, for example, when a perceptual set prohibits a person from using an object in a novel way. We do not eat peas with a knife, even if we can dip the knife in honey. These constraints can be much more profound, however, as in the examples in the preceding chapter where parents persist in patterns of unproductive first-order change. In fact, as Rubinstein notes, one's whole world view constrains one to certain types of perceptions and solutions to problems.

In Chapter 11 we saw that, almost by definition, second-order change is difficult to achieve. There are no surefire methods for escaping one's perceptual constraints. Rubinstein emphasizes the importance of flexibility and of maintaining an attitude in which you look for unusual views and solutions. Reading and talking with colleagues can also help in expanding your awareness of alternatives. Once you do bypass some perceptual constraint, a new set of solutions becomes possible. As you work with these solutions, you develop skill in this area of problem solving, an area that was previously unavailable to you.

Let me mention a few examples of unnecessary constraints that have frequently been present in how clinicians approach language-disordered children. First, we have often focused intervention on vocabulary and syntax as ends in themselves, rather than as means for communication with other people. Another example stems from the linear cause-and-effect model. We may view "bad" behavior as representing emotional states within the child, rather than as relationship communication in response to the clinician's relationship tactics. Poor attention provides a third example. We can think of a child as having an attentional deficit, or we can think of a clinician as having a saliency deficit. In each of these examples, there is nothing specifically wrong with the first view, but it constrains the clinician to certain approaches. The second view increases the options available in developing possible solutions to the problem.

Guidelines for Problem Solving

Rubinstein (1975) suggests several principles in seeking solutions to problems. To begin with, get a general picture of the problem before exploring all the detail. One is reminded of the clinician who has many test scores, detailed information on which grammatical morphemes the child is using, and so on, but no understanding of the child as a communicating human being. In contrast, recall the sequence of assessment procedures described in Chapter 7. We begin with a very broad question: Is there a language impairment present? Assuming the answer is yes, we then explore in more detail through language sampling and perhaps additional standardized tests. On the basis of these results, we assess specific areas of difficulty through informal procedures. Finally, we attempt to understand these areas through exploratory teaching, in which we aim to tune our intervention to the child's behavior. All along, the sequence is one in which a more general picture guides the clinician to relevant details.

Rubinstein's second suggestion is to withhold judgment for a period of time. Avoid deciding on a course of action too early in the game. I have performed occasional "instant cures," where nonverbal children have flowered into talking in only a couple weeks of my magic method. Clearly, I had decided too quickly that these children needed intervention in the first place. In some work settings there may be temptation not to withhold judgment long enough, because of pressure to get the child evaluated and assigned to an intervention program. Exploratory teaching provides one safeguard here; the child can be tentatively placed, but assessment continues.

This observation brings us to another principle: a change in representation may help in problem solving. If we can change our perspective on a problem, see it in a new way, then we can sidestep some of the unnecessary perceptual constraints discussed earlier. If we represent grammatical structures as options to mean, rather than as linguistic rules, we see more directly their relevance to communication. If we represent nonverbal behavior as iconic relationship communication, we have a new perspective in which to understand what it means.

I have argued for a change in representation for our whole approach to children's language disorders. Typically, we think of problem solving as follows. Some question or problem exists, and we analyze that situation in order to develop a solution. In effect, we study the problem from the outside. This picture certainly fits the stereotype of problem solving in the sciences, or in detective novels, and in the use of standardized tests. A different representation of problem solving, however, is required in approaching language-impaired children and their parents, because the clinician is part of the problem. That is, part of their behavior is in response to us. That is why exploratory teaching looks both ways. More generally, the transactional model is a change in the representation of language problems from a linear cause-and-effect view. This change is paralleled by shifts in other fields, such as human development (Bronfenbrenner 1979) and family therapy (Keeney 1979).

Borrowing from Bertrand Russell, Rubinstein notes another important aspect of problem solving, namely, the will to doubt. Do not accept premises automatically. Consider the premises that all language-impaired children need to be taught vocabulary and grammar or that all clinical management should be based on structured contingency management. Similarly, think of the children mentioned in an earlier chapter who were identified as retarded and then treated on that premise, when actually they had hearing impairments. Again, consider the premise that most disadvantaged black youngsters are impoverished in language skills. Because of the will to doubt of various scholars and educators, that premise is now demonstrated to be false. In clinical work we must hold tentative our first impressions, our test results, and decisions about intervention. Notice that Rubinstein does not merely state that a potential for doubting exists. It is a *will* to doubt. We have a responsibility to question our premises and conclusions, especially when we are making decisions that affect other people's lives.

Models

Rubinstein strongly emphasizes the importance of models in problem solving. "A model is an abstract description of the real world; it is a simple representation of more complex forms, processes, and functions of physical phenomena or ideas" (1975, p. 192). Or, in a quote that speaks more directly to clinical problems, "A model is a simpler representation of the real world problem; it is supposed to help you" (1975, p. 15). A model, then, is a frame of reference for understanding some situation. It may be impossible to operate without some sort of model. That is, we construct our own individual views of reality. The perceptual sets and punctuations that we apply, then, may be considered models, even though we may not even be conscious of them. Given that it is not possible to behave without some sort of framework for viewing reality, it makes sense consciously and purposefully to develop the most powerful models we can regarding children's language disorders. If a model is helpful, we can employ it and refine it. If it turns out to be of little use, it will be discarded and we will begin again.

I have depended on models throughout this book, although they have taken different forms. Some have been represented through line drawings, such as the models of causation, the pragmatics model, and the model of communication space in Chapter 5. Others have been in the form of a table, such as the summary of the microcosmic matrix in Chapter 8. Still others have been stated more implicitly, such as the description of various types of concepts and rules in Chapter 1 and the family system in Chapter 12. Some models are downright vague, as in my references to the child's language-learning strategies.

Rubinstein notes that models may have two functions. They can help in understanding a problem, and they can help in prediction. Partly they accomplish these functions through simplifying. They help provide the general picture mentioned earlier. Consider an example of the first function, providing understanding. Language structure is complex, but I described it through Pike's simple model of function, class, and position. This model was then fleshed out through the microcosmic matrix. The result is not a grammar of English, but a model for approaching English grammar. However, grammar needs to be related to language use, which I have modeled as decision making. Accordingly, Pike's functions are modeled as options-to-mean, and meaning is modeled as differentiating among alternatives. All of these models oversimplify, but in so doing they highlight crucial aspects of language structure and use. We take whichever ones are relevant to the clinical problems at hand.

For a second example, take the referential communication paradigm. It is not intended as an intervention technique, although it has been used that way. Rather, it is a model in which to develop and evaluate different interventions. Note that it depends on the models of language in the preceding paragraph, but places them in a model of teacher-child interaction, with senders, receivers, and feedback. My goal, again, is to identify fundamental elements of language learning and instruction so that we can be aware of them in interventions of various types. The referential communication paradigm can also be related to a more idealized model of language learning and intervention, in which the child's performatory acts are matched by a responsive environment.

The second function of models discussed

305

by Rubinstein is prediction. A set of developmental milestones may be considered a predictive model. If individual children are achieving their milestones at appropriate ages, we make the prediction that they will continue to develop normally. I have emphasized that prediction is at the very heart of assessment and of choosing intervention strategies as well.

It should be clear that there can be more than one model for a given phenomenon, and that some models are better than others. We select models according to our values, a topic we will return to in a moment. I have my ideas about what is important in language intervention, and I have represented those ideas through models. Regardless of my values, however, a model is only good if it works. Thus, models are evaluated by applying them. If a model helps understanding or prediction, then it is a useful model. If one model helps more than another, then it is a better model, although this again relates to one's values, one's model of objective truth. Consequently, I urge you to take any of the models from this book and other sources and evaluate them in the context of your own work in language intervention. Look for models that help clarify things for *you*.

There is a danger with models, however, and that is that they can lead to unnecessary constraints such as those warned against earlier. For example, I have argued that the linear cause-and-effect model does just that. Ideally, we could develop a model for each situation. Perhaps we do so unconsciously, but there is not always the time to develop separate models for each occasion. Further, if a model is worth anything, it should be applicable in many situations. Consequently, I have emphasized models that are broad and flexible. Again I mention the transactional model, the pragmatics model,

and the referential communication paradigm. There is "room" in these models for many different solutions. What they do is clarify the issues to be dealt with. While they may imply general directions for intervention, they do not specify what should be done. That is the problem for the clinician to solve.

Values

One of the models of problem solving that Rubinstein (1975) discusses consists of three stages. In the first stage we describe the present state or situation. In the second stage, we define the goal state, the situation we would like to achieve. The third stage involves determining the processes that will bridge the gap between the present state and the goal state. This model of problem solving is also a reasonable model for language intervention. We describe the present status of the child, select appropriate intervention goals, and then decide which intervention strategies might be most effective. Of course, we also evaluate those strategies as we work with the child. In sum, we think of language intervention as a logical, rational process. We employ the scientific method: We gather data carefully, make hypotheses and decisions on the basis of that data, and evaluate our results with additional data.

As Rubinstein points out, however, much of this model depends not only on the scientific method, but also on values. How we define a child's present status, how we define goals and select intervention strategies, all of these derive ultimately from values that we hold. A value is usually defined in terms of benefit and utility. This benefit may be ethical, economic, esthetic, or it may be of value in other ways. Further, values may benefit the individual, or they may relate to larger segments of society.

Imagine that a mother and preschool child are playing together and that several people are watching. One observer might say, "Isn't that cute? I just love children." Another might say, "That child is very bright." Still another could say, "That mother sure loves her little boy." A language clinician who was watching would be likely to say something like, "Wow! Lotta good language there." Each of these observers interprets the situation from a different set of values. Similarly, as clinicians, our values direct our perceptions and our selection of models to work from. We make these choices on the basis of what we think is important and relevant, but importance and relevance are related to the values we hold.

Consider, for example, the definition of the term "children's language disorders." In the Introduction I said that a language disorder is a "significant impairment of the use of language," one that is "over and above (the) difficulties with language we all encounter . . ." (p. 4) Significant to whom? In what circumstances? How far over and above? These questions ultimately involve value judgments. We use the trappings of science, such as developmental norms and standardized tests, and we look at means and standard deviations in interpreting scores, but these techniques only help us make a value decision: How does one define "language disorder"?

We face other value decisions routinely. Of course we want to help all children maximize their development, but what does that mean? Should we adopt what I refer to as the missionary model and attempt to bring all children to perfection? Rubinstein states that, "Values are benefit oriented and can be assessed by a cost-benefit function in which cost represents effort and energy expended for the realization of a value" (1975, p. 475). How can we define this function

when we are talking about individuals who are impaired in language, an area that is so fundamental in human activity? Is it better to invest our energies in a larger number of moderately language-impaired children for whom the prognoses are good, or should we invest more of those energies in a smaller number of more severely impaired children with less optimistic prognoses? Is it fair to assume that an individual's prognosis is poor in the first place? Similarly, how do we determine when intervention should be concluded? Such questions exemplify the cost-benefit value judgments that we repeatedly face.

Behavioral science is a rich resource in developing intervention strategies. Even here, though, values are important, because they influence the types of strategies individual clinicians will choose. Some lean toward play, some get close to psychotherapy, others function more directly as teachers, and so on. While clinicians and trainers may develop data and theoretical arguments to support their positions, these positions stem ultimately from values those individuals hold. Behavior modification provides an example of how values influence the selection of intervention strategies. People who support this approach have produced miles of data demonstrating its power and success. Still, some individuals vigorously oppose contingency management and decry its pellet-popping paraphernalia. It should be clear that data are rarely the issue here; it is a question of values, of what one thinks is important in dealing with other people.

There have been occasional efforts to demonstrate that clinicians and researchers are really the same. Both gather data, make hypotheses and test them; both are committed to rigor, and so on. These arguments have merit, but they miss the point. The scientific method is not enough. Its purpose is to serve values. Let me put the matter in a different light. One time I participated in a series of discussions about whether clinical work is an art or a science. After due deliberation it was concluded that clinical work is a scientific enterprise. I remember accepting that decision as the common wisdom but having vague reservations about it. Over a year later it finally dawned on me why I had doubts: There is an art to being a good scientist.

I am certainly not arguing against behavioral science. Rather, I am trying to place it in a larger perspective. Through the scientific method we can measure differences among individuals. However, it is a value judgment to say that some of those differences are problems or disorders. The questions of dialect and bilingualism illustrate this situation nicely. Dialects can be described precisely through linguistic science. If a child is having difficulty in school that seems to be related to dialect or bilingualism, however, the decisions about what should be done will be based as much or more on values as on scientific information. It is not unusual that child, teacher, language clinician, and parent may all approach such decisions from quite different sets of values. Is it any wonder that discussions of dialect and bilingualism have often been so emotional?

We are led in one more direction. Values are the basis for the general policy decisions that result from our political process. These policy decisions include the allocation of resources to serve special populations and the identification and selection of those groups. I do not mean that we should lobby for language in some self-serving way. Rather, following Bronfenbrenner (1979), there is value in increased interaction be-

tween social policy makers and professionals who serve special groups.

Rubinstein refers to values succinctly as the problem of problems: What do we think is important? What problems should we tackle and how should we approach them? We must explore questions of value, of utility and relevance, with as much energy as those of science. Values are the ultimate basis for our decisions about language-impaired children and for our very existence as language clinicians.

DESIGNS FOR INTERVENTION

It follows from the previous section that my model of the language clinician is neither that of healer nor that of behavioral engineer. Rather, I see the clinician as a problem solver. This problem solving rests on the following foundation. First, we are guided by linear logic, including the principles of problem solving described above, and by various models, strategies, and techniques for language intervention. Second, we are guided by our intuitions about human behavior and human relationships. Finally, we are guided by values about what we should try to accomplish, what approaches are appropriate, and so on.

In this book I have discussed a variety of models and principles for understanding children's language disorders and for intervention. In addition, I have described various techniques illustrating possible applications of these models and principles. However, I have not presented a Monolithic Metamodel, an ultimate plan for intervention. Why? First, as has been indicated several times, individual differences among children are so great that it is hard to imagine an approach that would be effective with all. In my experience at least, a strategy that works beautifully with some children is likely to fail miserably with others. Second, there are also individual differences among clinicians and trainers, as discussed in the preceding section. Two clinicians may work with very similar children but treat them differently. Their choices of treatment are influenced by the values they hold. Both may still be successful, because of the principle of equifinality. Accordingly, I have presented different models and metaphors to guide intervention. While I see them as a coherent whole, other language clinicians may choose to emphasize one area more than another.

In other words, I leave the final decisions about the design of intervention to you. If you've read this far, however, it seems to me that you are entitled to my opinions on this matter. Following my own values, I base my interventions on two assumptions. My first premise is that children are active learners; given an appropriate context, they will learn on their own. At least, we do not have to teach everything. My second premise is that we can best understand how children develop as communicators through the transactional model. This view focuses attention on the reciprocal patterns between child and environment, rather than on the child alone; it denies the view that the language disorder is wholly within the child.

At this point I urge you to call up your will to doubt. Do these premises make sense? Are there situations where they do not apply?

Given these two premises, the goal of intervention is to devise transactional patterns in which the child will grow as a language user. Exploratory teaching is a good framework in which to pursue this goal. On a theoretical level, it provides a direct link between a model of causation and a model for intervention. From the problem-solving point of view, it allows us to withhold judgment as we explore various alternatives. On a practical level, it emphasizes the decision-making or problem-solving activity of the clinician, but places that problem solving in the context of the reciprocal influences between child and clinician. We can view this situation as one in which the clinician attempts to respond to the child in ways that enhance the child's language skill, rather than concentrating only on how the child responds to the clinician. Thus, the child changes as the clinician changes. In the same way, the clinician changes as the child changes. The clinician searches for changes that lead to language growth in the child. The child is searching, too.

Now let's look more specifically at the options for intervention that I've described: language as structure and content, language as relationship communication, and language as part of the family system. People all the way from Einstein to John Mitchell (President Nixon's Attorney General) have said: Watch what we do, not what we say. After viewing videotapes of my own work with language-impaired children, I'm afraid I have the same problem. I do not always do what I say I do. Nevertheless, let me attempt to outline the strategy I think I follow.

Relationships and Communication

I begin by concentrating on relationship factors, because relationship decisions are "meta" to linguistic decisions. We have to begin with a relationship context in which the child is willing to attend and to attempt to communicate. This focus has been known traditionally as building rapport. It may also be thought of as developing motivation. In any case, it is a reciprocal process; how the child behaves depends on how you behave. At first, this view seems to complicate matters, but ultimately it is a blessing. You can always change your behavior, using different activities, altering the amount of structure, and so forth. This is the nature of exploratory teaching. With many children there are no particular difficulties in developing an appropriate relationship context for language learning. If interacting with the clinician is autotelic for the child, a constructive relationship can usually be negotiated. With some children, however, it will be necessary to employ more powerful relationship tactics, such as reframing or contingency management.

Exploration of relationship factors raises another issue. There are several possibilities for intervention inherent in the transactional model. Can we accomplish change most effectively through working with the parents or the child or both? This decision will depend on each child's specific situation. Frequently, we cannot know which alternative would truly be best, and so we make a decision based partly on obtained information, but heavily on our own values. My prejudice is to work directly with parents. The younger the child is, the more important home intervention becomes. I want to enhance the parents' language-teaching strategies in order to stimulate and take advantage of the child's language-learning strategies.

But what is at the core of these parental strategies and child strategies? For the most part, they are not consciously aimed at language teaching or language learning. Their goal is successful communication. This is the reason that I emphasize ecological validity so much. It is why I do not want to train parents as mini-clinicians. *Effective communication is the best language teacher*. Language is learned in the service of communication, not the other way around. In addition, effective communication is self-validating. Consequently, I want to help parents to generate appropriate messages to their children and to "read" each child's behavior as insightfully as possible. Teaching parents facilitative play techniques is a useful way to approach this process. The choice of facilitative play, however, stems largely from my value system. Other possibilities exist. For example, it might be fruitful to begin with structured referential communication tasks between parent and child.

Again it is time to exercise the will to doubt. Establishing a certain kind of transactional pattern between parent and child or clinician and child will not guarantee language growth. It is your responsibility as clinician to monitor the child's communicative behavior carefully enough to know what effects you are having. With some children there may be little change, or a rate of change that is too slow to be acceptable. Judgments about what is appropriate change are difficult to make, however. As pointed out previously, even rapid language learning cannot necessarily be measured by the day or the week.

Training Specific Options

In any case, there will be children for whom you will want to provide more specific training of language options. Depending on their values, some clinicians will prefer to start with specific training in the first place, perhaps in addition to a relationship intervention. Others will add specific training in cases where they are dissatisfied with the child's rate of progress with a less focused approach or if it proves difficult to change the prevailing transactional patterns. Note that these "failures" could be described as situations in which the clinician could not see an appropriate second-order change. We cannot despair too long about these perceptual constraints, however. They are an inescapable aspect of human experience. As discussed earlier, we can overcome some of them through learning and practice.

In moving to more specific training, the same principle as above applies: Effective communication is the best language teacher. Therefore, in teaching vocabulary and grammatical options, I try to design my interventions around the referential communication paradigm. In this model, language learning arises from communication, because of the focus on using language options to differentiate among alternatives. As we have seen, the referential communication paradigm provides a basis for many varieties of language training. Our judgments about how training should be designed for a particular child will often end up a compromise between an emphasis on communication and ecological validity, and the amount of structure necessary to concentrate attention on specific aspects of language.

Here it is useful to note that structure is related to specificity of training. If we want to teach particular options such as modals or pronouns, then the transactions between clinician and child will have to be structured sufficiently that the focus is indeed on those options. In addition, however, structure is also related to the clinician's values. Some people need to know where they stand in their human relationships. In this regard, I value flexibility. I try to let the child's behavior lead me to establishing an appropriate level of structure. My perceptions are that I work with as little structure as I can and still be effective. If a child is not responding appropriately, however, and I

cannot think of a second-order change, I do not hesitate to move in with more direct control tactics as necessary.

It is time to invoke the will to doubt again. If a child's language use is not changing as a result of direct training, we obviously ask why. It is helpful here to review the ideals for intervention listed at the beginning of Chapter 10. Does the task have meaning and relevance to the child? Is there something in the transactional pattern we have negotiated that is getting in the way? Similarly, are the activities evoking active problem solving from the child? Are we providing an appropriately responsive environment for this activity by the child? Does the child find the activities appealing?

There are other possibilities as well. A child may not possess the concepts that are represented by the language options we are trying to teach. When I have doubts here, I turn to informal assessment and exploratory teaching. If it seems necessary to teach concepts, that will again involve active learning by the child and can be guided by the referential communication paradigm, so that conceptual development and language development enhance each other. In my judgment even very early cognitive skills, such as object permanence, can be taught this way. How many parents have not played games with their babies in which they hide an object, exclaiming, "All gone," and pop it out into view with, "Here it is!"

Finally we come to another set of possibilities—that the child is having difficulties with information processing and perceptual skills. I leave these areas till last because they are the most mysterious. As we have seen in Chapters 2 and 3, they are complex and poorly understood. Given this state of affairs, there can hardly be a clear-cut way to assess them, much less train them. The will to doubt enters in another way also. I have argued against viewing processing skills as distinct entities. To the extent that they become reified as explanatory principles, they put additional unnecessary constraints on our perceptions of children's language disorders. In my value system we are better off considering information processing and perception in the contexts in which they occur. What is important and relevant to me is how children use language in real communicative situations. In this context we are free to look at many possibilities in regard to a child who has difficulty with attention or memory span. At the same time, this perspective leads us back to the earlier steps in the problem-solving process I have been describing.

Summary

We have a variety of potential intervention goals, including emphasis on relationships, amount of talking, referential communication, and linguistic structures. The research on Head Start programs (summarized in Karnes and Teska 1975, Bronfenbrenner 1979, and elsewhere) is very instructive here. The conclusion of this research is essentially as follows: You get out what you put in. Programs that emphasize cognitive development are likely to produce gains in cognitive development. Those that highlight spontaneity and feelings of self-worth are inclined to produce gains in those areas. Head Start programs that stress academic skills similarly tend to enhance children's academic skills. Ultimately, then, the goals and success of any particular Head Start program are determined on the basis of values.

I believe that we are in a similar situation with children's language disorders. It follows that there will be different approaches to intervention as long as there are clinicians and trainers with different values. The question of the "best" approach must be seen in that light. First, what do you want to accomplish? Then, how best can you go about it? There are a lot of goals that I value, so I am led to experimenting with combinations of approaches. For example, a program might include a group situation emphasizing facilitative play, individual instruction focusing on referential communication, and a home program based on fostering transactional patterns that enhance language growth in the child. A combined approach has its own problems, however. In addition to the practical logistics involved, it is essential that the three components of the program truly complement each other, rather than acting independently, or even working against each other. The program would have to be flexible so that the relative weight of these three areas could vary with each child's situation. A preschooler might require heavier attention to home intervention. A language-impaired youngster in junior high school might need more individual instruction. Ultimately, however, both need not only increased skill with language. To be effective communicators, they also need opportunities, practice, and the desire to use that skill in dealing with other people in the world.

The will to doubt is particularly important in an imperfect process such as language intervention. No matter what intervention strategies you employ, keep one eye on the child's overall communicative behavior. No matter how structured and specific your procedures, stay aware of the broader picture. Is there any generalization of what the child is learning? Is whatever you are doing having any impact on how the child uses language in daily life?

CONCLUSIONS

One can legitimately ask if an integrated approach to children's language disorders is possible. Rubinstein (1975) notes that one difficulty in problem solving is that people may not use all the available information. Surely that must be the case with language clinicians. As I have outlined it, we are dealing with conceptual development, information processing, language structure, language function, human relationships, and the family system all at once. We have decision making by the child, problem solving by the clinician, the transactional model, the pragmatics model, and the referential communication paradigm. We have options-to-mean, differentiation among alternatives, and function, class, and position. There are iconic signs, validation, relational concepts, morphostatic processes, enmeshment, and disengagement. On and on. I see no way that anyone could be actively aware of so many variables at the same time.

My response to this situation is twofold. First, I take a systems view. The different factors involved in children's language disorders interact in various ways. We can look at subsets of factors, such as conceptual development, relationship tactics, or parental language teaching strategies. I have tried to develop metaphors to make clear the relations between these subsystems and language use. Second, I frankly do not try to be aware of everything at once. As already discussed, I view the clinician as a problem solver. In making decisions about intervention for a particular child, then, I consider one subsystem at a time. The sequence that I think I use was described in the preceding section. I thought of developing a flow chart to illustrate this sequence, but I decided not to because I did not want to make the process appear more formal or rigid than it really is. As Rubinstein also points out, flexibility is a key to successful problem solving. You may wish to develop some flow charts of your own. I encourage you to make several. Each should make sense, but perhaps from different sets of values. Indeed, how are we to integrate the many factors related to children's language impairments?

Language is at the heart of human experience. It involves all three of the great spheres through which we interact with the world: the sensate, the rational, and the emotional. It is sensate because it depends on and guides perception, the receiving and recognizing of information through the senses. It is rational both because it is a coherent linguistic system and because logic and reason depend on language. Finally, it is emotional, not only because we use language to express emotions, but because language use both forms human relationships and derives from human relationships. Childhood is the crucible in which these three ways to know the world develop in each individual. The study of children's language disorders is of value at two levels, then. First, we can explore the question of how best to serve language-impaired children and their families. Second, because disorders of language highlight the human processes in which they occur, we can learn a little more about ourselves. Let us begin.

CODA

One of my first experiences in working with families of language-impaired children was with a kindergarten boy who was severely language delayed and who also demonstrated a number of autistic characteristics. The child and his family lived in a modest home in a suburban area. A student trainee and I made several visits to the home. We worked primarily with the boy's mother, emphasizing general child management as well as language learning. The child made remarkable improvement, with a truly dramatic lessening of disruptive behavior, matched with equally impressive gains in language use. His mother developed much more successful ways of dealing with him and seemed to show a lot of insight into the situation. Our last visit had two major goals. We reviewed the procedures she had found effective, and we acknowledged and praised the accomplishments that both mother and son had achieved. As we were leaving, we stopped for a moment on the front porch. The mother, the trainee, and I all stood there congratulating and thanking each other. As I turned to go, the mother touched me on the arm and said, "You know, my boy is always worse when there's a full moon."

GLOSSARY

Note: Words appearing in italics are defined in their own entries in the glossary.

abstract concept. A concept based on relations among other concepts, rather than on physical characteristics. Synonymous with *relational concept.* Compare *concrete concept.*

adaptability. In family theory, the flexibility with which a family approaches problem solving and family functioning.

analysis-by-synthesis. A theory of perception emphasizing active processing by the individual; aspects of the stimulus and its context are combined with previous information in memory in recognizing stimuli and in anticipating upcoming stimuli.

aphasia. In adults, the loss or impairment of language functions due to brain damage.

auditory processing disorder. Inability to recognize, retain, comprehend, or otherwise deal with auditory stimuli; not due to hearing loss or mental retardation.

autotelic activity. Any activity in which the goals and rewards are intrinsic in the activity itself; activity that is done for its own sake rather than for some external purpose.

bottom-up processing. In perception, processes based on assigning meaning to a stimulus by beginning with the physical characteristics of that stimulus rather than more abstract knowledge of the stimulus and the situation. Compare *top-down processing.*

childhood aphasia. Impairment of language skills in children which is thought to be due to brain dysfunction present from infancy, but without clearly identifiable signs of brain damage; separate from mental retardation, emotional disturbance, and hearing loss. Compare *aphasia.*

chunking. In *information processing,* the tendency to group stimulus items together and then treat each group as one item.

clause. A group of words containing both a subject and a verb or predicate.

clause types. A subclassification of clauses in terms of different relations among subject, verb, and object, including *transitive, intransitive,* and *equative* clauses. Compare *clause variations.*

clause variations. A subclassification of clauses in terms of form of statement to a listener, including declarative, interrogative, and imperative clauses. Compare *clause types.*

clinical method. Procedures for assessment (derived from Piaget's work) in which the techniques for eliciting and evaluating responses vary with the child and the examiner; the goal is to insure that the child has had opportunities to adequately demonstrate knowledge in the area being assessed. Compare *standardized testing.*

closed system. In *general systems theory,* a *system* which is self-contained; it operates without being influenced by other systems around it. Compare *open system.*

cognitive strategy. Any technique used by an individual for processing information in perception, memory, and problem solving; these techniques may be consciously employed, or they may be used without awareness.

cohesion. In family theory, the degree of closeness and support that the members of a family demonstrate toward each other.

complement. In *grammar,* a word or words that fill out or complete another grammatical structure such as a subject or verb.

concrete concept. A concept based on the physical characteristics of some type of object. Compare *core concept* and *relational concept.*

constraint. In human relations, any activity by one person that limits or interrupts the activity of another.

contextualized speech. Speech that is related to, or dependent on, the nonverbal situation in which it takes place. Compare *decontextualized speech.*

contingency management. A set of procedures for changing specific behaviors by controlling the events that occur before and after those behaviors, especially through the use of reinforcement.

continuous system. In communication theory, a *system* in which each symbol blends or grades into the next, rather than each being uniquely different from the others. Compare *discrete system.*

contrast set. In referential meaning, the group of items from which one item is being identified; these items may be physically present or only implied.

coordination. Any grammatical process in which grammatical structures are joined, but both structures remain at the same grammatical level, rather than one performing a grammatical function within the other. Compare *subordination.*

core concept. A concept developing from the use of some type of object, rather than from that object's appearance or other physical characteristics. Compare *concrete concept.*

criterial attribute. Any characteristic of a concept that must be present in an object in order for that object to be classified as a member of that particular concept.

decontextualized speech. Talking that is independent of the nonverbal situation in which it occurs. Compare *contextualized speech.*

defining context. A situation in which some type of object is used so that the relations between the object and the situation can be seen, thus allowing the development of a core concept for that object. See *core concept.*

denotation. In *semantics,* the concept or concepts regularly represented by a word; denotation is general, rather than being specific to individual utterances. Compare *reference* and *sense.*

discrete system. In communication theory, a *system* in which each symbol is clearly distinguishable from each other symbol. Compare *continuous system.*

discursive system. In communication theory, a *system* in which all senders and receivers share approximately the same knowledge of what each symbol in the system means. Compare *nondiscursive system.*

ecological validity. The importance or relevance of something to a person's life; in language training, the degree to which the training situation parallels the child's life situation, and the degree to which specific items that are trained are relevant and useful in the child's daily life.

episodic memory. Memory of an entire event or stimulus as a whole, rather than through analyzing its parts or reconstructing it in memory. Compare *semantic memory.*

equative. A clause in which subject and *complement* are joined by a linking verb, such as a form of BE; subject and complement are equated in some way.

equifinality. In *general systems theory,* the idea that the same outcome can derive from different beginnings, and the same beginning can lead to different outcomes.

explanatory principle. An idea that is used to explain various phenomena, but which is not well understood itself, for example, gravity.

exploratory teaching. An approach to assessment in which different procedures are used with a child in order to evaluate both the child's skill and knowledge, and the effectiveness of each procedure with that child; assumes that child's knowledge can be inferred from the response to teaching.

extinction. In *contingency management,* the elimination of a response in an individual, especially through a process of witholding rewards for that response.

facilitative play. An approach for encouraging talking, based on following the child's lead in play and minimizing *constraint.*

family homeostasis. In family theory, the tendency of a family to maintain a balance among its members, and maintain the family *system.*

general systems theory. The view that physical, biological, and social *systems* can all be understood with the same set of principles; a description of those principles; and the view that most events can only be understood in relation to the *system(s)* in which they occur.

generative transformational grammar. An approach to linguistics emphasizing the speaker's intuitions about language, rather than objective observation; stresses theoretical analysis rather than

description. Compare *structural linguistics* and *semantically based grammar.*

grammar. Commonly used in linguistics to refer to the combination of both *morphology* and *syntax* in the study of how utterances are structured.

grammatical morpheme. A *morpheme* which represents a grammatical function more than an area of semantic content. Compare *lexical morpheme.*

grammatical operator. Any device that helps show the relations among the components of an utterance, such as melodic contour, stress, and *grammatical morphemes.*

Hubbell's law. People take themselves too seriously.

iconic sign. A message whose physical form is parallel in some way with its meaning, such as a map or a smile; the relationship between an iconic sign and its meaning is one of similarity, rather than the arbitrary relationship between a word and its meaning.

information processing. Human abilities involved in receiving, interpreting, remembering, and transmitting stimuli.

intentional memory. Purposely attempting to retain some information in memory. Compare *involuntary memory.*

intransitive. A verb or *clause* that does not take an object; the action or thought of the verb does not take effect on some object or person. Compare *transitive.*

interactional model. A view of the cause of developmental disorders in which the disorder is the result of a combination of specific factors in the environment and the child's constitution. Compare *linear cause-and-effect model* and *transactional model.*

intuitive information. Knowledge gained without the conscious application of rational logic, as in emotions and meditative states. Compare *linear knowledge.*

involuntary memory. Retaining information in memory without any purposeful attempt to do so; also called automatic memory. Compare *intentional memory.*

language sample. An excerpt of a child's talking used for assessment, primarily of grammatical skills.

lexical morpheme. A *morpheme* that represents some area of semantic content, rather than grammatical function. Compare *grammatical morpheme.*

linear cause-and-effect model. A view of the cause of developmental disorders in which there is a direct relationship between specific precipitating factors (causes) and specific disorders (effects). The cause may be in the child's constitution or in the environment. Compare *interactional model* and *transactional model.*

linear knowledge. Information of the rational, logical type exemplified by western science. Compare *intuitive information.*

long-term memory. Retention of information in memory for long periods of time, or permanently. Compare *short-term memory.*

major sentence. In *language sampling,* any utterance which is likely to reflect some of the child's knowledge of grammatical structure; an utterance that is grammatically productive. Compare *minor sentence.*

mediation. In memory, any process in which one type of stimulus is used to represent another type; for example, names of objects may be retained rather than images of the objects themselves.

metacommunication. Communication about other communication; usually refers to signals about how messages should be interpreted, or about the human relationships in which those messages are being communicated.

metarule. A higher-level rule that governs the use of one or more lower-level rules.

microcosmic matrix. The *system* used in this text for analyzing grammatical skill through *language sampling;* it focuses on a microcosm or miniature grammar of essential aspects of English structure; this miniature *grammar* provides a matrix or framework for further language learning.

minor sentence. In *language sampling,* any utterance which probably does not reflect the child's knowledge of grammatical structure, such as an interjection or a stereotyped phrase; an utterance that is not grammatically productive. Compare *major sentence.*

mnemonic device. Any technique purposely used to aid retention of information in memory.

model. (1) A framework or perspective for understanding some situation or set of situations. (2) A stimulus presented to a child with the intent that the child learn that stimulus, such as a particular utterance. (3) The individual who demonstrates that stimulus, for example, the person who says the utterance to be learned.

morpheme. A minimal unit of meaning or grammatical pertinence in a language; may be a word, or an affix such as tense or plural markers.

morphogenic process. In *general systems theory,* any influence that tends to cause change in a *system.* Compare *morphostatic process.*

morphology. In linguistics, the study of *morphemes,* the minimal units of meaning and grammatical pertinence in language.

morphostatic process. In *general systems theory,* any influence that tends to maintain a *system* in the same state. Compare *morphogenic process.*

negotiated meaning. A process in which, through repeated use, symbols or communicative acts develop specific meanings shared by two or more persons; these meanings may or may not be apparent to a casual observer.

nondiscursive system. In communication theory, a *system* in which the meanings of the symbols used by the sender are not standardized or shared by the receiver. Compare *discursive system.*

open system. In *general systems theory,* a *system* whose functions are influenced by other systems around it. Compare *closed system.*

perceptual attribute. Any physical characteristic of an object that can be apprehended through one or more of the senses.

performatory act. Any behavior in which the child interacts with the environment in ways that reveal alternatives that are available in the environment.

phonology. In linguistics, the study of speech sounds and sound systems in language.

picture-utterance match. A type of task commonly used in psycholinguistic research and in language assessment and training in which the subject must equate particular utterances with particular pictures.

pragmatics. (1) In linguistics, the study of language use, rather than the study of language forms in the abstract; pragmatics relates the structure of utterances to their contexts and the intentions of the speaker. (2) The effects of communication on behavior.

punctuation. In human relations, the tendency of each individual to view an interaction or situation from his or her own perspective, rather than as a complex whole.

reference. In *semantics,* the use of an utterance by a speaker to designate a particular relationship, object, or event; reference is always specific to an individual utterance and situation. Compare *denotation* and *sense.*

referential communication. Interaction in which one person talks about particular stimuli so that a second person can determine precisely which stimuli the first speaker has in mind.

reframing. In psychotherapy, a strategy in which the behavior or attitudes of the client are interpreted or described in such a way that the client is forced to change his or her view of that behavior or situation.

reification. Treating an abstraction as if it were a real thing or concrete entity.

relational concept. A concept based on relations among other concepts, rather than on physical characteristics; synonymous with *abstract concept.* Compare *concrete concept.*

relationship tactic. Verbal or nonverbal behavior used by one person to influence other people's behavior or attitudes in a particular relationship; may or may not be consciously employed.

responsive environment. A situation which maximizes the child's opportunities to learn by participating in or interacting with that situation; encourages and clarifies the child's learning in the situation.

retrieval. Active attempts to recall information from memory.

rule. A statement of a relationship among a set of concepts; may or may not be descriptive of some aspect of human behavior.

saliency. The strength of a stimulus in attracting and holding the attention of an observer.

semantically based grammar. An approach to linguistic analysis in which grammatical structures are derived from the relations among underlying semantic functions, or *semantic roles.* Compare *structural linguistics* and *generative transformational grammar.*

semantic memory. Remembering an event

or stimulus by reconstructing it in memory; this reconstruction depends on previously learned concepts and language. Compare *episodic memory.*

semantic role. In *semantically based grammars,* an area of meaning that can be expressed through the *grammar,* such as agent, action, or location; a fundamental category of meaning in language.

semantics. In linguistics, the study of meaning as it relates to language.

sense. In *semantics,* the meaning of a word in terms of its relations with other words, rather than its relations with concepts outside the language *system.* Compare *reference* and *denotation.*

short-term memory. Retention of information in memory for brief periods of time, usually a few minutes or less. Compare *long-term memory.*

standardized testing. Procedures for assessment in which the techniques for eliciting responses from the child and the methods for evaluating those responses are specified in advance and are the same for all children. Compare *clinical method.*

structural linguistics. An approach to linguistics based on objective observation of utterances; emphasizes description and classification, but minimizes abstract interpretation. Compare *generative transformational grammar* and *semantically based grammars.*

subordination. Any process in which grammatical structures are combined, such that one structure performs a grammatical function within another structure. Compare *coordination.*

syntax. In linguistics, the study of sentence formation.

system. A group of things, ideas, or other entities and the relations among them; the group and the relations among its members are seen as a unified whole.

top-down processing. In perception, those processes based on predicting what a stimulus might be, filling in the details of a stimulus, and in general constructing perceptions from previous knowledge. Compare *bottom-up processing.*

transactional model. A view of the cause of developmental disorders in which a specific outcome evolves from continuing reciprocal influences between the child and the environment over time; these influences are not simply additive, but change each other as time goes on. Compare *linear cause-and-effect model* and *interactional model.*

transactional pattern. A characteristic way of relating among individuals, especially in families; these patterns are developed and maintained over time, and are specific to individual families and their members.

transitive. A verb or *clause* that takes an object; the action or thought of the verb takes effect on some object or person. Compare *intransitive.*

validation. In family theory, the process of recognizing and encouraging growth, maturity, and personal worth in one person by another.

wholeness. In *general systems theory,* the idea that each part of a *system* influences other parts, so that change in one part of a system is always associated with change elsewhere in the system.

REFERENCES

Allen, L. 1965. Toward autotelic learning of mathematical logic by the *WFF'N PROOF* games. In Mathematical Learning, eds., Morrisett, L., and Vinsonhaler, J. *Monographs of the Society for Research in Child Development,* 30, serial no. 99.

Anderson, B. 1975. *Cognitive Psychology.* New York: Academic Press.

Annett, J. 1969. *Feedback and Human Behavior.* Baltimore: Penquin Books.

Apter, M. 1970. *The Computer Simulation of Behavior.* New York: Harper and Row.

Arlt, P., and Goodban, M. 1976. A comparative study of articulation acquisition as based on a study of 240 normals, aged three to six. *Language, Speech and Hearing Services in Schools,* 7, 173–180.

Asher, J. 1977. Children learning another language: a developmental hypothesis. *Child Development,* 48, 1040–1048.

Baldwin, T., McFarlane, P., and Garvey, C. 1971. Children's communication accuracy related to race and socioeconomic status. *Child Development,* 42, 345–357.

Baltaxe, C., and Simmons, J. 1975. Language in childhood psychosis: A review. *J. Speech and Hearing Disorders,* 40, 439–458.

Bandler, R., and Grinder, J. 1975. *The Structure of Magic.* Palo Alto, Cal.: Science and Behavior Books.

Bandura, A. 1969. *Principles of Behavior Modification.* New York: Holt, Rinehart and Winston.

Bandura, A., and Harris, M. 1966. Modification of syntactic style. *J. Experimental Child Psychology,* 4, 341–352.

Baratz, J. 1968. Language in the economically disadvantaged child: a perspective. *Asha,* 10, 143–145.

Baratz, J., and Shuy, R. 1969. *Teaching Black Children to Read.* Washington, D.C.: Center for Applied Linguistics.

Bateson, G. 1972. *Steps to an Ecology of Mind.* New York: Ballantine.

Battig, W. 1975. Within-individual differences in "cognitive" processes. In *Information Processing and Cognition,* ed., Solso, R. Hillsdale, New Jersey: Lawrence Erlbaum Associates.

Bayles, K. 1974. The Effects of Constraint and Nonconstraint on the Verbal Behavior of Preschool Children. Unpublished Master's Thesis, Arizona State University.

Bedrosian, J., and Prutting, C. 1978. Communicative performance of mentally retarded adults in four conversational settings. *J. Speech and Hearing Research,* 21, 79–95.

Beilin, H. 1976. Constructing cognitive operations linguistically. In *Advances in Child Development and Behavior,* Vol. 11, ed., Lipsitt, L. New York: Academic Press.

Belmont, J., and Butterfield, E. 1969. The relations of short-term memory to development and intelligence. In *Advances in Child Development and Behavior,* Vol. 4, eds., Lipsitt, L., and Reese, H. New York: Academic Press.

Belmont, J., and Butterfield, E. 1971. What the development of short-term memory is. *Human Development,* 14, 236–248.

Berko-Gleason, J. 1958. The child's learning of English morphology. *Word,* 14, 150–177.

Bernstein, B. 1970. A sociolinguistic approach to socialization: with some reference to educability. In *Language and Poverty: Perspectives on a Theme,* ed., Williams, F. Chicago: Markham.

Bernstein, B. 1973. *Class Codes and Control.* London: Routledge and Kegan Paul.

Berry, M. 1969. *Language Disorders of Children.* Englewood Cliffs, N.J.: Prentice-Hall.

Bertalanffy, L., von. 1968. *General Systems Theory: Foundations, Development, Application.* New York: G. Braziller.

Bever, T. 1970. The cognitive basis for linguistic structure. In *Cognition and the Development of Language,* ed., Hayes, J. New York: John Wiley and Sons.

Birch, H., and Belmont, L. 1965. Auditory-visual integration, intelligence and reading ability in school children. *Perceptual and Motor Skills,* 20, 295–305.

Birch, H., and Lefford, A. 1963. Intersensory development in children. *Monographs of the Society for Research in Child Development,* 28, serial no. 89.

Blank, M. 1975. Eliciting verbalization from young children in experimental tasks: a methodological note. *Child Development,* 46, 254–257.

Bloom, L. 1970. *Language Development: Form and Function in Emerging Grammars.* Cambridge, Mass.: MIT Press.

Bloom, L. 1974. Talking, understanding, and thinking. In *Language Perspectives—Acquisition, Retardation, and Intervention,* eds., Schiefelbusch, R., and Lloyd, L. Baltimore: University Park Press.

Bloom, L., and Lahey, M. 1978. *Language Development and Language Disorders.* New York: John Wiley and Sons.

Bloom, L., Lightbown, P., and Hood, L. 1975. Structure and variation in child language. *Monographs of the Society for Research in Child Development,* 40, serial no. 160.

Bohannon, J., and Marquis, A. 1977. Children's control of adult speech. *Child Development,* 48, 1002–1008.

Bolinger, D. 1975. *Aspects of Language,* 2nd edition, New York: Harcourt Brace Jovanovich.

Braine, M. 1976. Children's first word combinations. *Monographs of the Society for Research in Child Development,* 41, serial no. 164.

Briggs, D. 1970. *Your Child's Self Esteem: The Key to His Life.* Garden City, N.Y.: Doubleday.

Broen, P. 1972. The verbal environment of the language-learning child. *Asha Monographs,* no. 17.

Bronfenbrenner, U. 1974. Experimental human ecology: A reorientation to theory and research on socialization. Paper presented at the 82nd Annual Convention of the American Psychological Association, New Orleans.

Bronfenbrenner, U. 1975. Nature with nurture: A reinterpretation of the evidence. In *Race and IQ,* ed., Montague, A. New York: Oxford University Press.

Bronfenbrenner, U. 1979. *The Ecology of Human Development.* Cambridge, Mass.: Harvard University Press.

Brown, A. 1975. The development of memory: knowing, knowing about knowing, and knowing how to know. In *Advances in Child Development and Behavior,* Vol. 10, ed., Reese, H. New York: Academic Press.

Brown, R. 1973. *A First Language.* Cambridge, Mass.: Harvard University Press.

Brown, R., and Bellugi, U. 1964. Three processes in the acquisition of syntax. *Harvard Educational Review,* 34, 133–151.

Brown, R., and Hanlon, C. 1970. Derivational complexity and order of acquisition in child speech. In *Cognition and the Development of Language,* ed., Hayes, J. New York: John Wiley and Sons.

Bruner, J. 1966. On cognitive growth. In *Studies in Cognitive Growth,* eds., Bruner, J., Oliver, R., and Greenfield, P. New York: John Wiley and Sons.

Bruner, J. 1972. Nature and uses of immaturity. *American Psychologist,* 27, 687–708.

Bruner, J. 1975. The ontogenesis of speech acts. *J. Child Language,* 2, 1–19.

Bruner, J., Goodnow, J., and Austin, G. 1956. *A Study of Thinking.* New York: John Wiley and Sons.

Bruner, J., Jolly, A., and Sylva, K. 1976. *Play: Its Role in Development and Evolution.* New York: Basic Books.

Buckley, W. 1967. *Sociology and Modern Systems Theory.* Englewood Cliffs, N.J.: Prentice-Hall.

Buium, N., Rynders, J., and Turnure, J. 1974. Early maternal linguistic environment of normal and Down's syndrome language-learning children. *American Journal of Mental Deficiency,* 79, 52–58.

Buros, O. 1972. *Mental Measurements Yearbook,* Seventh Edition, New Brunswick, N.J.: Rutgers University Press.

Butterfield, E., and Belmont, J. 1975. Assessing and improving the cognitive functions of mentally retarded people. In *Psychological Issues in Mental Retardation,* eds., Bialer, I., and Sternlicht, M. Chicago: Aldine.

Butterfield, E., Wambold, C., and Belmont, J. 1973. On the theory and practice of improving short-term memory. *American Journal of Mental Deficiency,* 77, 654–669.

Byrne, M. 1978a. Appraisal of child language acquisition. In *Diagnostic Methods in Speech Pathology,* Second Edition, eds., Darley, F., and Spriestersbach, D. New York: Harper and Row.

Byrne, M. 1978b. Supplementary case history outline: language development and its disorders. In *Diagnostic Methods in Speech Pathology,* Second Edition, eds., Darley, F., and Spriestersbach, D. New York: Harper and Row.

Byrne, M., and Shervanian, C. 1977. *Introduction to Communicative Disorders.* New York: Harper and Row.

Caldwell, B. 1978. *Home Observation for Measurement of the Environment.* Little Rock, Ark: University of Arkansas at Little Rock, mimeographed.

Carrow, E. 1973. *Test for Auditory Comprehension of Language,* Fifth Edition. Austin, Tex.: Learning Concepts.

Cazden, C. 1970. The Situation: A neglected source of social class differences in language use. *J. Social Issues,* 26, 35–60.

Chafe, W. 1970. *Meaning and the Structure of Language.* Chicago: University of Chicago Press.

Chafe, W. 1972. Discourse structure and human knowledge. In *Language Comprehension and the Acquisition of Knowledge,* eds., Carroll, J., and Freedle, R. Washington, D.C.: V.H. Winston & Sons.

Chalfant, J., and Scheffelin, M. 1969. *Central Processing Dysfunctions in Children,* Bethesda, Md.: U.S. Department of Health, Education and Welfare.

Chandler, M., Greenspan, S., and Barenboim, C. 1974. Assessment and training of role-taking and referential communication skills in institutionalized emotionally disturbed children. *Developmental Psychology,* 10, 546–553.

Chapman, R., and Miller, J. 1975. Word order in early two- and three-word utterances: does production precede comprehension? *J. Speech and Hearing Disorders,* 18, 355–371.

Chomsky, C. 1969. *The Acquisition of Syntax in Children from Five to Ten.* Cambridge, Mass.: MIT Press.

Chomsky, N. 1957. *Syntactic Structures.* Paris: Mouton.

Chomsky, N. 1965. *Aspects of the Theory of Syntax.* Cambridge, Mass.: MIT Press.

Chomsky, N. 1972a. *Language and Mind, enlarged ed.* New York: Harcourt Brace Jovanovich.

Chomsky, N. 1972b. *Studies on Semantics in Generative Grammar.* Paris: Mouton.

Clevenger, T., and Matthews, J. 1971. *The Speech Communication Process.* Glenview: Scott, Foresman.

Condon, W., and Ogston, W. 1967. A segmentation of behavior. *J. Psychiatric Research,* 5, 221–235.

Condon, W., and Sander, L. 1974. Neonate movement is synchronized with adult speech: interactional participation and language acquisition. *Science,* 183, 99–101.

Cook-Gumperz, J. 1977. Situated instructions: language socialization of school age children. In *Child Discourse,* eds., Ervin-Tripp, S., and Mitchell-Kernan, C. New York: Academic Press.

Cooper, F. 1972. How is language conveyed by speech? In *Language by Ear and by Eye,* eds., Kavanagh, J., and Mattingly, I. Cambridge, Mass.: MIT Press.

Cooper, J., and Ferry, P. 1978. Acquired auditory verbal agnosia and seizures in childhood. *J. Speech and Hearing Disorders,* 43, 176–184.

Courtright, J., and Courtright, I. 1976. Imitative modeling as a theoretical base for instructing language-disordered children. *J. Speech and Hearing Research,* 19, 655–663.

Courtright, J., and Courtright, I. 1979. Imitative modeling as a language intervention strategy: The effects of two mediating variables. *J. Speech and Hearing Research,* 22, 389–402.

Craik, F., and Lockhart, R. 1972. Levels of processing: A framework for memory research. *J. Verbal Learning and Verbal Behavior,* 11, 671–684.

Craik, F., and Tulving, E. 1975. Depth of processing and the retention of words in episodic memory. *J. Experimental Psychology: General,* 104, 268–294.

Cramblit, N., and Siegel, G. 1977. The verbal environment of a language-impaired child. *J. Speech and Hearing Disorders,* 42, 474–482.

Crystal, D., Fletcher, P., and Garman, M. 1976. *The Grammatical Analysis of Language Disability.* New York: Elsevier.

Curtis, J. 1970. Segmenting the stream of speech. In *The First Linconland Conference on Dialectology,* eds., Griffith, J., and Miner, L. University, Ala. University of Alabama Press.

Curtiss, S. 1977. *Genie: A Psycholinguistic Study of a Modern-Day "Wild Child."* New York: Academic Press.

Dale, P. 1976. *Language Development,* Second Edition, New York: Holt, Rinehart and Winston.

Darley, F. 1978. The case history. *In Diagnostic Methods in Speech Pathology,* Second Edition, eds., Darley, F., and Spriestersbach, D. New York: Harper and Row.

Darley, F, ed. 1979. *Evaluation of Appraisal Techniques in Speech and Language Pathology.* Reading, Mass.: Addison-Wesley.

Denes, P., and Pinson, E. 1973. *The Speech Chain.* Garden City, N.Y.: Anchor Books.

Denney, D. 1973. Modification of children's information processing behaviors through learning: A review of the literature. *Child Study Journal Monographs,* 3, 1–22.

Deutsch, M. 1965. The role of social class in language development and cognition. *American Journal of Orthopsychiatry,* 35, 78–88.

Dever, R. 1972. A comparison of the results, of a revised version of Berko's Test of

Morphology with the free speech of mentally retarded children. *J. Speech and Hearing Research,* 15, 169–178.

Dever, R. 1978. *TALK: Teaching the American Language to Kids.* Columbus: Ohio: Charles E. Merrill.

Dickson, W., Hess, R., Miyake, N., and Azuma, H. 1979. Referential communication accuracy between mother and child as a predictor of cognitive development in the United States and Japan. *Child Development,* 50, 53–59.

Donaldson, M., and Wales, R. 1970. On the acquisition of some relational terms. In *Cognition and the Development of Language,* ed., Hayes, J. New York: John Wiley and Sons.

Duchan, J., and Erickson, J. 1976. Normal and retarded children's understanding of semantic relations in different verbal contexts. *J. Speech and Hearing Research,* 19, 767–776.

Dumont, M. 1968. *The Absurd Healer: Perspectives of a Community Psychiatrist.* New York: Viking Press.

Dunn, L. 1965. *Peabody Picture Vocabulary Test.* Circle Pines, Minn.: American Guidance Service.

Eimas, P. 1974. Linguistic processing of speech by young infants. In *Language Perspectives—Acquisition, Retardation and Intervention,* eds., Schiefelbusch, R., and Lloyd, L. Baltimore: University Park Press.

Eisenson, J. 1972. *Aphasia in Children.* New York: Harper and Row.

Elardo, R., Bradley, R., and Caldwell, B. 1977. A longitudinal study of the relation of infants' home environments to language development at age three. *Child Development,* 48, 595–603.

Elias, M. 1973. Disciplinary barriers to progress in behavior genetics: defensive reactions to bits and pieces. *Human Development,* 16, 119–132.

Ervin-Tripp, S. 1977. Wait for me, roller skate! In *Child Discourse,* eds., Ervin-Tripp, S., and Mitchell-Kernan, C. New York: Academic Press.

Ervin-Tripp, S., and Mitchell-Kernan, C. 1977. Introduction. In *Child Discourse,* eds., Ervin-Tripp, S., and Mitchell-Kernan, C. New York: Academic Press.

Farber, B. 1960. Family organization and crisis: Maintenance of integration in families with a severely mentally retarded child. *Monographs of the Society for Research in Child Development,* 25, serial no. 75.

Feuerstein, M., Ward, M., and LeBaron, S. 1979. Neuropsychological and neurophysiological assessment of children with learning and behavior problems: a critical appraisal. In *Advances in Clinical Child Psychology,* Vol. 2, eds., Lahey, B., and Kazdin, A. New York: Plenum Press.

Fillmore, Charles. 1968. The case for case. In *Universals in Linguistic Theory,* eds., Bach, E., and Harms, R. New York: Holt, Rinehart and Winston.

Fishbein, H., and Osborne, M. 1971. The effects of feedback variations on referential communication of children. *Merrill-Palmer Quarterly,* 17, 243–250.

Flavell, J. 1970. Developmental studies of mediated memory. In *Advances in Child Development and Behavior.* Vol. 5, eds., Reese, H., and Lipsitt, L. New York: Academic Press.

Fodor, J., Bever, T., and Garrett, M. 1974. *The Psychology of Language.* New York: McGraw-Hill.

Frankenburg, W., and Dodds, J. 1967. The Denver Developmental Screening Test. *J. of Pediatrics,* 71, 181–191.

Fromberg, D. 1976. Syntax model games and language in early education. *J. of Psycholinguistic Research,* 5, 245–260.

Fromberg, D. 1977. *Early Childhood Education: A Perceptual Models Curriculum.* New York: John Wiley and Sons.

Fry, D. 1970. Speech reception and perception. In *New Horizons in Linguistics,* ed., Lyons, J. Baltimore: Penguin Books.

Furth, H. 1970. *Piaget for Teachers.* Englewood Cliffs, N.J.: Prentice-Hall.

Furth, H., and Wachs, H. 1974. *Thinking Goes to School: Piaget's Theory in Practice.* New York: Oxford University Press.

Gagné, R. 1970. *The Conditions of Learning,* Second Edition. New York: Holt, Rinehart and Winston.

Gallagher, J. 1975. Perception. In *The Application of Child Development Research to Exceptional Children,* ed., Gallagher, J. Reston, Va.: The Council for Exceptional Children.

Garfinkel, R., and Thorndike, R. 1976. Binet item difficulty then and now. In *Child Development,* 47, 959–965.

Gesell, A. 1940. *The First Five Years of Life: A Guide to the Study of the Preschool Child.* New York: Harper and Row.

Glucksberg, S., and Danks, J. 1975. *Experimental Psycholinguistics, An Introduction.* Hillsdale, New Jersey: Lawrence Erlbaum Associates.

Glucksberg, S., Hay, A., and Danks, J. 1976. Words in utterance contexts: Young children do not confuse the meanings of *same* and *different. Child Development,* 47, 737–741.

Glucksberg, S., and Krauss, R. 1967. What do people say after they have learned to talk? Studies of the development of referential communication. *Merrill-Palmer Quarterly,* 13, 309–316.

Glucksberg, S., Trabasso, T., and Wald, J. 1973. Linguistic structures and mental operations. *Cognitive Psychology,* 5, 338–370.

Goffman, E. 1967. *Interaction Ritual.* Garden City, N.Y.: Anchor Books.

Goldstein, K., and Scheerer, M. 1941. Abstract and concrete behavior: an experimental study with special tests. *Psychological Monographs,* 53, no. 239.

Gonzales, R. 1975. Towards an analysis of English-Spanish intrasentential code switching in Tucson. Unpublished paper.

Goodnow, J. 1972. Rules and repertoires, rituals and tricks of the trade: Social and informational aspects to cognitive and representational development. In *Information Processing in Children,* ed., Farnham-Diggory, S. New York: Academic Press.

Gotts, E. 1973. Some determinants of young children's attribute attending. *Merrill-Palmer Quarterly,* 19, 261–273.

Greenspan, S., Burka, A., Zlotlow, S., and Barenboim, C. 1975. A manual of referential communication games. *Academic Therapy,* 11, 97–106.

Grinder, J., and Bandler, R. 1976. *The Structure of Magic II.* Palo Alto, Cal.: Science and Behavior Books.

Guralnick, M., and Paul-Brown, D. 1977. The nature of verbal interactions among handicapped and nonhandicapped preschool children. *Child Development,* 48, 254–260.

Haas, W., and Wepman, J. 1974 Dimensions of individual difference in the spoken syntax of school children. *J. Speech and Hearing Research,* 17, 455–469.

Hagen, J., Jongeward, R., and Kail, R. 1975. Cognitive perspectives on the development of memory. In *Advances in Child Development and Behavior,* Vol 10, ed., Reese, H. New York: Academic Press.

Haley, J. 1963. *Strategies of Psychotherapy.* New York: Grune and Stratton.

Haley, J. 1976. *Problem Solving Therapy.* San Francisco: Jossey-Bass.

Haley, J., and Hoffman, L. 1967. *Techniques of Family Therapy.* New York: Basic Books.

Hall, A., and Fagen, R. 1956. Definition of system. *General Systems,* 1, 18–28. Reprinted in *Modern Systems Research for the Behavioral Scientist,* ed., Buckley, W. Chicago: Aldine, 1968.

Halliday, M. 1973. *Explorations in the Functions of Language.* London: Edward Arnold.

Halliday, M. 1975. Learning how to mean.

In *Foundations of Language Development: A Multidisciplinary Approach,* Vol. I, eds., Lenneberg, E., and Lenneberg, E. New York: Academic Press.

Harris, S. 1975. Teaching language to nonverbal children—with emphasis on problems of generalization. *Psychological Bulletin,* 82, 565–580.

Hayakawa, S. 1949. *Language in Thought and Action.* New York: Harcourt Brace Jovanovich.

Hayes, J. 1972. The child's conception of the experimenter. In *Information Processing in Children.* ed., Farnham-Diggory, S. New York: Academic Press.

Hedrick, D., Prather, E., and Tobin, A. 1975. *Sequenced Inventory of Communication Development.* Seattle: University of Washington Press.

Hockett, C. 1960. The origins of speech. *Scientific American,* 203, 88–96.

Hodgson, W. 1969. Misdiagnosis of children with hearing loss. *J. of School Health,* 39, 570–575.

Holland, A. 1975. Language therapy for children: some thoughts on context and content. *J. Speech and Hearing Disorders,* 40, 514–523.

Horowitz, F. 1969. Learning, developmental research, and individual differences. In *Advances in Child Development and Behavior,* Vol. 4, eds., Lipsitt, L., and Reese, H. New York: Academic Press.

Howe, C. 1976. The meanings of two-word utterances in the speech of young children. *J. Child Language,* 3, 29–47.

Hubbell, R. 1973. A study of verbal feedback in families with young children. Paper presented at the annual convention of the American Speech and Hearing Association, Detroit, Michigan.

Hubbell, R. 1977. On facilitating spontaneous talking in young children. *J. Speech and Hearing Disorders,* 42, 216–231.

Hunt, K. 1965. *Grammatical Structures Written at Three Grade Levels.* Champaign, Ill.: National Council of Teachers of English, Research Report No. 3.

Hunt, E. 1971. What kind of a computer is man? *Cognitive Psychology,* 2, 57–98.

Huttenlocher, J. 1974. The origins of language comprehension. In *Theories in Cognitive Psychology: The Loyola Symposium,* ed., Solso, R. Potomac, Md.: Lawrence Erlbaum.

Huttenlocher, J., and Burke, D. 1976. Why does memory span increase with age? *Cognitive Psychology,* 8, 1–31.

Ingram, D. 1974. The relationship between comprehension and production. In *Language Perspectives: Acquisition, Retardation, and Intervention,* eds., Schiefelbusch, R., and Lloyd, L. Baltimore: University Park Press.

Irwin, J., and Marge, M., eds. 1972. *Principles of Childhood Language Disabilities.* New York: Meredith.

Itard, J. 1962. *The Wild Boy of Aveyron.* Englewood Cliffs, N.J.: Prentice-Hall.

Jackson, D. 1965. The study of the family. *Family Process,* 4, 1–20.

Jackson, D. 1967. The eternal triangle. In *Techniques of Family Therapy,* eds., Haley, J., and Hoffman, L. New York: Basic Books.

Jenkins, J. 1971. Second discussant's comments: What's left to say? *Human Development,* 14, 279–286.

Johnson, K. 1970. *Teaching the Culturally Disadvantaged.* Palo Alto, Cal.: Science Research Associates.

Johnson, N. 1970. The role of chunking and organization in the process of recall. In *The Psychology of Learning and Motivation,* Vol. 4, ed., Bower, G. New York: Academic Press.

Johnson, W. 1946. *People in Quandaries: The Semantics of Personal Adjustment.* New York: Harper and Row.

Johnson-Laird, P. 1970. The perception and memory of sentences. In *New Horizons in Linguistics,* ed., Lyons, J. Baltimore, Md.: Penguin Books.

Johnson-Laird, P. 1974. Experimental psycholinguistics. In *Annual Review of Psy-*

chology, Vol. 25, eds., Rosenzweig, M., and Porter, L. Palo Alto, Cal.: Annual Reviews.

Jordan, T. 1978. Influences on vocabulary attainment: a five-year prospective study. *Child Development,* 49, 1096–1106.

Kagan, J. 1965. Impulsive and reflective children: The significance of conceptual tempo. In *Learning and the Educational Process,* ed., Krumboltz, J. Chicago: Rand McNally.

Karnes, M., and Teska, J. 1975. Children's response to intervention programs. In *The Application of Child Development Research to Exceptional Children,* ed., Gallagher, J. Reston, Va.: Council for Exceptional Children.

Katz, J., and Fodor, J. 1964. The structure of a semantic theory. In *The Structure of Language,* eds., Fodor, J., and Katz, J. Englewood Cliffs, N.J.: Prentice-Hall.

Keeney, B. 1979. Ecosystemic epistemology: An alternative paradigm for diagnosis. *Family Process,* 18, 117–129.

Kelly, E. 1967. *Assessment of Human Characteristics.* Belmont, Cal.: Brooks/Cole.

Kirk, S., and Kirk, W. 1971. *Psycholinguistic Learning Disabilities.* Urbana: University of Illinois Press.

Kirk, S., McCarthy, J., and Kirk, W. 1968. *Illinois Test of Psycholinguistic Abilities,* Revised Edition. Urbana: University of Illinois Press.

Kleffner, F. 1973. Hearing losses, hearing aids, and children with language disorders. *J. Speech and Hearing Disorders,* 38, 232–239.

Knobloch, H., and Pasamanick, B. 1974. *Gesell and Amatruda's Developmental Diagnosis,* Third Edition. New York: Harper and Row.

Knobloch, H., Stevens, F., and Malone, A. 1980. *Manual of Developmental Diagnosis.* Hagerstown, Md.: Harper and Row.

Korzybski, A. 1948. *Science and Sanity; An Introduction to Non-Aristotelian Systems and General Semantics,* Third Edition. Lakeville, Conn.: International Non-Aristotelian Library Publishing Co.

Koupernick, C., MacKeith, R., and Francis-Williams, J. 1975. Neurological correlates of motor and perceptual development. In *Perceptual and Learning Disabilities in Children,* Vol. 2, eds., Cruickshank, W., and Hallahan, D. Syracuse, N.Y.: Syracuse University Press.

Krauss, R., and Glucksberg, S. 1977. Social and nonsocial speech. *Scientific American,* 236, 100–105.

Kuczaj, S., II, and Maratsos, M. 1975. On the acquisition of *front, back* and *side. Child Development,* 46, 202–210.

Labov, W. 1969. *The Study of Nonstandard English.* Washington, D.C.: Center for Applied Linguistics.

Labov, W. 1972a. *Language in the Inner City.* Philadelphia: University of Pennsylvania Press.

Labov, W. 1972b. *Sociolinguistic Patterns.* Philadelphia: University of Pennsylvania Press.

Lahey, M., and Bloom, L. 1977. Planning a first lexicon: which words to teach first. *J. Speech and Hearing Disorders,* 42, 340–350.

Laing, R. 1970. *Knots.* New York: Random House.

Leach, E. 1972. Adult-child dialog: some diagnostic implications. *Acta Symbolica,* 3, 46–49.

Lee, L. 1969. *The Northwestern Syntax Screening Test.* Evanston, Ill.: Northwestern University Press.

Lee, L. 1974. *Developmental Sentence Analysis.* Evanston, Ill.: Northwestern University Press.

Lee, L., Koenigsknecht, R., and Mulhern, S. 1975. *Interactive Language Development Teaching: The Clinical Presentation of Grammatical Structure.* Evanston, Ill.: Northwestern University Press.

Lempert, H. 1978. Extrasyntactic factors affecting passive sentence comprehension by young children. *Child Development,* 49, 694–699.

Lenneberg, E. 1967. *Biological Foundations of Language.* New York: John Wiley and Sons.

Leonard, L. 1974. A preliminary view of generalization in language training. *J. Speech and Hearing Disorders,* 39, 429–436.

Leonard, L. 1975. Relational meaning and the facilitation of slow-learning children's language. *American Journal of Mental Deficiency,* 80, 180–185.

Leonard, L., Prutting, C., Perozzi, J., and Berkley, R. 1978. Nonstandard approaches to the assessment of language behaviors. *Asha,* 20, 371–379.

Levenstein, P. 1970. Cognitive growth in preschoolers through verbal interaction with mothers. *American Journal of Orthopsychiatry,* 40, 426–432.

Lewis, J., Beavers, W., Gossett, J., and Phillips, V. 1976. *No Single Thread: Psychological Health in Family Systems.* New York: Brunner-Mazel.

Lewis, M. 1975. The development of attention and perception in the infant and young child. In *Perceptual and Learning Disabilities in Children, Vol. 2:* eds., Cruickshank, W., and Hallihan, D. Syracuse, N.Y.: Syracuse University Press.

Lewis, M., and McGurk, H. 1972. Evaluation of infant intelligence. *Science,* 178, 1174–1177.

Liberman, A. 1970. The grammars of speech and language. *Cognitive Psychology,* 1, 301–323.

Lieberman, P. 1975. *On the Origin of Languages: An Introduction to the Evolution of Human Speech.* New York: Macmillan.

Lindsay, P., and Norman, D. 1972. *Human Information Processing.* New York: Academic Press.

Loban, W. 1963. *The Language of Elementary School Children.* Champaign, Ill.: National Council of Teachers of English, Research Report No. 1.

Loban, W. 1968. *Language Development During the School Years.* Lawrence, Kan.: University of Kansas Publications.

Lobitz, W., and Johnson, S. 1975. Parental manipulation of the behavior of normal and deviant children. *Child Development,* 46, 719–726.

Lovaas, O., Varni, J., Koegel, R., and Lorsch, N. 1977. Some observations on the non-extinguishability of children's speech. *Child Development,* 48, 1121–1127.

Lyons, J. 1968. *Introduction to Theoretical Linguistics.* Cambridge: Cambridge University Press.

Lyons, J. 1977. *Semantics,* Vol. I. Cambridge: Cambridge University Press.

McDavid, R. 1970. The sociology of education. In *Linguistics in School Programs,* ed., Marckwardt, A. Chicago: National Society for the Study of Education.

MacDonald, J. and Horstmeier, D. 1978. *Environmental Language Intervention Program.* Columbus, Ohio: Charles E. Merrill.

MacDonald, J., and Blott, J. 1974. Environmental language intervention: the rationale for a diagnostic and training strategy through rules, context, and generalization. *J. Speech and Hearing Disorders,* 39, 244–256.

MacDonald, J., Blott, J., Gordon, K., Spiegel, B., and Hartmann, M. 1974. An experimental parent-assisted treatment program for preschool language-delayed children. *J. Speech and Hearing Disorders,* 39, 395–415.

Madden, J., Levenstein, P., and Levenstein, S. 1976. Longitudinal IQ outcomes of the mother-child home program. *Child Development,* 47, 1015–1025.

Mahoney, G. 1975. Ethological approach to delayed language acquisition. *American Journal of Mental Deficiency,* 80, 139–148.

Marshall, N., Hegrenes, J., and Goldstein, S. 1973. Verbal interactions: mothers and their retarded children vs. mothers and their nonretarded children. *American*

Journal of Mental Deficiency, 77, 415–419.

Marslen-Wilson, W. 1975. Sentence perception as an interactive parallel process. *Science,* 189, 226–228.

Marslen-Wilson, W., and Welsh, A. 1978. Processing interactions and lexical access during word recognition in continuous speech. *Cognitive Psychology,* 10, 29–63.

Martin, B. 1975. Parent-child relations. In *Review of Child Development Research,* Vol. 4, ed., Horowitz, F. Chicago: University of Chicago Press.

Matthews, J. 1957. Speech problems of the mentally retarded. In *Handbook of Speech Pathology,* ed., Travis, L. Englewood Cliffs, N.J.: Prentice-Hall.

Meichenbaum, D. 1977a. *Cognitive Behavior Modification: An Integrative Approach.* New York: Plenum Press.

Meichenbaum, D. 1977b. Teaching children self control. In *Advances in Clinical Child Psychology,* Vol. 2., eds., Lahey, B., and Kazdin, A. New York: Plenum Press.

Meichenbaum, D., and Goodman, J. 1971. Training impulsive children to talk to themselves: a means of developing self control. *J. Abnormal Psychology,* 77, 115–126.

Mein, R. 1961. A study of the oral vocabularies of severely sub-normal patients II: grammatical analysis of speech samples. *J. Mental Deficiency Research,* 5, 52–59.

Menyuk, P. 1969. *Sentences Children Use.* Cambridge, Mass.: MIT Press.

Messer, S. 1976. Reflection-impulsivity: a review. *Psychological Bulletin,* 83, 1026–1052.

Miller, G. 1956. The magical number seven, plus or minus two: some limits on our capacity for processing information. *Psychological Review,* 63, 81–96.

Miller, G., Galanter, E., and Pribram, K. 1960. *Plans and the Structure of Behavior.* New York: Holt, Rinehart and Winston.

Miller, G., Heise, G., and Lichten, W. 1951. The intelligibility of speech as a function of the context of the test materials. *J. Experimental Psychology,* 41, 329–335.

Miller, G., and Isard, S. 1963. Some perceptual consequences of linguistic rules. *J. Verbal Learning and Verbal Behavior,* 2, 217–228.

Miller, J., and Yoder, D. 1974. An ontogenetic language teaching strategy for retarded children. In *Language Perspectives: Acquisition, Retardation and Intervention,* eds., Schiefelbusch, R., and Lloyd, L. Baltimore: University Park Press.

Miller, L. 1978. Pragmatics and early childhood language disorders: communicative interactions in a half-hour sample. *J. Speech and Hearing Disorders,* 43, 419–436.

Miller, W. 1964. The acquisition of grammatical rules by children. Paper presented at the annual meeting of the Linguistic Society of America, New York. Reprinted in *Studies of Child Language Development,* eds., Ferguson, C., and Slobin, D. New York: Holt, Rinehart and Winston, 1973.

Minuchin, S. 1974. *Families and Family Therapy.* Cambridge, Mass.: Harvard University Press.

Minuchin, S., Rosman, B., and Baker, L. 1978. *Psychosomatic Families—Anorexia Nervosa in Context.* Cambridge, Mass.: Harvard University Press.

Moerk, E. 1976. Processes of language teaching and training in the interactions of mother-child dyads. *Child Development,* 47, 1064–1078.

Moore, O. 1966. Autotelic responsive environments and exceptional children. In *Experience, Structure, and Adaptability,* ed., Harvey, O. New York: Springer.

Moore, O., and Anderson, A. 1968. The responsive environments project. In *Early Education,* eds., Hess, R., and Bear, R. Chicago: Aldine.

Moore, O., and Anderson, A. 1969. Some principles for the design of clarifying educational environments. In *Handbook of Socialization Theory and Research,* ed., Goslin, D. Chicago: Rand McNally.

Morehead, D., and Ingram, D. 1973. The development of base syntax in normal and linguistically deviant children. *J. Speech and Hearing Research,* 16, 330–352.

Morse, P. 1974. Infant speech perception: a preliminary model and review of the literature. In *Language Perspectives: Acquisition, Retardation and Intervention,* eds., Schiefelbusch, R., and Lloyd, L. Baltimore: University Park Press.

Moulton, W. 1970. The study of language and human communication. In *Linguistics in School Programs,* ed., Marckwardt, A. Chicago: National Society for the Study of Education.

Muma, J. 1978. *Language Handbook: Concepts, Assessment, Intervention.* Englewood Cliffs, N.J.: Prentice-Hall.

Murrell, S., and Stachowiak, J. 1965. The family group: development, structure, and therapy. *J. Marriage and the Family,* 27, 13–18.

Mysak, E. 1976. *Pathologies of Speech Systems.* Baltimore: Williams and Wilkins.

Naremore, R., and Dever, R. 1975. Language performance of educable mentally retarded and normal children at five age levels. *J. Speech and Hearing Research,* 18, 82–95.

Nation, J., and Aram, D. 1977. *Diagnosis of Speech and Language Disorders.* Saint Louis: C. V. Mosby.

National Society for Autistic Children. 1973. Working definition of autistic children. Brochure. Albany, New York: National Society for Autistic Children.

Nelson, K. 1973. Structure and strategy in learning to talk. *Monographs of the Society for Research in Child Development,* 38, serial no. 149.

Nelson, K. 1977. Facilitating children's syntax acquisition. *Developmental Psychology,* 13, 101–107.

Newell, A., and Simon, H. 1972. *Human Problem Solving.* Englewood Cliffs, N.J.: Prentice-Hall.

O'Donnell, R., Griffin, W., and Norris, R. 1967. *Syntax of Kindergarten and Elementary School Children: A Transformational Analysis.* Champaign, Ill.: National Council of Teachers of English, Research Report No. 8.

Olson, D. H., Sprenkle, D., and Russell, C. 1979. Circumplex model of marital and family systems: I. Cohesion and adaptability dimensions, family types and clinical applications. *Family Process,* 18, 3–28.

Olson, D. R. 1970a. *Cognitive Development.* New York: Academic Press.

Olson, D. R. 1970b. Language and thought: aspects of a cognitive theory of semantics. *Psychological Review,* 77, 257–273.

Olson, D. R., and Filby, N. 1972. On the comprehension of active and passive sentences. *Cognitive Psychology,* 3, 361–381.

Olswang, L., and Carpenter, R. 1978. Elicitor effects on the language obtained from young language-impaired children. *J. Speech and Hearing Disorders,* 43, 76–88.

Opie, I., and Opie, P. 1959. *The Lore and Language of School Children.* Oxford: The Clarendon Press.

Ornstein, R. 1972. *The Psychology of Consciousness.* San Francisco: W. H. Freeman.

Palmer, F. 1971. *Grammar.* Baltimore: Penguin Books.

Pasamanick, B., Knobloch, H., and Lilienfeld, A. 1956. Socioeconomic status and some precursors of neuropsychiatric disorders. *American Journal of Orthopsychiatry,* 26, 594–601.

Patel, P. 1973. Perceptual chunking, processing time and semantic information. *Folia Linguistica,* 6, 152–166.

Patterson, G., and Cobb, J. 1971. A dyadic analysis of aggressive behaviors. In *Minnesota Symposia on Child Psychology,*

Vol. 5, ed., Hill, J. Minneapolis: University of Minnesota Press.

Patterson, G., and Cobb, J. 1973. Stimulus control for classes of noxious behaviors. In *The Control of Aggression: Implications from Basic Research,* ed., Knutson, J. Chicago: Aldine.

Phillips, J. 1973. Syntax and vocabulary of mothers' speech to young children: age and sex comparisons. *Child Development,* 44, 182–185.

Piaget, J., and Inhelder, B. 1969. *The Psychology of the Child.* New York: Basic Books.

Pick, A., Frankel, D., and Hess, V. 1975. Children's attention: the development of selectivity. In *Review of Child Development Research,* Vol. 5, ed., Hetherington, E. Chicago: University of Chicago Press.

Pike, K. 1967. *Language in Relation to a Unified Theory of the Structure of Human Behavior. The Hague: Mouton.*

Prutting, C. 1979. Process \ 'präˌses \ n: The action of moving forward progressively from one point to another on the way to completion. *J. Speech and Hearing Disorders,* 44, 3–30.

Prutting, C., Gallagher, T., and Mulac, A. 1975. The expressive portion of the NSST compared to a spontaneous language sample. *J. Speech and Hearing Disorders,* 40, 40–48.

Rapaport, D., Gill, M., and Schafer, R. 1968. *Diagnostic Psychological Testing,* Revised Edition. New York: International Universities Press.

Raph, J. 1965. Language characteristics of culturally disadvantaged children: review and implications. *Review of Educational Research,* 35, 373–400.

Reed, E. 1975. Genetic anomalies in development. In *Review of Child Development Research,* Vol. 4, ed., Horowitz, F. Chicago: University of Chicago Press.

Rees, N. 1973. Auditory processing factors in language disorders: the view from Pro-

crustes' bed. *J. Speech and Hearing Disorders,* 38, 304–315.

Reitan, R. 1975. Assessment of brain-behavior relationships. In *Advances in Psychological Assessment,* Vol. 3, ed., McReynolds, P. San Francisco: Jossey-Bass.

Reitan, R., and Heineman, C. 1968. Interactions of neurological deficits and emotional disturbances in children with learning disorders: methods for differential assessment. In *Learning Disorders,* Vol. 3. Seattle: Special Child Publications.

Richer, J. 1975. Unwilling to relate. *New Behavior,* 17, 98–101.

Ridberg, E., Parke, R., and Hetherington, E. 1971. Modification of impulsive and reflective cognitive styles through observation of film-mediated models. *Developmental Psychology,* 3, 369–377.

Rommetveit, R. 1971. Words, contexts, and verbal message transmission. In *Social Contexts of Messages,* eds., Carswell, E., and Rommetveit, R. New York: Academic Press.

Rosch, E. 1973. On the internal structure of perceptual and semantic categories. In *Cognitive Development and the Acquisition of Language,* ed., Moore, T. New York: Academic Press.

Rosenthal, R., and Jacobson, L. 1968. Teacher expectations for the disadvantaged. *Scientific American,* 218, 19–23.

Rubinstein, M. 1975. *Patterns of Problem Solving.* Englewood Cliffs, N.J.: Prentice-Hall.

Ruesch, J. 1951. Communication and human relations: an interdisciplinary approach. In *Communication, the Social Matrix of Psychiatry,* Ruesch, J., and Bateson, G. New York: W. W. Norton.

Ruesch, J., and Bateson, G. 1951. *Communication, The Social Matrix of Psychiatry.* New York: W. W. Norton.

Ruesch, J., and Kees, W. 1956. *Nonverbal Communication.* Berkeley, Cal.: University of California Press.

Russell, C. 1979. Circumplex model of

marital and family systems: III. empirical evaluation with families. *Family Process,* 18, 29–45.

Rutter, M. 1979. Maternal deprivation, 1972–1978: New findings, new concepts, new approaches. *Child Development,* 50, 283–305.

Sameroff, A. 1975. Early influences on development: fact or fancy? *Merrill-Palmer Quarterly,* 21, 267–294.

Sameroff, A., and Chandler, M. 1975. Reproductive risk and the continuum of care-taking casualty. In *Review of Child Development Research,* Vol. 4, ed., Horowitz, F. Chicago: University of Chicago Press.

Sanders, D. 1977. *Auditory Perception of Speech: An Introduction to Principles and Problems.* Englewood Cliffs, N.J.: Prentice-Hall.

Satir, V. 1967. *Conjoint Family Therapy,* Revised Edition. Palo Alto, Cal.: Science and Behavior Books.

Scarr-Salapatek, S. 1975. Genetics and the development of intelligence. In *Review of Child Development Research,* Vol. 4, ed., Horowitz, F. Chicago: University of Chicago Press.

Scheflen, A. 1972. *Body Language and Social Order.* Englewood Cliffs, N.J.: Prentice-Hall.

Scheflen, A. 1974. *How Behavior Means.* Garden City, New York: Anchor Press.

Schlesinger, I. 1971. Production of utterances and language acquisition. In *The Ontogenesis of Grammar,* ed., Slobin, D. New York: Academic Press.

Scott, C., and Taylor, A. 1978. A comparison of home and clinic gathered language samples. *J. Speech and Hearing Disorders,* 43, 482–495.

Seitz, S. 1975. Language intervention—changing the language environment of the retarded child. In *Down's Syndrome: Research, Prevention, and Management,* eds., Koch, R. and Cruz, F. de la. New York: Bruner-Mazel.

Seitz, S., and Hoekenga, R. 1974. Modeling as a training tool for retarded children and their parents. *Mental Retardation,* 12, 28–31.

Seitz, S., and Marcus, S. 1976. Mother-child interactions: a foundation for language development. *Exceptional Children,* 42, 445–449.

Seitz, S., and Riedell, G. 1974. Parent-child interactions as the therapy target. *J. Communication Disorders,* 7, 295–304.

Sharf, D. 1972. Some relationships between measures of early language development. *J. Speech and Hearing Disorders,* 37, 64–74.

Shatz, M., and Gelman, R. 1973. The development of communication skills: modifications in the speech of young children as a function of listener. *Monographs of the Society for Research in Child Development,* 38, serial no. 152.

Shipley, E., Smith, C., and Gleitman, L. 1969. A study in the acquisition of language: free responses to commands. *Language,* 45, 322–342.

Siegel, G. 1963a. Adult verbal behavior in 'play therapy' sessions with retarded children. *J. Speech and Hearing Disorders Monograph Supplement,* No. 10, 34–38.

Siegel, G. 1963b. Verbal behavior of retarded children assembled with pre-instructed adults. *J. Speech and Hearing Disorders Monograph Supplement,* No. 10, 47–53.

Siegel, G. 1967. Interpersonal approaches to the study of communication disorders. *J. Speech and Hearing Disorders,* 32, 112–120.

Siegel, G., and Harkins, J. 1963. Verbal behavior of adults in two conditions with institutionalized retarded children. *J. Speech and Hearing Disorders Monograph Supplement,* No. 10, 39–46.

Sigel, I., and McBane, B. 1967. Cognitive competence and level of symbolization among five-year-old children. In *Disadvantaged Child,* Vol. 1, ed., Hellmuth, J. Seattle: Special Child Publications.

Simon, H. 1969. *The Sciences of the Artificial.* Cambridge, Mass.: MIT Press.

Simon, H. 1972. On the development of the processor. In *Information Processing in Children,* ed., Farnham-Diggory, S. New York: Academic Press.

Simon, H. 1974. How big is a chunk? *Science,* 183, 482–488.

Skeels, H. 1966. Adult status of children with contrasting early life experiences. *Monographs of the Society for Research in Child Development,* 31, no. 105.

Skeels, H., and Dye, H. 1939. A study of the effects of differential stimulation on mentally retarded children. *Proceedings and Addresses of the American Association on Mental Deficiency,* 44, 114–136.

Skeels, H., Updegraff, R., Wellman, B., and Williams, H. 1938. A study of environmental stimulation: an orphanage preschool project. *University of Iowa Studies in Child Welfare,* 15, no. 4.

Sloan, W. 1954. Progress report on special committee on nomenclature of the American Association on Mental Deficiency. *American Journal of Mental Deficiency,* 59, 345–351.

Slobin, D. 1973. Cognitive prerequisites for the development of grammar. In *Studies of Child Language Development,* eds., Ferguson, C., and Slobin, D. New York: Holt, Rinehart and Winston.

Sluzki, C. 1979. Migration and family conflict. *Family Process,* 18, 379–390.

Sluzki, C., and Verón, E. 1971. The double bind as a universal pathogenic situation. *Family Process,* 10, 397–410.

Snow, C. 1972. Mother's speech to children learning language. *Child Development,* 43, 549–565.

Snyder, L., and McLean, J. 1977. Deficient acquisition strategies: a proposed conceptual framework for analyzing severe language deficiency. *American Journal of Mental Deficiency,* 81, 338–349.

Snyder-McLean, L., and McLean, J. 1978. Verbal information gathering strategies: the child's use of language to acquire language. *J. Speech and Hearing Disorders,* 43, 306–325.

Starr, S. 1975. The relationship of single words to two-word sentences. *Child Development,* 46, 701–708.

Stremel, K., and Waryas, C. 1974. A behavioral-psycholinguistic approach to language training. In *Developing Systematic Procedures for Training Children's Language,* ed., McReynolds, L. *Asha Monographs,* 18.

Szasz, T. 1961. *The Myth of Mental Illness.* New York: Dell.

Taub, H., Goldstein, K., and Caputo, D. 1977. Indices of neonatal prematurity as discriminators of development in middle childhood. *Child Development,* 48, 797–805.

Templin, M. 1957. *Certain Language Skills in Children: Their Development and Interrelationships.* Minneapolis: University of Minnesota Press.

Torgesen, J. 1975. Problems and Prospects in the Study of Learning Disabilities. In *Review of Child Development Research,* Vol. 5, ed., Hetherington, E. Chicago: University of Chicago Press.

Turner, P. 1973. *Bilingualism in the Southwest.* Tucson, Ariz.: University of Arizona Press.

Turnure, J., Buium, N., and Thurlow, M. 1976. The effectiveness of interrogatives for prompting verbal elaboration productivity in young children. *Child Development,* 47, 851–855.

Tyack, D., and Gottsleben, R. 1974. *Language Sampling, Analysis and Training.* Palo Alto, Cal.: Consulting Psychologists Press.

Vasta, R., and Liebert, R. 1973. Auditory discrimination of novel prepositional constructions as a function of age and syntactic background. *Developmental Psychology,* 9, 78–82.

Washington, D., and Naremore, R. 1978. Children's use of spatial prepositions in two- and three-dimensional tasks. *J. Speech and Hearing Research,* 21,

151–165.

Watzlawick, P. 1976. *How Real Is Real?* New York: Random House.

Watzlawick, P. 1978. *The Language of Change.* New York: Basic Books.

Watzlawick, P., Beavin, J., and Jackson, D. 1967. *Pragmatics of Human Communication.* New York: W. W. Norton.

Watzlawick, P., Weakland, J., and Fisch, R. 1974. *Change: Principles of Problem Formation and Problem Resolution.* New York: W. W. Norton.

Webster, E. 1966. Parent counseling by speech pathologists and audiologists. *J. Speech and Hearing Disorders,* 31, 331–340.

Webster, E., ed. 1976. *Professional Approaches with Parents of Handicapped Children.* Springfield, Ill.: Charles C. Thomas.

Weiner, P., and Hoock, W. 1973. The standardization of tests: criteria and criticisms. *J. Speech and Hearing Research,* 16, 616–626.

Weir, R. 1962. *Language in the Crib.* The Hague: Mouton.

Weisberg, R. 1969. Sentence processing assessed through intrasentence word associations. *J. Experimental Psychology,* 82, 332–338.

Wepman, J., Jones, L., Bock, R., and Van Pelt, D. 1960. Studies in aphasia: background and theoretical formulations. *J. Speech and Hearing Disorders,* 25, 323–332.

Werner, E., Bierman, J., and French, F. 1971. *The Children of Kauai.* Honolulu: University of Hawaii Press.

Whitehurst, G. 1976. The development of communication: changes with age and modeling. *Child Development,* 47, 473–482.

Whitehurst, G., Novak, G., and Zorn, G. 1972. Delayed speech studied in the home. *Developmental Psychology,* 7, 169–177.

Whorf, B. 1956. *Language, Thought, and Reality.* Cambridge, Mass.: MIT Press.

Wiig, E., and Semel, E. 1976. *Language*

Disabilities in Children and Adolescents. Columbus, Ohio: Charles E. Merrill.

Wilcox, M., and Leonard, L. 1978. Experimental acquisition of wh- questions in language-disordered children. *J. Speech and Hearing Research,* 21, 220–239.

Williams, R., and Wolfram, W. 1977. *Social Dialects: Differences vs. Disorders.* Rockville, Md.: American Speech-Language-Hearing Association.

Winitz, H. 1973. Problem solving and the delaying of speech as strategies in the teaching of language. *Asha,* 15, 583–586.

Winitz, H., and Reeds, J. 1975. *Comprehension and Problem Solving as Strategies for Language Training.* The Hague: Mouton.

Woodworth, R., and Schlosberg, H. 1954. *Experimental Psychology,* Revised Edition. New York: Henry Holt.

Wright, J., and Vlietstra, A. 1975. The development of selective attention: from perceptual exploration to logical search. In *Advances in Child Development and Behavior,* Vol. 10, ed., Reese, H. New York: Academic Press.

Wulbert, M., Inglis, S., Kriegsmann, E., and Mills, B. 1975. Language delay and associated mother-child interactions. *Developmental Psychology,* 11, 61–70.

Yendovitskaya, T. 1971. Development of memory. In *The Psychology of Preschool Children,* eds., Zaporozhets, A., and Elkonin, D. Cambridge, Mass.: MIT Press.

Zelniker, T., and Jeffrey, W. 1976. Reflective and impulsive children: strategies of information processing underlying differences in problem solving. *Monographs of the Society for Research in Child Development,* 41, serial no. 168.

Zlatin, M., and Phelps, H. 1975. Structure, function and content of parents' child-directed language: a comparison within and among couples. Paper presented at the Annual Convention of the American Speech and Hearing Association, Washington, D.C.

AUTHOR INDEX

SUBJECT INDEX

Abstract concepts, 13–14. *See also* Relational concepts.
Acting out tasks, 149–51
Action: *See* Semantic roles.
Active learning, 206. *See also* Language learning strategies.
Adaptability: *See* Family system.
Adjectivals: *See* Noun phrases.
Adverbials, 166, 185
Agent: *See* Semantic roles.
Analysis-by-synthesis, 42–45; in comprehension, 198
Anoxia, 105–06
Aphasia: acquired in children, 108, 125; adult, 5, 137. *See also* Childhood aphasia.
Assessment: areas of, 131, 134–38; and child's problem-solving, 148–49; clinical method (Piaget), 144, 149, 151, 158 cognitive and relationship aspects, 158; of comprehension, 149–50; conceptual development, 136–37—of object-sorting tasks, 151; continuing, 132–33; of culturally different children, 156–57; of exploratory teaching, 151–56, 158–59; of expression, 149–50; general communicative functioning, 145–46; of grammatical skills, 144–45, 148–50; informal, 144–51, 158—of language, 148–51, techniques, 149–51; of information-processing skills, 137; interpretation of behavior, 261, 263–64, 302; and language sample, 148; language skills, 137–38; and linear cause-and-effect model, 158; perceptual skills, 137; physiological factors, 135–36; pragmatics, 138; prediction in, 133–34, 157; problem solving, 133, 303–04; relationship factors, 134–35, 158; relationship tactics, 146, 261, 302; sources of information, 139–40; techniques, 138–151; and transactional patterns, 138; and unresponsive child, 146; vocabulary, 144–45
At-risk factors, 281–82. *See also* Causation of language impairment.
Attention, 25–27; deficits in, 303; determinants of, 26; and exploration, 26–27; and family processes, 281; human information processing, 2; and human relationships, 202; levels of, 25–26; and saliency, 26; set to attend, 25
Attention span: impaired, 25; and relationship communication, 261, 263
Auditory processing disorders, 124–25; and minimal brain damage, 126–27;

and transactional model, 127
Autism, 123–24; and iconic signs, 90; and nondiscursive communication, 85
Automatic memory: and language training, 227
Autotelic activities, 219, 211–13; and play, 257

BE to be, 167–68; and Black English vernacular, 191
Behavior: changes in context, 153; determinants of, 140; interpretation of, 140–41; limits on, 152–53, 156; and problem solving, 140; as selection from repertoire, 140–41. *See also* Relationship communication.
Behavior modification. *See* Contingency management. *Be spontaneous* paradox, 250–52, 260; and facilitatve play, 256
Bilingualism, 100–102; and human relationships, 100; language sampling, 161; and values, 308. *See also* Culturally different children.
Black English vernacular. *See* Non-standard dialect.
Bottom-up processing, 316; and expression, 205

Causation of language impairment: anoxia, 105–6; at-risk factors, 105–7; constitutional factors, 108; delivery complications, 105–6; environmental factors, 105–11; and general systems theory, 128–29; heridity, 108, 111, 113; interactional model, 111, 318; linear cause-and-effect model, 107–11, 128—and assessment, 158 and punctuation, 119–20, and reification, 120; models of causation, 107–17; and prediction of development, 127–28; prematurity, 105–06, 111; research in, 105–7, 112. See also Transactional Model.
Chaotic systems: *See* Family systems.
Childhood aphasia, 108, 124–25; and minimal brain damage, 126–27; and transactional model, 127
Children's language disorders: definition of, 4–6—and values, 307; and emotional disturbance, 5; and family system, 270, 272–73, 278–87; and hearing loss, 5; and iconic signs, 89–90; and learning disabilities, 5; and mental retardation, 5; and sensory systems, 25. *See also* Language delay, Language learning, Childhood aphasia.
Chunking. *See* Memory.

Class, grammatical, 66–69, 80
Clause: constructions, summary of, 171; coordination, 185–87, 188; declarative, 170; dependent, 185–88; equative, 16–17; imperative, 170; infinitive, 185—early occurring, 185; intransitive, 166, 168; as learning matrix, 164, 171; obligatory elements, 166; optional elements, 166; questions, 170–71, 175—and discourse rules, 204; relative, 185; subordination, 185–88; transitive, 166–67; types, 165–69, 171; variations, 165, 169–71, 175
Closed systems, 117
Cognitive strategies: in comprehension, 199; development of, 38; and human information processing, 2, individual differences, 38–39; memory, 37–39; and metarules, 37–38; nature of, 37–38; and problem solving, 207–08; teaching of, 40, 207–09. *See also* Decision making.
Cognitive style, 38
Cohesion. *See* Family system.
Communication: content, 91–92; continuous, 84–87; dimensions of, 84–87; discrete and discursive, 84–87—and behavior modification, 253, and conceptual-semantic decisions, 265; and home intervention, 310; intuitive, 85–87, 116—and linear logic, 274, and relationship communication, 264, 290, and relationship tactics, 260; levels of, 91–96; linear, 116;—and behavior modification, 253, and conceptual-semantic decisions, 265; of linear knowledge, 85–87; nondiscursive, 85–87, 116—and autism, 85, and relationship communication, 264; nonverbal, 87–91—conventional gestures, 87–88, and expression, 203–04, idiosyncratic, 90, interpretation of, 92–95, and language, 68, 88, and language training, 87–91, levels of, 87–91, regulating social interaction, 88–89, relationship tactics, 261; and reality, 9; and transactional model, 128–29. *See also* Human relationships; Iconic signs; Metacommunication; Relationship communication.
Complement, 167. *See also* Semantic roles.
Completion tasks, 149–51
Comprehension: acceptance of message, 203; assessment of, 149–50; and expression, 198, 201–02, 206, 216, 235; and human